AF556387

ENCYCLOPAEDIA OF PHARMACY

Encyclopaedia of
Pharmacy

Rajeev Verma

ANMOL PUBLICATIONS PVT. LTD.
NEW DELHI - 110 002 (INDIA)

ANMOL PUBLICATIONS PVT. LTD.
H.O.: 4374/4B, Ansari Road, Daryaganj
New Delhi - 110 002
Ph.: 23278000, 23261597
B.O.: No. 1015, Ist Main Road, BSK III Stage
III Phase, III Block
Bangalore - 560 085 (India)
Visit us at: www.anmolpublications.com

Encyclopaedia of Pharmacy

© Reserved

First Published, 2006

ISBN 81-261-3028-8

[Responsibility for the facts stated, opinions expressed, conclusions reached and plagiarism, if any, in this volume is entirely that of the Editor/Author. The Publishers bear no responsibility for them, whatsoever.]

PRINTED IN INDIA

Printed at Mehra Offset Press, Delhi

Preface

The field of Pharmacy has grown so vast in the last few years, that to cover every term is impossible. We have therefore compiled a volume, which is appropriate for all medical workers. This Encyclopaedia of Pharmacy covers accurate and latest definitions of terms being used in latest context and also the current usage. It covers all aspect of Pharmacy.

Definitions are comprehensive, include drugs, procedures and pharmacology and are explained with illustrations. All fields of pharmacy are covered. This Encyclopaedia will prove a valuable reference for practitioners, specialists, consultants and students. Terms are concisely presented and explained in a very lucid manner. Pharmacy students in general will find the Encyclopaedia indispensable.

Users of this Encyclopaedia will find it easy to understand the various terms as they are explained in a very lucid manner It will benefit not only students, but also professionals, researchers, and scholars. We owe a great debt to all those scholars and authors in this field whose work we have consulted and who have influenced our understanding of the field. Author is especially thankful to Anmol Publications Pvt. Ltd. New Delhi for shaping this book in its final form. Suggestions for further improvement of this book are not only welcome but also greatly appreciated.

Author

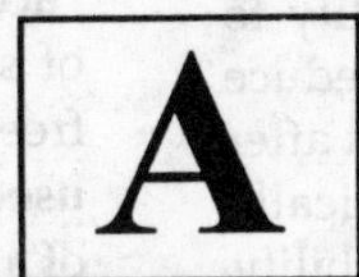

A An amount of drug or chemical in units of mass such as milligrams. Special attributes of the amount are indicated by subscripts: A0, the amount of drug in the body at "zero-time;" AB, the amount of drug in the body; AU, the amount of drug recovered in the urine, etc. The amount of drug in the drug's volume of distribution is equal to the concentration of the drug times the volume: $A = C \cdot Vd$.

A/G Ratio Albumin value divided by the globulin value.

A33 Monoclonal antibody A type of monoclonal antibody used in cancer detection or therapy. Monoclonal antibodies are laboratory-produced substances that can locate and bind to cancer cells.

Abacavir (ABC, Ziagen) Indications: Treatment of HIV infection in combination with other agents.

Contraindications: Known or suspected hypersensitivity.

Dosage: 300 mg po bid. Also available as Trizivir, a fixed dose combination of ZDV 300 mg, 3TC 150 mg, and abacavir 300 mg.

Toxicity: Four percent of patients develop a hypersensitivity reaction, usually within 6 weeks of initiating therapy. It is manifested by fever, constitutional or respiratory symptoms, gastrointestinal intolerance, and/or rash. Stopping the drug leads to rapid resolution of symptoms. Never rechallenge a patient thought to have had a hypersensitivity reaction to abacavir as severe reactions and death have been reported.

Other side effects include nausea, vomiting, diarrhea, headache, malaise.

Abarelix A drug used to reduce the amount of testosterone made in patients with advanced symptomatic prostate cancer for which no other treatment options are available. It belongs to the family of drugs called gonadotropin-releasing hormone (GnRH) antagonists. Also called Plenaxis.

ABI 007 A substance that is being studied in the treatment of cancer. It is a special form of the anticancer drug paclitaxel that may have fewer side effects and may be able to be given in higher doses. It belongs to the families of drugs called mitotic inhibitors and taxanes.

Ablation In medicine, the removal or destruction of a body part or tissue or its function. Ablation may be performed by surgery, hormones, drugs, radiofrequency, heat, or other methods.

Absorption Before a compound can exert a pharmacological effect in tissues, it has to be taken in to the bloodstream—usually via mucous surfaces like the digestive tract (intestinal absorption). Uptake into the target organs or cells needs to be ensured, too. This can be a serious problem at some natural barriers like the blood-brain barrier. Factors such as poor compound solubility, chemical instability in the stomach, and inability to permeate the intestinal wall can all reduce the extent to which a drug is absorbed after oral administration. Absorption critically determines the compound's bioavailability

ABT 510 A substance that is being studied in the treatment of cancer. It belongs to the family of drugs called angiogenesis inhibitors.

ABT 751 A substance that is being studied in the treatment of cancer. It belongs to the family of drugs called sulfonamides.

ABX-EGF A monoclonal antibody that is being studied in the diagnosis and treatment of some types of cancer. Monoclonal antibodies are made in the laboratory and can locate and bind to cancer cells. Also called panitumumab.

Acceptance criteria The criteria a software productmust meet to successfully complete a test phase or to achieve delivery requirements.

Acclimatization The biological process whereby an organism adapts to a new environment. One example is the process of developing microorganisms that degrade toxic wastes in the environment.

Accommodation schedule Defines all areas that can influence unit operations required for manufacturing, and relationships and flows between them.

Account policy Specifies how passwords must be defined and employed for all user accounts on a system. It specifically addresses the issues of password aging, password uniqueness, and locking a user account because of invalid logon attempts.

Accuracy The use of the word "accurate" - free of error - in referring to a scientific observation or scientific method sometimes obscures the fact that even the best methods and observations are only relatively free from error. The use of the single word "accurate" also hides the fact that a number of separate elements contribute to over-all freedom from error. "Accurate" is frequently used to refer indiscriminately to the effect of any of these elements, or to the combined effects of all of them on the freedom from error of a system. Effective use of a method or observation requires that we know the ways and degrees to which the data are free of error, not that we know only that the data are "accurate" or "inaccurate".

The elements to be taken into account in a complete evaluation of a method or system can be derived from the properties of the quantitative relationship between the "input" and the "output" for the system. The input-output relationship, for all its generality, has specific application—and specific names—in different scientific fields and for different kinds of experimental or observational systems. In physics and engineering, the "stress-strain diagram" is a special representation of the input-output relationship; in pharmacology, the "dose-effect curve" is an example of the input-output relationship. In quantitative chemical analyses, the "calibration curve" is an example of the input-output relationship. Generally, "input" can be looked on as the measured value of an independent variable or "measurand"; "output" can be viewed as a measurement made under non-standard or test conditions.

"Accuracy", as formally defined, and the elements that contribute to it can be only briefly outlined here.

ACE inhibitors Are drugs that inhibit ACE (angiotensin converting enzyme). An enzyme needed for the production of the peptide angiotensin II, which causes arteries to constrict and therefore raises the blood pressure. ACE inhibitors lower the blood pressure by inhibiting the formation of angiotensin II. This relaxes the arteries and thus lowers blood pressure. Relaxing the arteries also helps to improve the pumping efficiency of a failing heart and therefore increase cardiac output in patients with heart failure. ACE inhibitors are used in the treatment of hypertension (high blood pressure) and congestive heart failure. ACE inhibitors currently in use include: benazepril, captopril, lisinopril, quinapril, and ramipril.

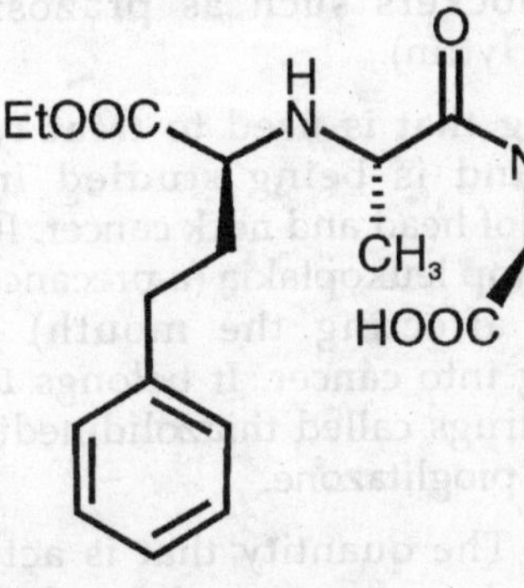

Acetaminophen A pain reliever and fever reducer. Brand name: Tylenol. The exact mechanism of action of acetaminophen is not known. Acetaminophen relieves pain by elevating the pain threshold (that is, by requiring a greater amount of pain to develop before it is felt by a person). Acetaminophen reduces fever through its action on the heat-regulating center (the "thermostat") of the brain.

Acetylcysteine A drug usually used to reduce the thickness of mucus and ease its removal. It is also used to reverse the toxicity of high doses of acetaminophen. Also called N-acetyl-L-cysteine.

Acid A compound of an electronegative element or radical with hydrogen; it form salts by replacing all or part of the hydrogen with an electropositive element or radical. Or, a hydrogen-containing substance that when dissolved in water dissociates to produce one or more hydrogen ions (H+).

Acid feed Injection of an acid into a liquid stream to make it less alkaline (pH adjustment).

Acrylonitrile A substance used to make plastics, rubber, and textiles. Being exposed to acrylonitrile may increase the risk of developing certain cancers, such as lung, brain, or prostate cancer.

Action levels Levels or ranges distinct from product specificationswhich, when deviated from, signal a drift from normal operatingconditions and which require actions.Alert or Warning Levels: Levels or ranges which, when deviated from,signal a potential drift from normal operating conditions but which donot necessarily require action.

Action point A value set to identify when a parameter has drifted outside the operating range (Acceptance Criteria). A documented response is usually required.

Activase A protein that is made by the body and that helps dissolve blood clots. It can also be made in the laboratory and is used in the treatment of heart attack and stroke. It is also being studied in the treatment of cancer. Activase belongs to the family of drugs called systemic thrombolytic agents. Also called tissue plasminogen activator (tPA), recombinant tissue plasminogen activator (r-tPA), and Alteplase.

Activated carbon Material used to adsorb organic impurities from water. Derived from wood, lignite, pulp-mill char, blood, etc. The source material is initially charred at high temperature to convert it to carbon. The carbon is then "activated" by oxidation from exposure to high temperature steam. It comes in granular or powdered form.

Active center The location in an enzyme where the specific reaction takes place.

Active immunity The formation of an antibody that can be stimulated by infection or vaccination.

Active ingredient Any component that is intended to furnish pharmacological activity or other direct effect in the diagnosis, cure, mitigation, treatment, or prevention of disease, or to affect the structure or any function of the body of man or other animals. The term includes those components that may undergo chemical change in the manufacture of the drug product and are present in the drug product in a modified form intended to furnish the specified activity or effect.

Active site The region of a protein molecule that binds the specific substrate and chemically modifies it into the new product (in an enzyme) or interacts with it (in a receptor).

Active substance A basic active substance which is the bearer of the drug effects.

Active transport Energy-requiring transport of a solution across a membrane in the direction of increasing concentration.

Activity, intrinsic The property of a drug which determines the amount of biological effect produced per unit of drug-receptor complex formed. Two agents combining with equivalent sets of receptors may not produce equal degrees of effect even if both agents are given in maximally effective doses; the agents differ in their intrinsic activities and the one producing the greater maximum effect has the greater intrinsic activity. Intrinsic activity is not the same as "potency" and may be completely independent of it. Meperidine and morphine presumably combine with the same receptors to produce analgesia, but regardless of dose, the maximum degree of analgesia produced by morphine is greater than that produced by meperidine; morphine has the greater intrinsic activity. Intrinsic activity - like affinity - depends on the chemical natures of both the drug and the receptor, but intrinsic activity and affinity apparently can vary independently with changes in the drug molecule

Benign prostrate hypertrophy (hyperplasia) is an enlargement of the prostrate gland. This can often compress the urethra and partially block urine flow. Prostate enlargement adversely affects about half the men in their 60s and close to 80 percent of men in their 80s. The presence or absence of prostate gland enlargement is not related to the development of prostate cancer. Treatment: Alpha1 blockers such as prazosin or terazosin (Hytrin).

Actos A drug that is used to treat type 2 diabetes and is being studied in the prevention of head and neck cancer. It may be able to stop leukoplakia (a precancerous condition affecting the mouth) from developing into cancer. It belongs to the family of drugs called thiazolidinediones. Also called pioglitazone.

Actual yield The quantity that is actually produced at any appropriate phase of manufacture, processing, or packaging of a particular drug product.

Acupressure The application of pressure or localized massage to specific sites on the body to control symptoms such as pain or nausea. It is a type of complementary and alternative medicine.

Acute Refers to intense, short-term symptoms or illnesses that either resolve or evolve into long-lasting, chronic disease manifestations.

Acyclovir A substance used to prevent or treat cytomegalovirus and herpes simplex infections that may occur when the body is immunosuppressed. It belongs to the family of drugs called antivirals.

AD 32 A drug that is used to treat bladder cancer that does not respond to BCG (Bacillus Calmette Guerin). It is an anthracycline and belongs to the family of drugs called antitumor antibiotics. Also called valrubicin.

Addiction A maladaptive pattern of substance use leading to clinically significant impairment or distress as manifested by three (or more) of the following, occurring at any time in the same 12-month period:

* Substance is often taken in larger amounts or over longer period than intended

* Persistent desire or unsuccessful efforts to cut down or control substance use

* A great deal of time is spent in activities necessary to obtain the substance (e.g., visiting multiple doctors or driving long distances), use the substance (e.g., chain smoking), or recovering from its effects

* Important social, occupational or recreational activities given up or reduced because of substance abuse

* Continued substance use despite knowledge of having a persistent or recurrent psychological, or physical problem that is caused or exacerbated by use of the substance

* Tolerance, as defined by either: (a) need for increased amounts of the substance in order to achieve intoxication or desired effect; or (b) markedly diminished effect with continued use of the same amount

* Withdrawal, as manifested by either: (a) characteristic withdrawal syndrome for the substance; or (b) the same (or closely related) substance is taken to relieve or avoid withdrawal symptoms"

Additive Additives are substances enabling processing of the active substance itself resulting in a medical preparation of a characteristic drug form, while ensuring the required stability and quality of the drug, they may influence, for example, the release of an active substance from the drug form and its absorption, they correct sensual perception, etc. Additives may cause an allergy in certain individuals; the content of additives must be carefully monitored even necessitating a certain type of diet. Additives include stabilizers, dyes and antioxidants.

Adenine (A) A purine base, 6-aminopurine, occurring in RNA (ribonucleic acid) and DNA (deoxyribonucleic acid) and as a component of adenosine triphosphate.

Adjunct agent In cancer therapy, a drug or substance used in addition to the primary therapy.

Adjunctive therapy Another treatment used together with the primary treatment. Its purpose is to assist the primary treatment.

Adjuvant A material that enhances the action of a drug or antigen

Adjuvant chemotherapy The use of one or more chemotherapy drugs following the removal of a tumor or after radiotherapy. The aim is to kill any remaining cancer cells.

Adjuvant therapy Cancer treatment used in addition to the main treatment, such as surgery. Adjuvant therapy usually refers to hormonal therapy, chemotherapy, radiation therapy, or immunotherapy added after surgery to increase the chances of curing the disease or minimizing symptoms.

ADME Absorption Distribution Metabolism Excretion studies (pharmacokinetics).

Admission criteria Basis for selecting target population for a clinical trial. Subjects must be screened to ensure that their characteristics match a list of admission criteria and that none of their characteristics match any single one of the exclusion criteria set up for the study.

ADR (Regarding marketed medicinal products) A response to a drug that is noxious and unintended and that occurs at doses normally used in man for prophylaxis, diagnosis, or therapy of diseases or for modification of physiological function.

Adrenaline A hormone and neurotransmitter. Also called epinephrine.

Adriamycin An anticancer drug that belongs to the family of drugs called antitumor antibiotics. It is an anthracycline. Also called doxorubicin.

Adsorption Adhesion of the molecules of a gas, liquid or dissolved substance to a surface because of chemical or electrical attraction - typically accomplished with granular activated carbon to remove dissolved organics and chlorine. The attachment of charged particles to the chemically active groups on the surface and in the pores of an ion exchanger.

Adult T cell leukemia/lymphoma ATLL. An aggressive (fast-growing) type of T-cell non-Hodgkin's lymphoma caused by the human T-cell leukemia virus type 1 (HTLV-1). It is marked by bone and skin lesions, high calcium levels, and enlarged lymph nodes, spleen, and liver.

Adverse agents Undesired effects or toxicity due to exposure (often but not limited to a drug or medical device).

Adverse drug reaction (ADR) In the pre-approval clinical experience with a new medicinal product or its new usages, particularly as the therapeutic dose(s) may not be established: all noxious and unintended responses to a medicinal product related to any dose should be considered adverse drug reactions. The phrase responses to a medicinal product means that a causal relationship between a medicinal product and an adverse event is at least a reasonable possibility, i.e. the relationship cannot be ruled out. Regarding marketed medicinal products: a response to a drug which is noxious and unintended and which occurs at doses normally used in man for prophylaxis, diagnosis, or therapy of diseases or for modification of physiological function .

Adverse effect An unwanted side effect of treatment.

Adverse effects of drugs The adverse effects of drugs are represented by any adverse or unwanted consequence of the drug administration; certain adverse effects can be subjectively sensed by the patient, however, others require various medical examinations. Some adverse effects will fade away with time; if there is any serious change in the health condition which might be connected with the drug administration it is necessary to stop using the drug and to consult the physician on what to do next; adverse effects often experienced by patients include headache, nausea, impaired digestion, increased fatigue, reduced concentration, skin symptoms, etc.

Adverse event (AE) An AE is any untoward medical occurrence in a patient or clinical investigation subject administered a pharmaceutical product and that does not necessarily have a causal relationship with this treatment. An AE can therefore be any unfavorable and unintended sign (including an abnormal laboratory finding), symptom, or disease temporally associated with the use of a medicinal (investigational) product, whether or not related to the medicinal (investigational) product.

Adverse reaction See adverse drug reaction.

Advisory alarm An alarm indicating a drift of a monitored parameter toward an out-of-spec condition. It is advisory in that no GMP violation has occurred, and is used to advise corrective action before an action alarm can happen.

AE 941 A substance made from shark cartilage that is being studied for its ability to prevent the growth of new blood vessels to solid tumors. It belongs to the family of drugs called angiogenesis inhibitors.

Aerobe An organism that can live and grow only in the presence of oxygen.

1. Facultative aerobe: one which normally thrives in the absence of oxygen, but which may acquire the faculty of living in the presence of oxygen.

2. Obligate aerobe: one that cannot live without air.

Aerobia The plural of aerobe.

Aerobic bacteria Bacteria capable of growing in the presence of Oxygen.

Aerobic Living in air.

Aerosol 1. In general, a fine mist or spray which contains minute particles.

2. In medicine, a spray administered by a nebulizer and inhaled for treatment.

3. In medicine, a mist that causes disease as, for example, the hantavirus pulmonary syndrome.

4. In the environment, particles emitted into the air naturally as in volcanic eruptions and through human action such as burning fossil fuel.

5. In the environment, the pressurized gas used to propel substances out of a container.

Aerosol photometer Light-scattering mass concentration indicating instrument with a threshold sensitivity of at least 10 to the negative third power microgram per liter for 0.3μm diameter DOP (Dioctyl Phthalate) concentrations over a range of 10 to the fifth power times the threshold sensitivity. Photometers may include hand-held remote meter probes that can scan for airborne contaminants in HEPA filters, in penetrations around frames, seals and plenums, and in hoods and work stations.

Aerosolize In medicine, to turn a liquid drug into a fine mist that can be inhaled.

AES see: Auger Electron Spectroscopy

Afferent nerves A nerve, which transmits impulses from the peripheral tissues and organs to the brain and spinal cord (for example sensory nerve).

Affinity (drug) The equilibrium constant of the reversible reaction of a drug with a receptor to form a drug-receptor complex; the reciprocal of the dissociation constant of a drug-receptor complex. Under the most general conditions, where there is a 1:1 binding interaction, at equilibrium the number of receptors engaged by a drug at a given drug concentration is directly proportional to their affinity for each other and inversely related to the tendency of the drug-receptor complex to dissociate. Obviously, affinity depends on the chemical natures of both the drug and the receptor. "Affinity" is not the same as "duration of action".

Affinity The equilibrium constant of the reversible reaction of a drug with a receptor to form a drug-receptor complex; the reciprocal of the dissociation constant of a drug-receptor complex. Under the most general conditions, where there is a 1:1 binding interaction, at equilibrium the number of receptors engaged by a drug at a given drug concentration is directly proportional to their affinity for each other and inversely related to the tendency of the drug-receptor complex to dissociate. Obviously, affinity depends on the chemical natures of both the drug and the receptor.

Aflatoxin A harmful substance made by certain types of mold (Aspergillus flavus and Aspergillus parasiticus) that is often found on poorly stored grains and nuts. Consumption of foods contaminated with aflatoxin is a risk factor for primary liver cancer.

AFP Alpha-fetoprotein. A protein normally produced by a developing fetus. AFP levels are usually undetectable in the blood of healthy nonpregnant adults. An elevated level of AFP suggests the presence of either a primary liver cancer or germ cell tumor.

AG 013736 A substance that is being studied in the treatment of cancer. It belongs to the families of drugs called angiogenesis inhibitors and protein tyrosine kinase inhibitors.

AG2037 A substance that is being studied in the treatment of cancer. It belongs to the family of drugs called glycinamide ribonucleotide formyl transferase inhibitors.

AG3340 A substance that is being studied in the treatment of cancer. It is a matrix metalloproteinase inhibitor and belongs to the family of drugs called angiogenesis inhibitors. Also called prinomastat.

AG337 A substance that is being studied in the treatment of liver cancer. It belongs to the family of drugs called thymidylate synthase inhibitors. Also called Thymitaq and nolatrexed.

Agar A complex mixture of polysaccharides obtained from marine red algae, used as an emulsion stabilizer in foods, as a sizing in fabrics, as a gelling agent and as a solid substrate or media for the laboratory culture of microorganisms. Agar melts at 100°C and when cooled below 44°C forms a stiff and transparent gel. Microorganisms are seeded and grown on the surface of the gel.

Agarose A highly purified form of agar.

Agarose gel electrophoresis A method used to separate, identify, and purify molecules of different molecular weight and/or structure. It is specifically applied to the separation of protein or DNA fragments where it is rapid, simple, and accurate, and the separated molecules can be visualized directly by staining with dyes. The electrophoretic migration rate of molecules through agarose gel is dependent on the following parameters: 1. Molecular size: molecules pass through the gel at rates that are inversely proportional to the log of their molecular weight.

2. Agarose concentration: a molecule of a given size migrates at different rates through gels containing different concentrations of agarose.

3. Molecular conformation: a molecule of the same molecular weight but of a different conformation will migrate at different rates. Generally, closed circular or globular forms will migrate faster than linear forms.

4. Electric current: at low voltages the rate of migration is proportional to the voltage, but as the voltage is increased the rate of migration of high molecular weight fragments is increased differentially.

Age related macular degeneration (AMD) Is a disease that progressively destroys the central portion of the retina, which is called the macula. AMD is the leading cause of severe vision loss in people aged 50 and over in the Western World. As many as 30-million people throughout the world are thought to suffer from the condition. There are two types of AMD - the wet type and the milder and more common dry type. Although the wet form of AMD accounts for just 10-15% of all cases of AMD, it is responsible for 90% of severe vision loss associated with the disease. Some research suggests that taking supplements of zinc and the antioxidants vitamin C, vitamin E, and beta-carotene may help to slow the progression of wet AMD.

Agene Nitrogen Trichloride (NCl3).

Agent study In cancer prevention clinical trials, a study that tests whether taking certain medicines, vitamins, minerals, or food supplements can prevent cancer. Also a called chemoprevention study.

Agglomerate Suspended solids clustered together to form larger clumps or masses that are easier to remove by filtration or settling.

Agglutination The sticking together of insoluble antigens such as bacteria, viruses or erythrocytes by a particular antibody.

Agglutination assays are used to type human blood before a transfusion.

Aging Inhibition of acetycholinesterase (AchE) with organophosphates results in a increase in Ach levels. If allowed to associate with AchE for certain period of time a phenomenon called 'aging' occurs, involving the loss of a group attached to phosphorus and leading to the formation of a negatively charged irreversibly phosphorylated AchE enzyme. The aging process can be very short (ie. nerve gases, secs) or longer (ie. pesticides, hrs). Pralidoxime (2-PAM) can regenerate AchE from the organophosphate but only before the 'aging' process.

Agonist(s) An endogenous substance or a drug that can interact with a **receptor** and initiate a physiological or a pharmacological response characteristic of that receptor (contraction, relaxation, secretion, enzyme activation, etc.)

Agonist, full A full agonist is an agonist that produces the largest maximal response of any known agonist that acts on the same receptor.

Agonist, inverse An inverse agonist is a ligand that by binding to a receptor reduces the fraction of receptors in an active conformation, thereby reducing basal activity. This can occur if some of the receptors are in the active form in the absence of a conventional agonist.

Agonist, partial A partial agonist is an agonist that produces a maximal response that is less than the maximal response produced by another agonist acting at the same receptors on the same tissue, as a result of lower intrinsic activity.

AHF (Antihemophilic factor) In the clotting of blood it is also known as Factor VIII.

AIDS Acquired immune deficiency syndrome.

Air change rate The number of times the total air volume of a defined space is replaced in a given unit of time. This is computed by dividing the total volume of the subject space (in cubic feet) into the total volume of air exhausted from (or supplied to) the space per unit of time.

Air cleaners Filtration systems that may be freestanding or installed in a ceiling or wall to remove contaminants such as bacteria, viruses, and dust from the air. Air cleaners may incorporate HEPA filters.

Air lift bioreactor A reactor in which the source of agitation is air sparged upwards through a draft tube - most widely used for cell culture applications and monoclonal antibody production.

Air velocity meters/monitors Meters to measure and indicate the force and speed of airflow. Meters may use a variety of probes for measuring near HEPA filters and at right angles. Monitors check and record air velocity.

Airborne particulate cleanliness classes Statistically allowable number of particles equal to, or larger than 0.5μm in size per cubic foot of air. According to ISO 14644-1, a classification number, N, shall designate airborne particulate cleanliness.

Airflow visualization Using chemical smoke or fog to visualize flow patterns in a cleanroom or clean space.

Airlock A room or space designed to act as a means of segregating areas of different air classification or quality. It may contain a method to remove particulate contamination from clean room garments as personnel pass through, and usually includes HEPA filtered air supply and interlocking doors. Airlocks pressure will "float" between those of the spaces being protected. With all doors closed, the airlock pressure will be somewhere between that of the highest adjoining room and that of the lowest adjoining room as air flows through it from room to room. "Ventilated airlocks" are in neutral ducted air balance (supply CFM = return CFM).

Alanine aminopeptidase AAP. An enzyme that is used as a biomarker to detect damage to the kidneys, and that may be used to help diagnose certain kidney disorders. It is found at high levels in the urine when there are kidney problems.

Alanine transferase An enzyme found in the liver and other tissues. A high level of alanine transferase released into the blood may be a sign of liver damage, cancer, or other diseases. Also called serum glutamate pyruvate transaminase or SGPT.

Alanosine A substance that is being studied in the treatment of cancer. It belongs to the family of drugs called antimetabolites. Also called SDX-102.

Alarms Audible or visual signals used to warn of unacceptable conditions at monitored sites. They may be buzzers, horns, speakers, bells, or warning lights. They can be Advisory, Alert, or Action alarms. The first two are for operation and maintenance information, to alert of abnormal situations that do not compromise product SISPQ. The Action alarm is for GMP records, indicating that product SISPQ may have been compromised, but Alert alarms are also usually recorded.

Albumin Commonly, the white of egg is a simple protein widely distributed throughout the tissues and fluid of plants and animals. Soluble in pure water it is also precipitable from a solution by mineral acids, and coagulable by heat in acid or neutral solution.

Albuminoid Resembling albumin, a simple protein present in horny and cartilaginous tissues, insoluble in neutral solvents. Keratin, elastin, and collagen are albuminoids.

Alcohol Unless otherwise specified, ethyl alcohol (ethanol). Concentration is normally in percent by volume. "Dehydrated alcohol", or "Absolute alcohol" is 100%.

Aldesleukin A laboratory-made colony-stimulating factor that stimulates the production of blood cells, especially platelets, during chemotherapy. It is a cytokine that belongs to the family of drugs called hematopoietic (blood-forming) agents. Also called interleukin-2 or IL-2.

Aldosterone Aldosterone is secreted by the zona glomerulosa of the adrenal gland. It causes the body to retain sodium and secrete potassium. It effects the distal tubule and collecting ducts of the kidney. It also effects the sweat and saliva glands. Its secretion is stimulated by...

ACTH adrenocorticotropic hormone.

angiotensin II.

elevated blood potassium levels.

Alemtuzumab A type of monoclonal antibody used in the treatment of leukemia. Monoclonal antibodies are laboratory-produced substances that can locate and bind to cancer cells. Also called Campath-1H.

Alendronate sodium A drug that affects bone metabolism. It is used in treating osteoporosis and Paget's disease, and is being studied in the treatment of hypercalcemia (abnormally high levels of calcium in the blood) and in treating and reducing the risk of bone pain caused by cancer. Alendronate sodium belongs to the family of drugs called bisphosphonates.

NH_2

H_2PO_3 — PO_3H_2

OH

Alert point Used in determining when a parameter is drifting toward extremes of the operating range.

Algorithm Step-by-step procedure for solving a mathematical problem; also used to describe step-by-step procedures for making a series of choices among alternative decisions to reach an outcome.

Alimta A drug that is used to treat malignant pleural mesothelioma and advanced non-small cell lung cancer and is being studied in the treatment of other types of cancer. It belongs to the family of drugs called enzyme inhibitors. Also called pemetrexed disodium and LY231514.

Aliquot Of, pertaining to, or designating an exact divisor or factor of a quantity, specially of an integer. To divide out a sample to multiple containers for multiple analytical tests.

Alkaline phosphorus A material found in the blood related to liver and bone.

Alkalinity An expression of the total amount of basic anions (hydroxyl groups) present in a solution. In water analysis, it also represents the presence of carbonate, bicarbonate, and occasionally borate, silicate, and phosphate salts that react to produce hydroxyl groups. Bicarbonate and carbonate ions are expected to be in most waters. Hydroxide may occur in water that has been softened by the lime soda process or has been in contact with fresh concrete. Alkalinity furnishes a guide in choosing appropriate treatment of either raw water or plant effluents.

Alkeran A drug that is used to treat multiple myeloma and ovarian epithelial cancer and is being studied in the treatment of other types of cancer. It belongs to the family of drugs called alkylating agents. Also called melphalan.

Alkylating agent A drug that is used in the treatment of cancer. It interferes with the cell's DNA and inhibits cancer cell growth.

Allantoic fluid The clear white portion of an egg. In influenza vaccine manufacturing, the virus is propagated in the embryonic chick and sloughed into the allantoic fluid that is harvested to produce the vaccine.

Allele Alternative form of a genetic locus; a single allele for each locus is inherited separately from each parent (e.g., at a locus for eye color the allele might result in blue or brown eyes)

Allergenic extract An extract in a solvent of a substance that causes an allergic reaction. They are relative crude drugs by contemporary standards and are manufactured by specialty companies and in some cases, by a practicing allergist. Also, allergenic extracts are generally difficult to filter since they most frequently are extracts of natural substances such as foods, house dust, animal hair, etc.

Allergic Response Some drugs may act as haptens or allergens in susceptible individuals; re-administration of the hapten to such an individual results in an allergic response that may be sufficiently intense to call itself to the attention of the patient or the physician. The response may be so severe as to endanger the patient's life. The symptomatology of the allergic response is the result of the complex mechanism that is only "triggered" by the hapten. Hence, allergic responses to different haptens are fundamentally alike and qualitatively different from the pharmacologic effects the hapten-drugs manifest in normal subjects, i.e., patients not hypersensitive to the drug. Dose-effect curves obtained after administration of antigen to sensitized subjects usually reflect the dose-effect curves of the products of the allergic reaction even though the severity of the effects measured is proportional to the amount of antigen administered. Positive identification of a response as being allergic in nature depends on the demonstration of an antigen-antibody reaction underlying the response. In the case of specific patients, presumptive diagnoses of an allergic response must sometimes be made since no opportunity exists for formal identification of an antigen-antibody reaction; such diagnoses can be made and justified since the clinical symptomatology of allergic responses is usually characteristic and clear. Obviously, not all untoward effects of drugs are allergic in nature.

Allergy Allergies are inappropriate or exaggerated reactions of the immune system to substances that, in the majority of people, cause no symptoms. Symptoms of the allergic diseases may be caused by exposure of the skin to a chemical, of the respiratory system to particles of dust or pollen (or other substances), or of the stomach and intestines to a particular food.

Allodynia A state when a normally non-harmful, non-noxious stimulus induces pain.

Allometric scaling Allometric scalling is an empirical examination of the quantitative relationships between an extensive biological parameter, such as body size, body surface area or organ weight, and a intensive physiological or pharmacokinetic parameter, such as oxygen consumption rate or kidney filtration rate. The relationship is fitted to an exponential equation of the form:

$$\text{Log}(Y) = \text{Log}\, a + b \times \text{Log}(W)$$

Where Y is the intensive parameter

W is the extensive parameter

and parameters "a" and "b" are determined from the fit.

The usual purpose of allometric scaling is to predict human pharmacokinetic parameters, such as clearance rates or volume of distribution, by measuring the parameters in laboratory animals, such as rodents, monkeys and dogs.

Allopurinol A drug that lowers high levels of uric acid (a byproduct of metabolism) in the blood caused by some cancer treatments.

Allovectin 7A substance that is being studied as a gene therapy agent in the treatment of cancer. It increases the ability of the immune system to recognize cancer cells and kill them.

Aloe emodin A substance found in certain plants, including aloe vera. It belongs to a family of compounds called anthraquinones, which have shown anti-inflammatory and anticancer effects.

Alpha blocker Chemical substance, which blocks the effect on alpha-receptors. It relaxes the region of the urethra and simplifies the voiding of the bladder.

Alprazolam A benzodiazepine sedative that causes dose-related depression of the central nervous system. Alprazolam is useful in treating anxiety, panic attacks, insomnia, and muscle spasms.

Alteplase A protein that is made by the body and that helps dissolve blood clots. It can also be made in the laboratory and is used in the treatment of heart attack and stroke. It is also being studied in the treatment of cancer. Alteplase belongs to the family of drugs called systemic thrombolytic agents. Also called tissue plasminogen activator (tPA), recombinant tissue plasminogen activator (r-tPA), and Activase.

Alternative medicine Practices used instead of standard treatments. They generally are not recognized by the medical community as standard or conventional medical approaches. Alternative medicine includes dietary supplements, megadose vitamins, herbal preparations, special teas, acupuncture, massage therapy, magnet therapy, spiritual healing, and meditation.

Altretamine An anticancer drug that belongs to the family of drugs called alkylating agents.

Alum Aluminum sulfate, commonly added during municipal water treatment to cause insoluble colloids to coalesce into larger particles that can be removed by settling.

Aluminum sulfate A type of immune adjuvant (a substance used to help boost the immune response to a vaccine). Also called alum.

ALVAC CEA vaccine A cancer vaccine containing a canary pox virus (ALVAC) combined with the human carcinoembryonic antigen (CEA) gene.

Alzheimer's disease Also called SDAT (senile dementia Alzheimer's type). This disease is characterized by a general loss of intellectual ability and impairment of memory, judgment and abstract thinking, as well as changes in personality. Other symptoms include loss of speech, disorientation and apathy. Alzheimer's disease is the most common cause of dementia, rarely occurring before the age of 50. The disease takes from a few months to four or five years to progress to complete loss of intellectual function.

Ambien A drug used to treat insomnia (inability to sleep), and anxiety. It belongs to a family of drugs known as imidazopyridines (sedative hypnotics). Also called zolpidem.

Ambient The normal environment conditions such as temperature, relative humidity, or room pressure of a particular area under consideration.

Ames test This test for genotoxicity, developed in the 1970s, determines the reversion of a mutant his gene in Salmonella typhimurium when exposed to a genotoxic agent that causes base changes affecting the mutant gene.

Amethopterin A drug used to treat some types of cancers, including breast, head and neck, lung, blood, and bone, and other disorders. It belongs to the family of drugs called antimetabolites. Also called methotrexate.

AMG 706 A substance that is being studied in the treatment of some types of cancer. It belongs to the families of drugs called angiogenesis inhibitors and protein kinase inhibitors.

Amifostine A drug used as a chemoprotective drug to control some of the side effects of chemotherapy and radiation therapy.

Amikacin An antibiotic drug used to treat infection. It belongs to the family of drugs called aminoglycoside antibiotics.

Amiloride A drug that blocks sodium/proton antiport, used clinically as a potassium sparing diuretic.

Amine A substance that may be derived from ammonia by the replacement of one or more of the hydrogen atoms by hydrocarbon radicals.

Amino acids Any of a group of twenty hydrocarbon molecules (containing the radical group NH2) linked together in various combinations to form proteins in living things. Synthesized by living cells or obtained as essential components of the diet of human and animals, these twenty amino acids are divided into four (4) groups on the basis of their side-chain properties:

1. Neutral, hydrophobic side chains,
2. Neutral, hydrophilic side chains,
3. Acid, hydrophilic side chains,
4. Basic, hydrophilic side chains.

In addition to the twenty common amino acids there are less common derivatives (e.g. hydroxyproline, found in collagen) formed by the modification of a common amino acid.

Aminocamptothecin An anticancer drug that belongs to the family of drugs called topoisomerase inhibitors.

Aminoglutethimide An anticancer drug that belongs to the family of drugs called nonsteroidal aromatase inhibitors. Aminoglutethimide is used to decrease the production of sex hormones (estrogen in women or testosterone in men) and suppress the growth of tumors that need sex hormones to grow.

Aminoglycoside antibiotic A type of antibiotic that works against many types of bacteria and includes streptomycin, gentamicin, and neomycin. Aminoglycosides are used to treat bacterial infections.

Aminolevulinic acid A drug used in photodynamic therapy that is absorbed by tumor cells; when exposed to light, it becomes active and kills the cancer cells.

Aminopterin An anticancer drug that belongs to the family of drugs called antimetabolites.

Amiodarone A drug used to treat and prevent arrhythmias, part of a class of medications called antiarrhythmics. It works by relaxing an overactive heart. Causes significant and distinctive pulmonary toxicity.

Amitriptyline An antidepressant medication. In some patients with depression, abnormal levels of brain chemicals called neurotransmitters may relate to the depression. Amitriptyline elevates mood by raising the level of neurotransmitters in brain tissue. Amitriptyline is also a sedative that is useful for depressed patients with insomnia, restlessness, and nervousness. It is sometimes used to treat fibromyalgia and symptoms related to chronic pain.

Amonafide A substance that is being studied in the treatment of cancer. It belongs to the families of drugs called topoisomerase inhibitors and intercalating agents.

Amoxicillin An antibiotic drug used to treat infection. It belongs to the family of drugs called penicillins or penicillin derivatives.

Amphetamine and amphetamine type stimulants (ATS) From a chemical point of view all amphetamine-type stimulants are related to the ß-phenethylamin molecule (2-PEA). This molecule is the basic element of the body neurotransmitters (such as dopamine and adrenaline) that convey the neuronal information of the central and vegetative nervous system.

The relatively simple structure of 2-PEA can be designed in many ways, so that it is very difficult to calculate the exact number of all possible derivatives with similar pharmacological effects. .

Amphetamine itself might be called the prototype ('mother') psychostimulant. It was first synthesised in 1887 but was not used for medical purposes until the early 1930s, when it was found that it increased blood pressure, stimulated the central nervous system, cured bronchodilatation (asthma) and was useful in treating an epileptic seizure disorder.The abuse of this drug started at the same time.

Ampholyte Amphoteric electrolyte. Electrolyte that can either give up or take on a hydrogen ion and can thus behave as either an acid or a base.

Amphoteric Having two opposite characteristics.

Amphotericin B Indications: Pharmacist-prepared suspension for treatment of oral candidiasis; intravenous drug for treatment of systemic fungal infections.

Contraindications: Known hypersensitivity.

Dosage: Oral candidiasis: 1-5 ml of suspension po qid x 14 days.

Systemic fungal infections: intravenous doses range from 0.3-1.0 mg/kg/day depending on the pathogen and type of infection. Lipid complex preparations are less toxic but very expensive.

Toxicity: Oral suspension: nausea, vomiting, diarrhea, rash; intravenous drug: infusion-related chills, hypotension, nausea, vomiting, nephrotoxicity, hypokalemia, hypomagnesemia, hypocalcemia, anemia.

Ampicillin An antibiotic widely used in clinical treatment and rDNA research. It is a derivative of penicillin, which kills bacteria by interfering with the synthesis of the cell wall.

Amplification The amount of change in measured output per unit change in input. The slope of the input-output, or dose-effect, curve. (Engineers sometimes refer to "amplification" as "sensitivity".)

Ampoule or ampule A small glass vial sealed after filling and one of the earliest devices developed for safe storage of sterile injectable unit.

Amprenavir (Agenerase) Indications: Treatment of HIV infection in combination with other agents.

Contraindications: Known hypersensitivity.

Dosage: 1200 mg po bid. There are many potential drug interactions, some of which require dosage modification

Toxicity: Nausea, diarrhea, rash, headache, oral paresthesias.

Ampulla A sac-like enlargement of a canal or duct.

Amsacrine An anticancer drug that belongs to the family of drugs called topoisomerase inhibitors.

Amyloid plaque A build up of beta-amyloid protein. Amyloid plaques are one of the characteristic structural abnormalities found in the brains of Alzheimer patients. Upon autopsy, the presence of amyloid plaques and neurofibrillary tangles is used to positively diagnose Alzheimer's disease.

Amyotrophic lateral sclerosis An inherited, fatal degenerative nerve disorder, also known as Lou Gehrig's disease.

Anabolism The intracellular process involved in the synthesis of more complex compounds than those involved in catabolism (for example, glucose to glycogen) and requires energy.

Anaerobe A microorganism that thrives best, or only, when deprived of oxygen.

1. Facultative anaerobe: one able to grow in the presence or absence of free oxygen.

2. Obligate or obligatory anaerobe: one that will grow only in the absence of free oxygen.

Anaerobic bacteria Bacteria capable of growing in the absence of Oxygen.

Anaerobic Relating to an anaerobe.

Anaesthetics Drugs inducing anaesthesia; general anaesthetics are used for general anaesthesia (narcosis) while enabling major surgical and other operations to be performed; local anaesthetics are used for anaesthesia of a certain part of the body while performing minor surgical operations, such as wound sewing or tooth extraction; after their administration some individuals may experience an allergy.

Anagrelide A drug that is used to decrease the number of platelets in the blood in order to prevent blood clotting.

Anakinra A substance that is used to treat rheumatoid arthritis, and is being studied in the treatment of cancer. Anakinra blocks the action of interleukin 1 (IL-1). It belongs to the family of drugs called interleukin receptor antagonists. Also called Kinaret®.

Anal Having to do with the anus, which is the posterior opening of the large bowel.

Analgesia Loss of normal sensitivity to pain.

Analgesic A drug that reduces pain. Analgesics include aspirin, acetaminophen, and ibuprofen.

Analgesics antipyretics Drugs decreasing fever and acting as pain killers at the same time; the most frequently used contain acetylsalicylic acid and paracetamol; a series of analgesics-antipyretics is available without a prescription; the substances are available even in the form of combined preparations.

Analog A chemical compound that is structurally similar to another but differs slightly in composition, i.e. the replacement of one atom or functional group by another. In drug discovery, analogs of promising drug candidates are made and tested for increased efficacy and decreased side effect profiles.

Analyte specific reagents A new class of regulated product: analyte specific reagents. These products are usually a singular reagent, such as an antibody, which can be used toward developing a test by third parties, such as another company or a hospital. The manufacturer of this product is not planning to sell it as part of a kit, but only as an independent reagent. Therefore, if is of low risk to the user, it can be exempt from 501(k) [device] requirements, and by definition must be used "for identification and quantification of an individual chemical substance or ligand in biological substances."

Analytical data interchange (ANDI) A generic file format. It was common practice before CFR 21 Part 11 to save information from analytical instruments in this file format. The disadvantage now is that the approach does not allow replaying of data on a different system to yield the same result.

Analytical method Small scale process used to characterize and/or separate a mixture, a compound, or an unknown material into its constituent parts or elements.

Anaphylaxis Anaphylaxis, or anaphylactic shock, is a severe, frightening and life-threatening allergic reaction. The reaction, although rare, can occur after an insect sting or as a reaction to an injected drug - for example, penicillin or antitetanus (horse) serum. Less commonly, the reaction occurs after a particular food or drug has been taken by mouth.

Anaplastic thyroid cancer A rare, aggressive type of thyroid cancer in which the malignant (cancer) cells look very different from normal thyroid cells.

Anastrozole An anticancer drug that is used to decrease estrogen production and suppress the growth of tumors that need estrogen to grow. It belongs to the family of drugs called nonsteroidal aromatase inhibitors.

Ancestim A drug that is being studied for its ability to increase the number of stem cells in the blood. It belongs to the family of drugs called hematopoietic cell growth factors. Also called stem cell factor (SCF) and Stemgen.

Ancillary material Material used in preparing drugs that does not become a component of the drug (e.g. steam, air, N2, DI water).

Androgen A type of hormone that promotes the development and maintenance of male sex characteristics.

Androgen independent Describes the ability of tumor cells to grow in the absence of androgens (hormones that promote the development and maintenance of male sex characteristics). Many early prostate cancers require androgens for growth, but advanced prostate cancers are often androgen-independent.

Anemometer A device that measures air speed.

Anesthetic Literally an - without + aisthesis - perception by the senses (Gr.) A drug that causes loss of sensation. General anesthetics cause not only loss of sensation, but also loss of consciousness. Local anesthetics cause loss of sensation by blocking nerve conduction only in the particular area where they are applied.

Anetholtrithione A substance that is being studied in the treatment of cancer.

Angina pectoris A recurring pain or discomfort in the chest that happens when some part of the heart does not receive enough blood.

Angiogenesis Blood vessel formation. Tumor angiogenesis is the growth of blood vessels from surrounding tissue to a solid tumor. This is caused by the release of chemicals by the tumor.

Angiogenesis inhibitor A substance that may prevent the formation of blood vessels. In anticancer therapy, an angiogenesis inhibitor prevents the growth of blood vessels from surrounding tissue to a solid tumor.

Angiostatin A protein normally made by the body. It can also be made in the laboratory, and is being studied in the treatment of cancer. Angiostatin may prevent the growth of new blood vessels from the surrounding tissue to a solid tumor. It belongs to the family of drugs called angiogenesis inhibitors.

Angiotensin Angiotensin I is converted from angiotensinogen by renin. Angiotensin I is then converted to angiotensin II by angiotensin-converting enzyme (ACE). Angiotensin II is the active form. Its actions are...

vasoconstriction.

stimulates release of aldosterone.

stimulates release of ADH.

stimulates thirst.

Angiotensin converting enzyme (ACE) ACE converts angiotensin I to a biologically active form, angiotensin II. ACE is found in epithelial cells. Since the first major capillary bed the blood goes through after leaving the kidney is the lungs, most of the conversion takes place in the lungs epithelium. ACE inhibitors are used to combat hypertension.

Angiotensin converting enzyme inhibitor ACE inhibitor. A type of drug that is used to lower blood pressure. Angiotensin-converting enzyme inhibitors belong to the family of drugs called antihypertensives.

Angiozyme A substance that is being studied in the treatment of kidney cancer. It may prevent the growth of blood vessels from surrounding tissue to the tumor. It belongs to the families of drugs called VEGF receptor and angiogenesis inhibitors. Also called RPI.4610.

Angstrom (A°) A unit of length equal to one hundred-millionth of a centimeter (one ten-thousandth of a micron) used especially to specify radiation wavelengths.

Anhydrovinblastine An anticancer drug that belongs to the family of drugs called mitotic inhibitors.

Anidulafungin A drug that is used to treat infections caused by fungi. It belongs to the family of drugs called antifungals.

Anion A negatively charged particle or ion.

Anion exchange resin An ion exchange material that removes anions from solution by exchanging them with hydroxyl ions.

Annamycin A substance that is being studied in the treatment of cancer. It belongs to the family of drugs called anthracycline antibiotics.

Anneal The process by which the complementary base pairs in DNA strands combine.

Annealing A treatment process for steel in which the metal is heated and held at a suitable temperature and then cooled at a suitable rate for the purpose of reducing hardness, improving machinability, facilitating cold working, producing a desired microstructure, or obtaining desired mechanical, physical, or other properties.

Anodynes Drugs used to suppress strong pain, for example opiates (morphine, etc.).

Anorexia nervosa An eating disorder characterized by a misperception of body image. Individuals with anorexia nervosa often believe they are overweight even when they are grossly underweight.

Ansamycin An anticancer drug that belongs to the family of drugs called antineoplastic antibiotics.

Antacids Drugs neutralizing an extensive quantity of hydrochloric acid produced in the stomach; they are used for pyrosis, various digestive problems or in combination with ulcer healing drugs, followed by peptic ulcer healing. Antacids may reduce absorption when given at the same time as other drugs.

Antagonism The effect of two or more drugs such that the combined effect is less than the sum of the effects produced by each agent separately. The agonist is the agent producing the effect which is diminished by the administration of the antagonist. Antagonisms may be any of three general types:

1. Chemical: caused by combination of agonist with antagonist, with resulting inactivation of the agonist

2. Physiological: caused by agonist and antagonist acting at two independent sites and inducing independent, but opposite effects

3. Pharmacological: caused by action of the agonist and antagonist at the same site ie. epinephrine and propranolol at beta-receptors

Antagonist A drug or a compound that opposes the physiological effects of another. At the receptor level, it is a chemical entity that opposes the receptor- associated responses normally induced by another bioactive agent.

Anthracenedione An anticancer drug that belongs to the family of drugs called anticancer antibiotics.

Anthracycline A type of antibiotic that comes from the fungus

Anthraquinone A type of anticancer drug.

Anti agregancia Drugs reducing blood coagulation by impairing the function of platelets. They are administered to prevent a heart-attack while most frequently acetylsalicylic acid is administered in low dosage.

Anti anaemics Drugs used to prevent or improve anaemia; the most frequently prescribed preparations include folic acid, vitamin B12 and iron-containing drugs.

Anti arrhythmics Drugs administered for an impaired heart rate (arrhythmia).

Anti asthmatics A group of drugs used in the treatment of bronchial asthma; for example, represented by bronchodilators, substances affecting the vegetative nervous system, anti-histaminics, corticoids and others; they are available in a series of drug forms intended for both local and systemic application.

Anti CEA antibody An antibody against carcinoembryonic antigen (CEA), a protein present on certain types of cancer cells.

Anti coagulants Drugs used to prevent and treat excessive blood coagulation; they reduce blood coagulation.

Anti diabetics Drugs influencing the level of blood sugar in patients with diabetes mellitus; apart from insulin administered via injections, this group of drugs is also represented by tablets, so called oral anti-diabetics; when administering anti-diabetics it is necessary to follow precisely dosing and prescribed diet.

Anti diarhoics Drugs used in the treatment of diarrhoea, for example carbo medicinalis.

Anti emetics Drugs used to prevent or treat sensations of nausea and vomiting, for example nausea during travelling.

Anti epileptics A group of drugs used to prevent or treat attacks of epilepsy.

Anti hemorrhoidals Drugs used in the treatment of haemorrhoids, the majority of anti-haemorrhoidals are available in the form of ointments and suppositories.

Anti histaminics There are two types of anti-histaminics, i.e. drugs blocking the effect of histamine: the first being used to prevent or relieve symptoms of allergy, such as hay fever or rash (often anti-histaminics mean just this group concerned); while the second type is represented by so-called H2 anti-histaminics belonging to the ulcer healing drugs group.

Anti hypertension drugs Several groups of drugs reducing hypertension by various mechanisms, such as diuretics, vazodilatants, drugs affecting the vegetative nerve system and others; anti-hypertension drugs, sometimes also indicated as hypotensive drugs, are often combined in the treatment of hypertension.

Anti idiotype vaccine A vaccine made of antibodies that see other antibodies as the antigen and bind to it. Anti-idiotype vaccines can stimulate the body to produce antibodies against tumor cells.

Anti infective Something capable of acting against infection, by inhibiting the spread of an infectious agent or by killing the infectious agent outright.

Anti inflammatory drugs Anti-inflammatory drugs reduce the symptoms and signs of inflammation. Although not a drug, immunotherapy ("allergy shots") reduces inflammation in both allergic rhinitis and allergic asthma.

Anti interferon An antibody to an interferon. Used for the purification of interferons.

Anti muscarinic agent Pharmacological substance class which commits at muscarin-receptors. Anti-Muscarinic Agent tranquilizes the hyperactive muscles of the urinary bladder to regulate the activity of the bladder.

Anti parkinsonics Drugs used in the treatment of Parkinson's disease.

Anti phlogistics Anti-inflammation drugs.

Anti vertigo preparations Drugs used to prevent vertigo.

Anti viral preparations Drugs used in the treatment of virus-induced infections.

Antiandrogen therapy Treatment with drugs used to block production or interfere with the action of male sex hormones.

Antibiotics (ATB) Substances used in the treatment of infections induced by bacteria or other micro-organisms; there are several groups of antibiotics according to their chemical composition and effect in bacteria. The most important groups of ATB are represented by penicillin, tetracycline, cephalosporine, macrolide ATB, aminoglycosides, chinolons, peptide ATB; wide-spectrum ATB affect more types of bacteria at the same time, therefore, they are used in cases where it is unknown what bacteria has induced a disease; in order to achieve the required effect, as well as for the sake of safety and prevention of resistance of the bacteria it is necessary to use ATB regularly at specific time intervals while following the physician's advice.

Antibody A modified protein molecule present in the blood serum or plasma (and other body fluids), whose activity is associated chiefly with gamma globulin. Produced by the immune system in response to exposure to a foreign substance, it is the body's protective mechanism against infection and disease. An antibody is characterized by a structure complementary to the foreign substance, the antigen that provokes its formation, and is thus capable of binding specifically to the foreign substance to neutralize it.

Antibody affinity A measure of the binding strength between antibody and a simple hapten or antigen determinant. It depends on the closeness of stereochemical fit between antibody combining sites and antigen determinants, on the size of the area of contact between them, and on the distribution of charged and hydrophobic groups. It includes the concept of "avidity," which refers to the strength of the antigen-antibody bond after formation of reversible complexes.

Antibody therapy Treatment with an antibody, a substance that can directly kill specific tumor cells or stimulate the immune system to kill tumor cells.

Anticancer antibiotic A type of anticancer drug that blocks cell growth by interfering with DNA, the genetic material in cells. Also called an antitumor antibiotic or antineoplastic antibiotic.

Anticarcinogenic Having to do with preventing or delaying the development of cancer.

Anticholinergic A substance that blocks the parasympathetic nerves, which act to slow the heart rate, increase intestinal and gland activity, and relax sphincter muscles.

Anticoagulants Anticoagulants are drugs that prevent the formation of blood clots that can block blood flow to the brain.

Antidepressants A group of psychotropic drugs used for the treatment of various forms of depression.

Antiemetic A drug that prevents or reduces nausea and vomiting.

Antiestrogen A substance that blocks the activity of estrogens, the family of hormones that promote the development and maintenance of female sex characteristics.

Antifolate A substance that blocks the activity of folic acid. Antifolates are used to treat cancer. Also called folate antagonist.

Antifungal A drug that treats infections caused by fungi.

Antigen Any of various foreign substances such as bacteria, viruses, endotoxins, exotoxins, foreign proteins, pollen, and vaccines, whose entry into an organism induces an immune response (antibody production, lymphokine production, or both) directed specifically against that molecule. Response may be demonstrated as an increased reaction, such as hypersensitivity (usually protein or a complex of protein and polysaccharide, or occasionally a polysaccharide of high molecular weight), a circulating antibody that reacts with the antigen, or some degree of immunity to infectious disease if the antigen was a microorganism or its products.

Antigen presenting cell vaccine A vaccine made of antigens and antigen-presenting cells (APCs). Also called APC vaccine.

Antihistamine drugs Antihistamines are a group of drugs that block the effects of histamine, a chemical released in body fluids during an allergic reaction. In rhinitis, antihistamines reduce itching, sneezing, and runny nose.

Antihormone therapy Treatment with drugs, surgery, or radiation in order to block the production or action of a hormone. Antihormone therapy may be used in cancer treatment because certain hormones are able to stimulate the growth of some types of tumors.

Antimetabolite A drug that is very similar to natural chemicals in a normal biochemical reaction in cells but different enough to interfere with the normal division and functions of cells.

Antimicrotubule agent A drug that inhibits cell growth by stopping cell division. Antimicrotubule agents are used as treatments for cancer. Also called antimitotic agents, mitotic inhibitors, and taxanes. Docetaxel and paclitaxel are antimicrotubule agents.

Antimitotic agent A drug that inhibits cell growth by stopping cell division.

Antimitotic agents are used as treatments for cancer. Also called antimicrotubule agents, mitotic inhibitors, and taxanes. Docetaxel and paclitaxel are antimitotic agents.

Antimycotics Drugs against mycosis. They are applied locally to the affected place or, in the case of more extensive mycosis, also topically and even in the form of tablets.

Antineoplastic A substance that blocks the formation of neoplasms (growths that may become cancerous).

Antineoplastic antibiotic A type of anticancer drug that blocks cell growth by interfering with DNA, the genetic material in cells. Also called an anticancer antibiotic or antitumor antibiotic.

Antineoplaston A substance isolated from normal human blood and urine that is being tested as a type of treatment for some tumors and AIDS.

Antioxidant A nutrient or chemical that reacts with and neutralizes free radicals or chemicals that release free radicals. Antioxidants are also called free radical scavengers. Vitamins A, C, E and some of the B vitamins, beta-carotene, selenium and some key enzymes in your body are all antioxidants. By intercepting the free radicals, antioxidants prevent them from damaging molecular structures such as your DNA.

Antiparasitic A drug used to treat infections caused by bacteria and parasites. It is also used in the treatment of some cancers.

Antiplatelets Antiplatelets are drugs that stop blood platelets (substances in blood that promote clotting) from clumping together to form clots.

Antipsychotics A group of drugs used in the treatment of certain psychic and emotional conditions, including psychosis.

Antiretroviral therapy Treatment with drugs that inhibit the ability of the human immunodeficiency virus (HIV) or other types of retroviruses to multiply in the body.

Antirheumatic drugs Drugs against rheumatic diseases represented mainly by a group of so-called non-steroid antirheumatics (NSA) which, due to their effects also belong to the analgesic-antipyretics and anti-phlogistics groups; the most commonly used NSA contain acetylsalicylic acid, indometacine, ibuprophen, diclophenac; more extensively impaired inflammatory joints are additionally treated by salts of gold, corticoids, immunosuppressives and other drugs.

Antisense (molecule) An oligonucleotide or analog thereof that is complementary to a segment of RNA or DNA and that binds to it and inhibits its normal function.

Antisense c fos Synthetic genetic material that may slow or stop the growth of cancer cells.

Antisense DNA DNA that is complementary to the sense strand. (The sense strand has the same sequence as the mRNA transcript. The antisense strand is the template for mRNA synthesis.) Synthetic antisense DNAs are used to hybridize to complementary sequences in target RNAs or DNAs to effect the functioning of specific genes for investigative or therapeutic purposes.

Antisense molecules A sequence of nucleic acids, typically created in the lab, whose sequence is exactly complementary/ opposite to an mRNA molecule made by the body. mRNA molecules made by the body serve as templates for the synthesis of protein. Since the "antisense" mRNA molecule binds tightly to its mirror image, it can prevent a particular protein from being made.

Antisense oligonucleotides Short fragments of DNA or RNA that are used to alter the function of target RNAs or DNAs to which they hybridize.

Antiseptic Acting against sepsis. An antiseptic agent is one that has been formulated for use on living tissue such as mucous membranes or skin to prevent or inhibit growth or action of organisms. Antiseptics should not be used to decontaminate inanimate objects.

Antiserum The blood serum obtained from an animal after has been immunized with a particular antigen. It contains antibodies specific for that antigen as well as antibodies specific for any other antigens with which the animal has previously been immunized.

Antistatic cleaners Liquid cleaners that enhance surface conductivity of cleanroom tabletops, workstations, and other surfaces.

Antistatic Reducing static electric charges by retaining enough moisture to provide electrical conduction.

Antithrombotic therapy Treatment to prevent or interfere with the formation of thrombi, blood clots that form inside vessels and cause an obstruction to blood flow at the point of its formation.

Antithymocyte globulin A protein used to reduce the risk of or to treat graft-versus-host disease.

Antithyroid drugs Drugs used in the treatment of excessive activity of the thyroid gland.

Antitoxin An antibody that is capable of neutralizing the specific toxin that stimulated its production in the body. Antitoxins are produced in animals for medical purposes by injection of a toxin or toxoid, with the resulting serum being used to counteract the toxin in other individuals.

Antituberculosis Describes a drug or effect that works against tuberculosis (a contagious bacterial infection that usually affects the lungs).

Antitumor antibiotic A type of anticancer drug that blocks cell growth by interfering with DNA, the genetic material in cells. Also called an anticancer antibiotic or antineoplastic antibiotic.

Antiviral A drug used to treat infections caused by viruses.

Anxiolytics Drugs eliminating excessive nervousness, stress or anxiety.

APC vaccine A vaccine made of antigens and antigen-presenting cells (APCs). Also called antigen-presenting cell vaccine.

APC8015 Immune system cells that are collected from a patient with prostate cancer and treated in the laboratory with a molecule found on prostate cells. The treated cells are being studied for their ability to stimulate the immune system to kill prostate cancer cells.

API (Active pharmaceutical ingredient) Also called Drug Substance. Any substance or mixture of substances intended to be used in the manufacture of a drug (medicinal) product and that when used in the production of a drug becomes an active ingredient of the drug product. Such substances are intended to furnish pharmacological activity or other direct effect in the diagnosis, cure, mitigation, treatment, or prevention of disease or to affect the structure and function of the body.

API starting material A material used in the production of an API which is itself or is incorporated as a significant structural fragment into the structure of the API. A starting material may be an article of commerce, a material purchased from one or more suppliers under contract or commercial agreement, or it may be produced in-house. Starting materials are normally of defined chemical properties and structure.

Aplidine A substance that is being studied in the treatment of cancer. It is obtained from a marine organism.

Apoenzyme The protein moiety of an enzyme - determines the specifity of the enzyme reaction.

Apolipoprotein E (APOE) A gene situated on chromosome 19 that codes for a protein in lipoproteins that are normal constituents of blood plasma, for example HDL (high density lipoprotein), LDL (low density lipoprotein), and VLDL (very low density lipoprotein).

There are a number of common variations (alleles) of the APOE gene, the most common of which are known as: e2, e3, and e4. Research has shown that people who inherit one or more copies of the APOEe4 gene are at increased risk of developing Alzheimer's disease. Meanwhile, there is evidence to suggest that the relatively rare APOEe2 allele may offer some protection against the disease - it seems to be associated with a lower risk for Alzheimer's and a later age of onset if the disease does develop. APOEe3 is the most common form of the gene in the general population and is thought to have no effect on Alzheimer's risk.

Apolizumab A type of monoclonal antibody that is being studied as a treatment for hematologic (blood) cancers. Monoclonal antibodies are laboratory-produced substances that can locate and bind to cancer cells.

Apoptosis Or programmed cell death is a form of cell death in which a programmed sequence of events leads to the destruction of cells without releasing harmful substances into the surrounding area. Apoptosis plays an important role in health by eliminating aged cells, unnecessary cells, and unhealthy cells. A protein called bcl-2 prevents apoptosis in normal healthy cells. However, many cancer cells, which would normally be destroyed by apoptosis because they proliferate too quickly, produce high levels of bcl-2 in order to evade destruction.

Apparent permeability The apparent permeability coefficient (Papp) is a parameter that is determined in an in vitro or ex vivo transport assay system. It is referred to as apparent permeability because its value represents the composite effects of traversing all permeation pathways across the test system and does not represent the permeability across any single barrier, such as the unstirred water layer, the cell membrane or the tight junctions between epithelial cells. It is equal to (dQr/dt)/(A x Co), where dQr/dt is the cumulative amount of test compound appearing in the receiver compartment of the assay system vs. time, A is the area of absorption (cell monolayer or tissue), and Co is the initial concentration of the test compound in the donor compartment of the assay system.

Papp can be determined in either or both directions across an assay system. For cell monolayer assay systems the directions are referred to as apical to basolateral (A to B) and vice versa. For ex vivo tissue systems the directions are typically referred to as musocal to serosal and vice versa. A significant directional dependence in Papp values suggests that active absorption or efflux mechanisms mediate compound transport across the assay system. When determined in an appropriate assay system, such as Caco-2 cell monolayers or human intestinal tissue strips, the rank order of a compound's Papp value as compared to control reference compounds of known human absorption potential has been demonstrated to be predictive of the in vivo absorption classification of the same compound in humans

Applet A small application, typically downloaded from a server.

Applicable regulatory requirement(s) Any law(s) and regulation(s) addressing the conduct of clinical trials of investigational products of the jurisdiction where trial is conducted.

Application software (PMA CSVC) A program adapted or tailored to thespecific user requirements for the purpose of data collection, datamanipulation, data archiving or process control.

Appropriated login or impersonation Someone using the authorization code, usually user ID and password of another person to secure access to network resources for which he or she does not have privileges or authorization. Can be intentional or not. CFR 21 Part 11 mandates technical controls that prevent this.

Approval (in relation to institutional review boards) The affirmation decision of the IRB that the clinical trial has been reviewed and may be conducted at the institution site within the constraints set forth by the IRB, the institution, good clinical practice (GCP), and the applicable regulatory requirements. (ICH)

Aptamer A synthetic, specially- designed oligonucleotide with the ability to recognize and bind a protein ligand molecule or molecules with high affinity and specificity.

Aquifer An underground layer of permeable rock, sand, or gravel that contains water for wells or springs.

Arctigenin A substance found in certain plants, including burdock. It has shown antiviral and anticancer effects. Arctigenin belongs to a group of substances called lignans.

Arctiin A substance found in certain plants, including burdock. It has shown anticancer effects. Arctiin belongs to a group of substances called lignans.

Arginine butyrate A substance that is being studied in the treatment of cancer.

Arithmetic average roughness (Ra) The arithmetic average height of roughness component irregularities from the mean line measured within the sample length (L). This measurement conforms to ANSI/ASME B46.1 "Surface Texture - Surface Roughness, Waviness and Lay". Ra (formerly known as AA or Arithmetic Average in the U.S., and CLA Centerline Average in the U.K.) is usually expressed in microinches (µin), and performed by moving a stylus or profilometer in a straight line along the surface. A consistent and measurable surface finish can be specified for a desired roughness i.e., 9-11 microinch.

Aromatase inhibitor A drug that prevents the formation of estradiol, a female hormone, by interfering with an aromatase enzyme. Aromatase inhibitors are used as a type of hormone therapy for postmenopausal women who have hormone-dependent breast cancer.

Arrhythmia Any alteration in rhythm of the heartbeat either in time or force.

Ascites Abnormal build-up of fluid in the abdomen that may cause swelling. In late-stage cancer, tumor cells may be found in the fluid in the abdomen. Ascites also occur in patients with liver disease.

Ascomycetes A family of fungi marked by long spore-containing cells. Form sexual spores called ascospores, which are contained within a sac (a capsule structure). Ergot, truffles, some molds of the genera Neurospora and Aspergillus, and yeasts belong to this category.

Ascorbic acid A key nutrient that the body needs to fight infection, heal wounds, and keep tissues healthy, including the blood vessels, cartilage, ligaments, tendons, bones, muscle, skin, teeth, and gums. It is an antioxidant that helps prevent tissue damage caused by free radicals. The body does not make or store ascorbic acid, so it must be taken in every day. It is found in many fruits and vegetables, especially green peppers, citrus, strawberries, tomatoes, broccoli, leafy greens, potatoes, and cantaloupe. Also called vitamin C.

Asepsis A condition in which living pathogenic (causing or capable of causing disease) organisms are absent.

Aseptic Marked by or relating to asepsis.

Aseptic processing area Area in which sterile product is formulated, filled into containers, and sealed.

Aseptic transfer (in Isolators) The key issue in all contained aseptic environments. Aseptic transfer is essential for change parts, components, and even product to enter and exit an isolator system without sterility challenges. There are an increasing number of ways to make an aseptic transfer. The following is a brief list of some of the key techniques: 1. Alpha Beta Systems Double Door Systems: also called RTPs (Rapid Transfer Ports) and HCT (High Containment Transfer). When mated, the two ports act as one door, protecting the internal and external environments.

2. Alpha Beta Dry Heat Sterilized: similar to Alpha Beta port with the additional safeguard of a heat sterilized seal.

3. UV and Pulsed Light: light sterilization/ sanitization. Sterilizing the system by making use of a wide spectrum of light within the transfer chamber.

4. One Shot Systems: basically, two halves coming together. Similar to an Alpha Beta port but simpler, cheaper, and capable of only a single connection.

5. Heat Welded Bag Systems: passed in or passed out using a continuous polyethylene liner which is heat sealed and cut to maintain the integrity of the internal and external environments.

6. Steam Sterilized: the liquid component or powder path is clean steam sterilized after connection and prior to transfer.

7. Autoclave/Depyrogenation/Dryheat: pass through for batch. Use of conventional autoclave to sterilize a canister provided with an Alpha Beta port and filters to allow the passage of steam and safe aspiration on cooling. Depyrogenation/Dryheat uses dry heat to sterilize and at sufficient temperature depyrogenate components, typically glassware, in a batch oven

8. Depyrogenation Tunnel: standard volume glassware entry. Depyrogenation/Dry heat uses dry heat to sterilize and at sufficient temperature to depyrogenate components, typically glassware, in a tunnel allowing continuous input.

ASIC Acid-Sensing Ion Channel.

Asme bioprocessing equipment (BPE- 1997) An American National Standard that covers, either directly or by reference, requirements for materials, design, fabrication, examination, inspection, testing, certification (for pressure systems), and pressure relief (for pressure systems) of vessels and piping for bioprocessing systems, including sterility and cleanability (Part SD), dimensions and tolerances (Part DT), surface finish requirements (Part SF), material joining (Part MJ), and equipment seals (Part SG) for the bioprocessing systems in which the pressure vessels and associated piping are involved. This Bioprocessing Equipment (BPE) Standard does not address all aspects of these activities, and those aspects that are not specifically addressed should not be considered prohibited.

Requirements of this Standard apply to: 1. All parts that contact the product, raw materials, and/or product intermediates during manufacturing, process development, or scale-up.

2. All equipment or systems that are critical part of product manufacture, such as Water For Injection (WFI), clean steam, ultrafiltration, intermediate product storage, and centrifuges. ASME/ANSI B31 Code for Pressure Piping

A number of individually published Sections, each an American National Standard. Rules for each Section reflect the kinds of piping installations considered during its development, as follows: 1. B31.1 Power Piping: piping typically found in electric power generating stations, in industrial and institutional plants, geothermal heating systems, and central and district heating and cooling systems.

2. B31.3 Process Piping: piping typically found in petroleum refineries, chemical, pharmaceutical, textile, paper, semiconductor, and cryogenic plants, and related processing plants and terminals. Certain piping within a facility may be subject to other codes and standards, including but not limited to: (a) ANSI Z223.1 National Fuel Gas Code: piping for fuel gas from the point of delivery to the connection of each fuel utilization device. (b) NFPA Fire Protection Standards: fire protection systems using water, carbon dioxide, halon, foam, dry chemical, and wet chemicals. (c) NFPA 99 Health Care Facilities: medical and laboratory gas systems. (d) Building and plumbing codes, as applicable, for potable hot and cold water, and for sewer and drain systems.

3. B31.4 Pipeline Transportation Systems for Liquid Hydrocarbons and Other Liquids: piping transporting products that are predominately liquids between plants and terminals and within terminals, pumping, regulating, and metering stations.

4. B31.5 Refrigeration Piping: piping for refrigerants and secondary coolants.

5. B31.8 Gas Transportation and Distribution Piping Systems: piping transporting products that are predominately gas between sources and terminals, including compressor, regulating, and metering stations; gas gathering pipelines.

6. B31.9 Building Services Piping: piping typically found in industrial, institutional, commercial, and public buildings, and in multi-unit residences, which does not require the range of sizes, pressures, and temperatures covered in B31.1.

7. B31.11 Slurry Transportation Piping Systems: piping transporting aqueous slurries between plants and terminals and within terminals, pumping, and regulating stations.

Asparaginase An enzyme used in the treatment of cancer. It belongs to the family of drugs called antineoplastics.

Aspartate transaminase An enzyme found in the liver, heart, and other tissues. A high level of aspartate transaminase released into the blood may be a sign of liver or heart damage, cancer, or other diseases. Also called serum glutamic-oxaloacetic transaminase or SGOT.

Aspirin A drug that reduces pain, fever, inflammation, and blood clotting. Aspirin belongs to the family of drugs called nonsteroidal anti-inflammatory agents. It is also being studied in cancer prevention.

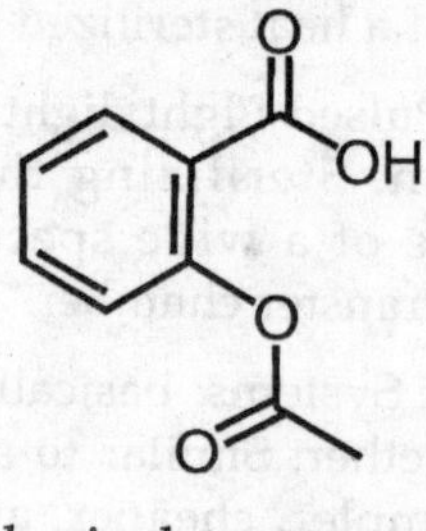

Assay A biological test, measurement or analysis done to determine whether a compound has the desired effect either in vivo, in situ or in vitro. A method to analyze or quantify a substance in a sample. An assay is an analysis done to determine either the presence of a substance and the amount of that substance of the biological or pharmacological potency of a drug. At Absorption Systems an assay is classified as either an Express Assay or a Custom Assay.

Assay assisted therapy A treatment program designed after laboratory analysis of an individual patient's tumor cells. The therapy plan is created taking into consideration the patient's response to chemotherapy regimens and combinations.

Assay, analysis Properly, an 'assay' determines how much of some particular material is in the sample (such as an assay for the Aspirin contentof Aspirin tablets). An 'analysis' generally determines (more or less) everything in the sample. An analysis of a rock would determine the content of calcium, magnesium, lithium, ... , and the length of the list would depend primarily on the sensitivity of the analysis.Both assays and analyses generally use similar procedures and instruments, but an analysis may be qualitative, reporting what is detected, or quantitative, reporting how much is found. An assay is always quantitative.

Assimilation The formation of cellular material utilizing small food molecules and energy.

AST/ALT Material found in the liver cells and muscle (heart) cells. Damage to these cells will increase values.

Asthma Asthma is a chronic, inflammatory lung disease characterized by recurrent breathing problems. People with asthma have acute episodes or when the air passages in their lungs get narrower, and breathing becomes more difficult. Sometimes episodes of asthma are triggered by allergens, although infection, exercise, cold air and other factors are also important triggers.

At rest HVAC room condition when unmanned, and without machinery operating. Previously called "static condition".

Atamestane A substance that is being studied in the treatment of cancer. Atamestane blocks the production of the hormone estrogen in the body. It belongs to the family of drugs called antiestrogens.

ATC group Anatomy-therapy-chemical drug classification according to the recommendation of the WHO (The World Health Organization). This is a group of drugs used for the same type of illness.

Atherosclerosis Atherosclerosis is the build-up of plaque (deposits of fat or cholesterol) in a blood vessel that eventually blocks the flow of blood through that vessel.

Atmospheric tank (fire code) A storage tank designed to operate at pressures from atmospheric through 0.5 pounds per square inch (psig) (3.4 kPa).

Atomic absorption spectrophotometry A highly sensitive instrumental technique for identifying and measuring metals in water.

Atovaquone (Mepron) Indications: Treatment (mild to moderate infection) and prophylaxis of PCP in patients unable to tolerate TMP-SMX or dapsone.

Contraindications: Known hypersensitivity.

Dosage: 750 mg of suspension po bid with food x three weeks for treatment. Same total daily dose for prophylaxis.

Toxicity: Gastrointestinal intolerance, rash, headache, fever.

ATP Adenosine triphosphate. A substance present in all living cells that provides energy for many metabolic processes and is involved in making RNA. ATP made in the laboratory is being studied in patients with advanced solid tumors to see if it can decrease weight loss and improve muscle strength.

Atrasentan A substance that is being studied in the treatment of cancer. It belongs to the family of drugs called endothelin-1 protein receptor antagonists.

Atrial fibrillation An abnormal, irregular heart rhythm characterized by chaotic electrical signals emanating from the atria, the upper chambers of the heart. Also known as atrial fib or a-fib.

Atrial naturetic hormone/factor/peptide (atriopeptin) Released by the atria in response to elevated blood pressure, ANH works to suppress aldosterone, and ADH. It also causes vasodilation. The net result is a decrease in blood pressure.

Atrial septal defect An inherited condition where an opening exists between the heart's two upper chambers. This allows oxygenated blood from the left atrium to return via the hole to the right atrium instead of flowing along its normal path to the left ventricle and then the body.

Atrophy Means the dying or death, normally referring to a gland or organ.

AUC The area under the plot of plasma concentration of drug (not logarithm of the concentration) against time after drug administration. The area is conveniently determined by the "trapezoidal rule": the data points are connected by straight line segments, perpendiculars are erected from the abscissa to each data point, and the sum of the areas of the triangles and trapezoids so constructed is computed. When the last measured concentration (Cn, at time tn) is not zero, the AUC from tn to infinite time is estimated by Cn/kel.

The AUC is of particular use in estimating bioavailability of drugs, and in estimating total clearance of drugs (ClT). Following single intravenous doses, AUC = D/ClT, for single compartment systems obeying first-order elimination kinetics; alternatively, AUC = C0/kel. With routes other than the intravenous, for such systems, AUC = F · D/ClT, where F is the bioavailability of the drug. The ratio of the AUC after oral administration of a drug formulation to that after the intravenous injection of the same dose to the same subject is used during drug development to assess a drug's oral bioavailability.

Auger electron spectroscopy (AES) An alternative surface analysis that can detect all elements with an atomic number greater than that of helium with the additional ability to analyze sub micron-diameter features. It is not as quantitative as ESCA and cannot determine the chemical state of an element. The primary advantage of Auger is that when combined with etching, a chemical depth profile can be measured rapidly and can image the distribution on the surface of spatial limitation resolution of 100 to 1,000 angstroms (depending on the equipment capability).

Augmerosen A substance that is being studied in the treatment of cancer. It may kill cancer cells by blocking the production of a protein that makes cancer cells live longer and by making them more sensitive to anticancer drugs. It belongs to the family of drugs called antisense oligodeoxyribonucleotides. Also called oblimersen, Genasense, and bcl-2 antisense oligodeoxynucleotide G3139.

Austenite A face-centered cubic crystal with high solubility for carbon (about 2%); an allotropic form of iron resulting from steel being heated above the transformation temperature.

Autegoneous weld A weld made by fusion of the base material without the addition of filler.

Authentication mechanisms Also known as authority checks, or authorized signers are mechanisms distinct from authorization that grants or denies access to a network resource, authentication programs are used by system administrators to establish and verify as conclusively as possible that a person logging in to the network is who he or she claims to be. department of health says that "authority checks" are to "ensure that only authorized individuals can use the system, electronically sign a record, access the operation or computer system, input or output device, alter a record, or perform operations".

Authentication The process of identifying a person, system, or company sufficiently to allow access to a system or part of a system.

Auto immune disease A disease in which the body produces an immunogenic response against self-antigens. In some cases, predominantly one organ is affected (e.g. hemolytic anemia and chronic thyroiditis); in others, the disease process is diffused through many tissues (e.g. SLE (Systemic Lupus Erythematosis)).

Autoclave An apparatus into which moist heat (steam) under pressure is introduced to sterilize or decontaminate materials placed within (e.g. filter assemblies, glassware, etc.). Steam pressure is maintained for pre-specified times and then allowed to exhaust. There are two types of autoclaves:

1. Gravity displacement autoclave: this type of autoclave operates at 121°C. Steam enters at the top of the loaded inner chamber, displacing the air below through a discharge outlet.

2. Vacuum autoclave: this type of autoclave can operate with a reduced sterilization cycle time. The air is pumped out of the loaded chamber before it is filled with steam.

Autoimmune disease Is a type of illness that occurs when the body tissues are attacked by its own immune system. People suffering from autoimmune diseases tend to have unusual antibodies circulating in their blood that target their own body tissues. Autoimmune diseases are more common in women than in men. Examples of autoimmune diseases include systemic lupus erythematosus (SLE or lupus), rheumatoid arthritis, multiple sclerosis, juvenile (type 1) diabetes, Addison disease, vitiligo, pernicious anemia, glomerulonephritis, and pulmonary fibrosis.

Automated system Term used to cover a broadrange of systems, including automated manufacturing equipment, controlsystems, automated laboratory systems, manufacturing execution systemsand computers running laboratory or manufacturing database systems. Theautomated system consists of the hardware, software and networkcomponents, together with the controlled functions and associateddocumentation. Automated systems are sometimes referred to ascomputerized systems; in this Guide the two terms are synonymous.

Automatic welding Welding with equipment that performs the welding operation without adjustment of the controls by a welding operator. The equipment may or may not perform the loading and unloading of the work.

Autonomic nervous system Innervation of smooth muscle, glands and visceral organs, which are not normally under voluntary control. Subdivided principally into the sympathetic and parasympathetic efferent systems. Autonomic reflexes are reflexes that act through these efferent systems; their afferent pathways may be either the same as pathways that subserve conscious perceptions (as with salivation) or they may be different (as with baroreceptor reflexes). The afferent pathways are not distinctive in any anatomical way, and are not usually described as 'autonomic' except by association with particular reflex actions

Autoradiography A technique that uses X-ray film to visualize radioactively labeled molecules or fragments of molecules; used in analyzing length and number of DNA fragments after they are separated by gel electrophoresis.

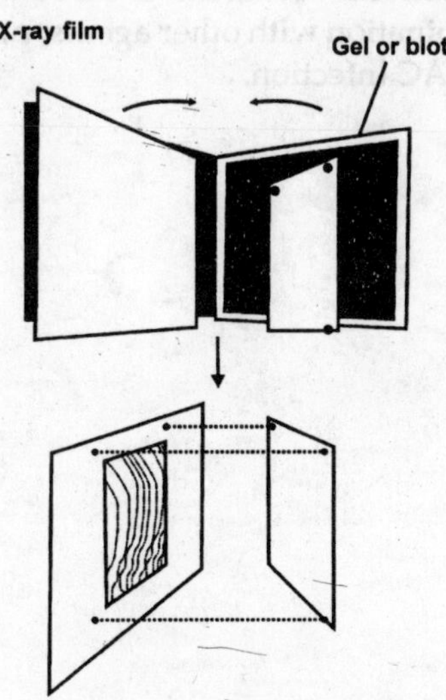

Fig. Autoradiography

Autosome A chromosome not involved in sex determination. The diploid human genome consists of 46 chromosomes, 22 pairs of autosomes, and 1 pair of sex chromosomes.

Autotrophs One of two categories in which microorganisms are classified on the basis of their carbon source. Autotrophs use carbon dioxide as a carbon source.

Avastin A monoclonal antibody used in the treatment of colorectal cancer that has spread. It is also being studied in the treatment of other types of cancer. It may prevent the growth of new blood vessels from surrounding tissue to a solid tumor. Also called bevacizumab.

AWP Average wholesale price of a drug.

Azacitidine An anticancer drug that belongs to the family of drugs called antimetabolites.

AZD2171 A substance that is being studied in the treatment of some types of cancer. It belongs to the families of drugs called angiogenesis inhibitors and vascular endothelial growth factor receptor (VEGFR) tyrosine kinase inhibitors.

Azithromycin (Zithromax)

Indications: Treatment of MAC infection in combination with other agents; prophylaxis of MAC infection.

Contraindications: Known hypersensitivity to macrolide antibiotics.

Dosage: MAC treatment: 600 mg po qd; prophylaxis: 1200 mg po weekly.

Toxicity: Gastrointestinal intolerance.

Azoxymethane A substance that is used in cancer research to cause colon tumors in laboratory animals. This is done to test new diets, drugs, and procedures for use in cancer prevention and treatment.

AZQ Diaziquone. An anticancer drug that is able to cross the blood-brain barrier and kill cancer cells in the central nervous system.

AZT A drug that inhibits the human immunodeficiency virus (HIV) that causes AIDS. Also called zidovudine.

O
HN
HO
O
N
HO
O
H
H
H
H
N
N
N

B

B The later segment of a biphasic plot of log C against t (following intravenous injection of a drug) represents the "elimination phase" of the drug's sojourn in the body, when eliminative, rather than distributive, processes dominate the rate at which plasma concentrations of drug decrease with the passage of time. b is used as a subscript for pharmacokinetic parameters appropriate to the elimination phase, e.g. t1/2b, Vdb, etc. For systems with more than two phases, the lower case Greek letters following b are used, in order, to designate the third, fourth, etc., phases.

B0 The slope of a linear plot of C (not the logarithm of C) against t; the slope of the linear plot of a zero-order reaction, in which, in equal time intervals, equal amounts of chemical undergo reaction.

BAC (Bacterial artificial chromosome) A vector used to clone DNA fragments (100-kb to 300-kb insert size; average, 150-kb) in E. Coli cells. Based on naturally occurring F-factor plasmid found in the bacterium E. coli.

Back up copy A magnetic copy of data, software, user-developed application, or operating parameters associated with an automated system and not considered the original.

Background contamination Contamination introduced accidentally in reagents, dilution water, solvents, rinse water, etc., which can be confused with constituents in samples being analyzed.

Background environment The environment that surrounds a critical area.

Backward compatibility A new version of a computer program that can use files and data created with an older version of the same program. A computer is said to be backward compatible if it can run the same software as the previous model. Backward compatibility is important because it eliminates the need to start over when you upgrade to a newer product, but is sometimes sacrificed in favor of a new technology.

Backwash The countercurrent flow of water through equipment, usually to clean or to recover performance, such as in a resin bed (flow-in at the bottom of the exchanger unit and out at the top) to clean and reclassify the bed after exhaustion. This process of reversing flow may also be applied to filters in order to force contaminants out of plugged pores and passages.

Bacteria The plural of Bacterium.

Bactericide An agent that kills vegetative bacteria but not mycobacteria or spores.

Bacteriophage A virus that exclusively infects bacteria. A protein coat surrounds the genome (DNA or RNA). One of the bacteriophages most extensively studied is the lambda phage, which is also one of the most important viral vectors used in rDNA work. Lambda promoters have been used to express eukaryotic proteins in E.coli.

Bacteriostatic Inhibiting growth of bacterial organisms without necessarily killing them or their spores.

Bacteriostatic water For Injection, U.S.P. Water that serves the same purposes as Sterile Water for Injection, it meets the same standards, with the exception that it may be packaged in either single-dose or multiple-dose containers of not larger than 30-mL size.

Bacterium Any of a large group of microscopic organisms having round, rod-shaped, spiral, or filamentous unicellular or noncellular bodies that are often aggregated into colonies, are enclosed by a cell wall or membrane (prokaryotes), and lack fully differentiated nuclei. Bacteria range in size from 0.4μm to 2.0μm and may exist as free-living organisms in soil, water, organic matter, or as parasites in the live bodies of plants. Some are disease producing, but most perform necessary functions such as digestion, fermentation, and nitrification. Most of the forms are variously grouped under generic names such as: Alcaligenes, Dialister, Escherichia, Klebsiella, Kurthia, Pasteurella, Salmonella, and Shigella.

Barometer Instrument used to measure atmospheric pressure.

Balanced study Trial in which a particular type of subject is equally represented in each study group.

Bandwidth An indicator of the throughput (speed) of data flow on a transmission path; the width of the range of frequencies on which a transmission medium carries electronic signals. All digital and analog signals have a bandwidth.

Bar code Bar code precisely determines a specific drug and packaging; once issued to the patient the bar code will ensure: allocation of the correct price of the drug, reference number for stock management and faster release.

Barbiturate A drug used to treat insomnia, seizures, and convulsions, and to relieve anxiety and tension before surgery. It belongs to the family of drugs called central nervous system (CNS) depressants.

Barium enema A procedure in which a liquid with barium in it is put into the rectum and colon by way of the anus. Barium is a silver-white metallic compound that helps to show the image of the lower gastrointestinal tract on an x-ray.

Baroreceptor reflex Baroreceptors found in the aorta arch and carotid sinuses, sense changes in blood pressure. As blood pressure goes up, the baroreceptors are stimulated and they deliver a higher rate of impulses to the vasomotor center of the brain. This causes a reduction in sympathetic tone and a stimulation of vagal tone. As a result, there is a reduction in heart rate, cardiac contractility, and vasodilation of blood vessels throughout the body which all contribute to lower blood pressure. If blood pressure goes down, baroreceptors reduce their rate of firing, causing the opposite effect. The baroreceptor reflex is more sensitive to rapidly changing pressure (standing up, or sitting down) than to a constantly elevated or depressed pressure. Baroreceptors will adapt to long term increased or decreased blood pressure.

Barrier isolator A containment device that utilizes barrier technology for the enclosure of a controlled workspace. There are two main types of isolator: 1. Type 1 Isolator: An isolator designed to protect the product from process-generated and external factors that would compromise its quality.

2. Type 2 Isolator: An isolator designed to protect the product from process-generated and external factors that would compromise its quality and to protect the operator from hazards associated with the product.

Barrier technology The technology of using separating environments, whether protecting the world from a product or the product from the world. Containment, barrier isolation and isolation all refer to the same technology, which is enclosing an environment. There are, however, some redefining terms that are gaining favor: 1. Containment - protect the world from the product (as in the case of highly potent compounds or a toxic).

2. Isolation - protect the product from the world (as in the case of a sterile product).

3. ISO 14644-7 "Minienvironments and Isolators" will define further levels of devices

Barriers to bioavailability Barriers to bioavailability are physicochemical or biological processes that reduce or prevent the systemic absorption of a drug following oral administration. At Absorption Systems we have a set of assays based on an in vivo rat model that can be used to help identify and quantify the causes of low oral bioavailability. These assays separately evaluate intestinal absorption, hepatic extraction, and site-dependent absorption. Also, concentration-dependence of saturable processes, such as hepatic extraction and carrier-mediated influx or efflux, can also be examined using these assays.

Base An electropositive element or radical that unites with an acid to form a salt. Or, a substance that when dissolved in water, dissociates to produce one or more hydroxyl ions (OH-).

Base pair (bp) Two nucleotides that are in different nucleic acid chains and whose bases pair by hydrogen bonding. In DNA, the nucleotide bases are adenine (A) that always pairs with thymine (T) and guanine (G) which pairs with cytosine (C). In RNA molecules, adenine (A) joins the uracil (U). Two strands of DNA are held together in the shape of a double helix by the bonds between these pairs.

Base sequence Analysis A method, sometimes automated, for determining the base sequence.

Baseline In some analytical procedures a sample is dissolved in water or combined with other reagents for analysis. A "blank" or standard consisting of the same reagents may be analyzed without sample present. This provides a comparative reference point, or baseline, so that the test results can be attributed solely to the sample itself.

Baseline assessment Assessment of subjects as they enter a trial and before they receive any treatment.

Baseline controlled studies In so-called baseline-controlled studies, the patient's state over time is compared with their baseline state. Although these studies are sometimes thought to use "the patient as his own control", they do not in fact have an internal control. Rather, changes from baseline are compared with an estimate of what would have happened to the patients in the absence of treatment with the test drug.

Baseline pharmaceutical engineering guides (ISPE) A series of industry publications developed in partnership with the US Food and Drug Administration (FDA). Each volume in the series is a collaborative effort of industry leaders representing a broad cross-section of manufacturers and other industry experts. The Guides document current industry practice for facilities and systems used for production of pharmaceutical products and medical devices. They are intended to:

Establish a baseline approach to new and renovated facility design, construction, commissioning, and qualification that is based upon clear understanding of the type of product and its manufacturing process.

Prioritize facility design features based upon the impact on product and process.

Avoid unnecessary spending on facility features that do not contribute to consistent production of quality products.

The Guides include five product manufacturing operation based guides (vertical guides), and three support system/ function based guides (horizontal guides):

1. Volume I - Bulk Pharmaceutical Chemicals (1996)
2. Volume II - Oral Solid Dosage Forms (1998)
3. Volume III - Sterile Manufacturing Facilities (1999)
4. Volume VI - Biotech (in progress)
5. Volume -Oral Liquids and Aerosols
6. Volume IV - Water and Steam Systems (in progress)
7. Volume V - Commissioning and Qualification Guide (in progress)
8. Volume VII - Packaging and Warehousing

Basic report A Basic Report contains:

the table of results for each assay specified in the project or study,

a list of specifications for the results,

if relevant, any observation about how test system, i.e., cell monolayers, animals, etc., reacted to the test compound(s),

if relevant, any observations about analytical method

A Basic Report is by default sent to the customer as a xls formatted file. Other formats such as pdf, or doc can be specified by the customer. The customer can also specify whether the reports are password protected.

Unlike a Standard Report a Basic Report does not include either a cover page or a description of the assay(s). Note that a description of the assay(s) can be found in the original proposal and any changes orders.

Examples of both a Basic Report and a Standard Report can be downloaded for this web site.

Basidiomycetes Reproduce by basidiospores, which are extended from the stalks of specialized cells called the basidia. The class comprises Photobasidiomycetes (smuts and rusts) and the Hymenomycetes (mushrooms and puffballs).

Basis of design A design document that describes what the purpose of a given system is and how the system will accomplish its required task. This document is created and approved before the issuance of bid specifications and is often used to develop them. Until the system is developed this is a conceptual document.

Batch A specific quantity of material produced in a process or series of processes so that is expected to be homogeneous within specified limits. In the case of continuous production a batch may correspond to a defined fraction of the production, characterized by its intended homogeneity. The batch size may be defined either by fixed quantity or the amount produced in a fixed time interval.

Batch fermentation The process in which a fixed volume of sterile medium in a vessel is inoculated with a desired organism. The broth is fermented for a defined period to completion, without further additions of media. After discharging the batch, the fermenter is cleaned and rebatched with medium for another cycle. Two other types of fermentation cycles are fed batch and continuous.

Batchwise Control The use of validated in-process sampling and testing methods such that results prove the process has done what it purports to do for the specific batch concerned, assuming control parameters have been appropriately maintained.

Batch number A unique combination of numbers and/or letters which specifically identify a batch or lot and from which the production and distribution history can be determined.

Batimastat An anticancer drug that belongs to the family of drugs called angiogenesis inhibitors. Batimastat is a matrix metalloproteinase inhibitor.

Bay 12-9566 An anticancer drug that belongs to the family of drugs called angiogenesis inhibitors.

Bay 43-9006 A substance that is being studied in the treatment of cancer. It belongs to the family of drugs called

Bay 56-3722 A substance that is being studied in the treatment of cancer. It belongs to the family of drugs called camptothecins.

Bay 59-8862 A substance that is being studied in the treatment of cancer. It belongs to the family of drugs called taxanes.

Bayesian statistics Statistical approach named for Thomas Bayes (1701–1761) that has among its features, giving a subjective interpretation to probability, accepting the idea that it is possible to talk about the probability of hypotheses being true and of parameters having particular values.

BB-10901 substance that combines a monoclonal antibody (huN901) with an anticancer drug (DM1), and is being studied in the treatment of certain cancers, including non-small cell lung cancer. Monoclonal antibodies are laboratory-produced substances that can locate and bind to cancer cells.

Beclomethasone A drug being studied in the treatment of graft-versus-host disease. It belongs to a family of drugs called corticosteroids.

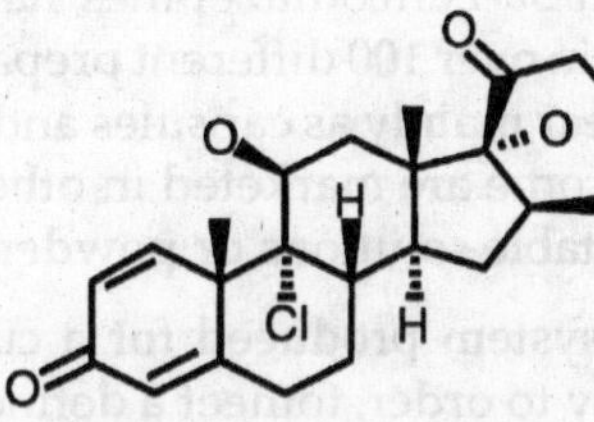

Bed Column of carbon, sand, chromatography, or ion exchange resins through which a liquid passes during operation.

Bed depth The height of the exchange or capture material in a column after proper backwashing for effective operation.

Bed expansion The effect produced during backwashing; resin particles separate and rise in the column. Regulating backwash flow may control bed expansion caused by the increase in space between resin particles.

Belladonna alkaloids Group of alkaloids, including atropine and scopolamine, found in plants such as belladonna and jimsonweed. They are used in medicine to dilate the pupils of the eyes, dry respiratory passages, prevent motion sickness, and relieve cramping of the intestines and bladder.

Beneficiary An individual who is either using or eligible to use health insurance benefits under an insurance contract.

Benign prostatic hyperplasia (BPH) Non-cancerous enlargement of the prostate.

Benign tumor A tumor or swelling that is not cancerous and remains in its site of origin and does not invade surrounding tissue or spread throughout the body. Benign tumors that contain normal cells can almost always be removed by surgery.

Benzodiazepines Benzodiazepines, therapeutically used as tranquillizers, hypnotics, anticonvulsants and centrally acting muscle relaxants, rank among the most frequently prescribed drugs. .

In 1960, the first benzodiazepine, chlordiazepoxide, was introduced. To date, more than 50 benzodiazepines have been marketed in over 100 different preparations. They appear mainly as capsules and tablets, however some are marketed in other forms such injectable solutions or powders.

Bespoke A system produced for a customer, specifically to order, tomeet a defined set of user requirements.

Beta blockers A large group of medications that are used in the of heart conditions such as angina, heart arrhythmias, high blood pressure and mitral valve prolapse. The drugs act to block specific receptors (beta-adrenergic receptors) in the nervous system, resulting in the slowing of the heart rate, reduction in blood pressure and reduced anxiety.

Bethanechol A substance generally used to increase muscle contraction along the gastrointestinal tract. It is used to treat gastroparesis and gastroesophageal reflux disease (GERD). It may cause hypotension, cardiac rate changes, and bronchial spasms.

Between-subject variation In a parallel trial design, differences between subjects are used to assess treatment differences.

Bexarotene n anticancer drug used to decrease the growth of some types of cancer cells. It belongs to the family of drugs called retinoids. Also called LGD1069.

Bexxar A monoclonal antibody in clinical trials as a treatment for B-cell Non-Hodgkin's Lymphoma.

Bexxar regimen Cmbination of monoclonal antibodies used to treat certain types of non-Hodgkin's lymphoma. The monoclonal antibody tositumomab is given with iodine I 131 tositumomab (a form of tositumomab that has been chemically changed by adding radioactive iodine). Monoclonal antibodies are laboratory-produced substances that can locate and bind to cancer cells.

Bezoar Usually a hard mass of entangled material, typically swallowed hair, fruit, or vegetable fibers or similar substances, sometimes found in the stomachs and intestines of animals or man. Bezoars can result from the hardening of food due to gastroparesis, and can cause nausea and vomiting. They are dangerous if they block the passage of food into the small intestine from the stomach.

Biafine cream topical preparation to reduce the risk of, and treat skin reactions to, radiation therapy.

Bias n a clinical trial, a flaw in the study design or method of collecting or interpreting information. Biases can lead to incorrect conclusions about what the study or trial showed.

BIBX 1382 Substance that is being studied in the treatment of cancer. It belongs to the family of drugs called epidermal growth factor receptor (EGFR) inhibitors.

Bicalutamide An anticancer drug that belongs to the family of drugs called antiandrogens.

Binary explosive An explosive material composed of separate components, each of which is safe for storage and transportation and would not in itself be considered as an explosive.

Binding site A specific region (or atom) in a molecular entity that is capable of entering into a stabilizing interaction with another molecular entity.

The reactive parts of a macromolecule that directly participate in its specific combination with another molecule.

Binding sites, antibody Local surface sites on antibodies which react with antigen determinant sites on antigens. They are formed from parts of the variable regions of the Fab fragment of the immunoglobulin.

Bioactivity A protein's ability to function correctly after it has been delivered to the active site of the body (in vivo).

Bioanalysis The quantitative measurement of an active drug or its metabolite(s) in both cell culture media and biological matrices such as plasma, serum, urine, feces, bile and tissues.

Bioanalytical assays Methods for quantitative measurement of a drug, drug metabolites, or chemicals in biological fluids.

Bioassay or biological assay "The determination of the potency of a physical, chemical or biological agent, by means of a biological indicator . . . The biological indicators in bioassay are the reactions of living organisms or tissues." Principles characterizing a bioassay include:

Potency is a property of the material to be measured, e.g., the drug, not a property of the response. Ordinarily, the relationship between changes in behavior of the indicator and differences in drug dose - (a dose-effect curve) - must be determined as a part of each assay.

Potency is relative, not absolute. The potency of one preparation (the "unknown") can be measured only in relationship to the potency of a second preparation (the "standard" or "reference drug") that elicits a similar biologic response. When the absolute amounts of standard used in the assay are known, the results of the assay can be used to estimate the amount - in absolute units - of biologically active material contained in the unknown preparation.

A bioassay provides only an estimate of the potency of the unknown; the precision of the estimate should always be determined, using the data of the assay.

Bioaugmentation A strategy involved in bioremediation that increases the activity of an organism to break down or metabolize a pollutant. This involves reseeding a waste site with bacteria as they die.

Bioavailability The percent of dose entering the systemic circulation after administration of a given dosage form. More explicitly, the ratio of the amount of drug "absorbed" from a test formulation to the amount "absorbed" after administration of a standard formulation. Frequently, the "standard formulation" used in assessing bioavailability is the aqueous solution of the drug, given intravenously.

The amount of drug absorbed is taken as a measure of the ability of the formulation to deliver drug to the sites of drug action; obviously - depending on such factors as disintegration and dissolution properties of the dosage form, and the rate of biotransformation relative to rate of absorption - dosage forms containing identical amounts of active drug may differ markedly in their abilities to make drug available, and therefore, in their abilities to permit the drug to manifest its expected pharmacodynamic and therapeutic properties.

"Amount absorbed" is conventionally measured by one of two criteria, either the area under the time-plasma concentration curve (AUC) or the total (cumulative) amount of drug excreted in the urine following drug administration. A linear relationship exists between "area under the curve" and dose when the fraction of drug absorbed is independent of dose, and elimination rate (half-life) and volume of distribution are independent of dose and dosage form. Alinearity of the relationship between area under the curve and dose may occur if, for example, the absorption process is a saturable one, or if drug fails to reach the systemic circulation because of, e.g., binding of drug in the intestine or biotransformation in the liver during the drug's first transit through the portal system.

Bioburden The level and type of microorganisms which may be present in raw materials, API (Active Pharmaceutical Ingredient) starting materials, intermediates, or APIs which have defined limits and should not affect the quality of the API. Bioburden should not be considered contamination unless the levels have been exceeded or defined objectionable organisms have been detected.

Biochemistry The study of chemical processes in living things. Despite the dramatic differences in the appearance of living things, the basic chemistry of all organisms is strikingly similar. Even tiny, one-celled creatures carry out essentially the same reactions that each cell of a complex organism, such as man, carries out.

Biocide An agent that can kill all pathogenic and non-pathogenic living organisms, including spores. More general than bacteriocide, biocide includes insecticides and any compound toxic to any living thing.

Biodegradable Material that can be broken down by biological action.

Bioequivalence Scientific basis on which generic and brand- name drugs are compared. To be considered bioequivalent, the bioavailability of two products must not differ significantly when the two products are given in studies at the same dosage under similar conditions. Some drugs, however, are intended to have a different absorption rate. department of health may consider a product bioequivalent to a second product with a different rate of absorption if the difference is noted in the labeling and doesn't affect the drug's safety or effectiveness or change the drug's effects in any medically significant way.

Bioequivalency A scientific basis on which generic and brand name drugs are compared with one another. Drugs are bioequivalent if they enter circulation at the same rate when given in similar doses under similar conditions.

Biofilms Are composed of populations or communities of microorganisms adhering to environmental surfaces. These micro-organisms are usually encased in an extracellular polysaccharide that they themselves synthesize. Biofilms may be found on essentially any environmental surface in which sufficient moisture is present.

Biogenerator A contained system, such as a fermentor, into which biological agents are introduced along with other materials so as to effect their multiplication or their production of other substances by reaction with the other materials. Biogenerators are generally fitted with devices for regulation, control, connection, material addition, and material withdrawal.

Biogenerics So far, drugs based on large biological molecules have been immune from copycat competition since most are still patent- protected and, critically, regulators in major markets have yet to set clear rules for approving generic versions.

Biohazard An infectious agent(s), or part thereof, presenting a real or potential risk to human, other animals, or plants, directly through infection or indirectly through disruption of the environment.

Bioinformatics The use of computers in the life sciences, electronic databases of genomes and protein sequences, and computer modeling of biomolecules and biologic systems.

Biologic A therapeutic agent derived from living things.

Biological availability The extent to which the active ingredient of a drug dosage form becomes available at the site of drug action or in a biological medium believed to reflect accessibility to a site of action.

Biological barrier An impediment (naturally occurring or introduced) to the infectivity and/or survival of a microbiological agent or eukaryotic cell once it has been released into the environment.

Biological equivalents Those chemical equivalents which, when administered in the same amounts, will provide essentially the same biological or physiological availability, as measured by blood levels, etc.

Biological impurities Impurities resulting from living matter (bacteria, virus, algae, protozoa, microfungi) and their by-products, including pyrogens (endotoxins).

Biological indicators Resistant microorganisms placed into or on various materials to confirm that a sterilization process is effective. They may for instance be placed within a filter in order to determine if a proposed autoclave cycle is effective. After autoclave, they are removed and culture tests are performed to see if the microorganisms were killed.

Biological reactivity tests, in vivo This classification is based on responses to a series of in vivo tests for which extracts, materials and routes of administration are specified. Six Plastic Classes are defined: 1. Class I - Uses a specified dosage of an extract of sample in Sodium Chloride Injection applied either intravenously or intracutaneously into a mouse or a rabbit.

2. Class II - Same as Class I but in addition uses an extract of sample in 1 in 20 Solution of Alcohol in Sodium Chloride Injection applied either intravenously or intracutaneously into a mouse or a rabbit.

3. Class III - Same as Class II but in addition uses an extract of sample in Polyethylene Glycol 400, and an extract of sample in Vegetable Oil, both applied either intraperitoneally or intracutaneously into a mouse.

4. Class IV - Same as Class II but in addition uses an extract of sample in Vegetable Oil applied intraperitoneally or intracutaneously into a mouse or a rabbit. Also uses implant strips of sample into a rabbit.

5. Class V - Same as Class II but in addition uses an extract of sample in Polyethylene Glycol 400, and an extract of sample in Vegetable Oil applied intraperitoneally or intracutaneously into a mouse or a rabbit.

6. Class VI - Same as Class V but in addition uses implant strips of sample into a rabbit.

These tests are designed to determine the biological response of animals to elastomerics, plastics and other polymeric material with direct or indirect patient contact, or by the injection of specific extracts prepared from the material under test. Three tests are described: 1. Systemic Injection Test - Designed to determine the systemic biological responses of animals to plastics and other polymers by the single-dose injection of specific extracts prepared from a sample.

2. Intracutaneous Test - Designed to determine the local biological responses of animals to plastics and other polymers by the single-dose injection of specific extracts prepared from a sample.

3. Implantation Test - Designed to evaluate the reaction of living tissue to the plastic and other polymers by the implantation of the sample (specimen under test) itself into animal tissue. With the exception of the Implantation Test, the procedures are based on the use of extracts that, depending on the heat resistance of the material, are prepared at one of the three standard temperatures: 50°, 70°, and 121°. Therefore, the class designation of a plastic must be accompanied by an indication of the temperature of extraction e.g., IV - 121°, which represents a class IV plastic extracted at 121°).

Biological response modifiers Substances that are used to boost the ability of the immune system to fight disease more effectively. The use of biological response modifiers in the treatment of cancer is an active and promising area of research. Types of biological response modifiers include interferons, interleukins and granulocyte colony-stimulating factor (G-CSF). The use of biological response modifiers is also known as immunotherapy.

Biological safety cabinets (BSCs) Bench-top or freestanding cabinets with unidirectional airflow used for handling materials that present a health hazard. The National Institutes of Health (NIH) Guidelines classify them as: 1. Class I - A negative pressure, ventilated cabinet for personnel protection having an inward flow of air away from the operator. The exhaust air is filtered through a HEPA filter (located at rear or top) either into the laboratory or to the outside. This cabinet is designed for general microbiological research with low and moderate risk agents (BL-2 and BL-3 agents), and is used in three operational modes: a) With a full width open front. The face velocity of the inward flow of air through the full width open front is at least 75' feet per minute. b) With an installed front closure panel (having four 6-inch diameter openings) without gloves. The face velocity of the inward flow of air through the openings will increase to approximately 150' feet per minute. c) With an installed front closure panel equipped with arm-length rubber gloves, and inlet air pressure relief for further protection. In this configuration, it is necessary to install a make-up air inlet fitted with a HEPA filter in the cabinet.

2. Class II - A ventilated cabinet for personnel and product protection having an open front with inward airflow for personnel protection (75' to 100' feet per minute), and HEPA filtered downward unidirectional airflow for product protection. The exhaust air is filtered through a HEPA filter for environmental protection. For selection and procurement of Class II cabinets refer to standards developed by the National Sanitation Foundation, Ann Arbor, Michigan. Cabinets are further classified as: a) Type A - Suitable for microbiological research in the absence of volatile or toxic chemicals and radionuclides (BL-2 and BL-3), with 70% recirculated air through HEPA. They are exhausted through HEPA into the laboratory or to the outdoors via a "thimble" connection to the building exhaust system. b) Type B - Hard ducted to the building exhaust system, contains negative pressure plena, and face velocity of 100' feet per minute. Type B cabinets are further sub-typed into types: B1 (30% recirculated air through HEPA; exhaust via HEPA and hard ducted. BL2 and BL-3), B2 (No recirculation; total exhaust via HEPA and hard ducted. BL-2 and BL-3), and B3 (same as IIA, but plena under negative pressure to room and exhaust air is ducted. BL-2 and BL-3).

Classes I and II should be located away from traffic patterns and doors, airflow from fans, room air supply louvers, and other air moving devices.

3. Class III - Closed-front ventilated cabinet of gas tight construction that provides the highest level of personnel protection from infectious aerosols, as well as protection of research materials from microbiological contaminants. The interior of the cabinet is protected from contaminants exterior to the cabinet. The cabinet is fitted with arm-length rubber gloves and is operated under negative pressure of at least 0.5 inches water gauge. All supply air is filtered through HEPA filters. Exhaust air is filtered through two HEPA filters in series or one HEPA filter and incinerator before being discharged to the outside environment. Class III cabinets are most suitable for work with hazardous agents that require Biosafety Level 3 or 4 containment. Cabinets must be connected to a double-door autoclave and/or chemical dunk tank used to sterilize or disinfect all materials exiting the cabinet, and to allow supplies to enter the cabinet.

Biological therapy The use of the body's immune system, either directly or indirectly, to fight cancer or to lessen side effects that may be caused by some cancer treatments. Also known as immunotherapy, biotherapy, or biological response modifier therapy.

Biologics Include blood, vaccines, tissue, allergenics and biological therapeutics.

Biologics, in contrast to drugs that are chemically synthesized, are derived from living sources (such as humans, animals, and microorganisms). Most biologics are complex mixtures that are not easily identified or characterized, and many biologics are manufactured using biotechnology. Biological products often represent the cutting- edge of biomedical research and, in time, may offer the most effective means to treat a variety of medical illnesses and conditions that presently have no other treatments available.

Veterinary biologics (vaccines, bacterins, diagnostics, etc, which are used to prevent, treat, or diagnose animal diseases) are regulated by the U.S. Department of Agriculture.

Biomass The entire assemblage of living organisms (both plant and animal), of a particular region, considered collectively.

Biometabolism Physical and chemical processes that occur within a cell or an organism, for example, the conversion of nutrients into energy.

Biometrics A method of verifying an individual's identity based on measurement of his/her physical feature(s) or repeatable action(s) where those features and/or actions are both measurable and unique to that individual. The main types of biometrics are: face recognition, finger scanning, hand geometry, finger geometry, iris recognition, palm, retina, signature, and voice recognition.

Bionics An interscience discipline for constructing artificial systems, which resemble or have the characteristics of living systems.

Biopharmaceuticals Biopharmaceuticals are generally complex macromolecules derived from recombinant DNA technology, cell fusion, or processes involving genetic manipulation. They include recombinant proteins, genetically engineered vaccines; therapeutic monoclonal antibodies; and nucleic acid based therapeutics, including gene therapy vectors.

Biopharmaceutics The science and study of the ways in which the pharmaceutical formulation of administered agents can influence their pharmacodynamic and pharmacokinetic behavior. Differences in pharmaceutical properties can cause substantial differences in the biologic properties - and therapeutic usefulness - of preparations which are identical with respect to their content of active ingredient. Pharmaceutical properties known to influence the therapeutic efficacy of drugs include: appearance and taste of the dosage form, solubility of the drug form used in the preparation, the nature of "fillers", binders, or menstrua in the dosage form, particle size, stability of the active ingredient, age of the preparation, thickness and type of coating of a dosage form for oral administration, the presence of impurities, etc.

Bioprocess engineering Process that uses complete living cells or their components (e.g., enzymes, chloroplast) to effect desired physical or chemical changes.

Bioprocessing The creation of a product utilizing a living organism.

Biopsy The gross and microscopic examination of tissues or cells removed from a living patient, for the purpose of diagnosis or prognosis of disease, or for the confirmation of normal conditions.

Biopure water Water that is sterile, pyrogen free and has a total solids content of less than 1 ppm.

Bioreactor A closed system used for bioprocessing (flask, roller bottle, tank, vessel, or other container), which supports the growth of cells, mammalian or bacterial, in a culture medium. A bacterial reaction usually is said to take place in a fermenter, and cell culture in a bioreactor.

Biosafety level The National Institutes of Health (NIH) specifies physical containment levels and defines Biosafety Levels in their "Guidelines for Research Involving Recombinant DNA Molecules" - Appendix G - May 1999. There are four biosafety levels for operations performed with infectious agents: 1. BL1: Practices, safety equipment, and facilities appropriate for work performed with defined and characterized strains of viable microorganisms not known to cause disease in healthy adult humans. The Basic Laboratory. This laboratory provides general space in which work is done with viable agents that are not associated with disease in healthy adults. Conventional laboratory designs are adequate. Areas known to be source of general contamination, such as animal rooms and waste staging areas, should not be adjacent to patient care activities. Public areas and general offices to which non-laboratory staff requires frequent access should be separated from spaces, that primarily support laboratory functions.

2. BL2: Practices, safety equipment, and facilities appropriate for work performed with a broad spectrum of moderate risk agents present and associated with human disease of varying severity. The Basic Laboratory. This laboratory provides general space in which work is done with viable agents that are not associated with disease in healthy adults. Conventional laboratory designs are adequate. Areas known to be sources of general contamination, such as animal rooms and waste staging areas, should not be adjacent to patient care activities. Public areas and general offices to which non-laboratory staff requires frequent access should be separated from spaces, which primarily support laboratory functions.

3. BL3: Practices, safety equipment, and facilities appropriate for work performed with indigenous or exotic agents where the potential for infection by aerosols is real and the disease may have serious or lethal consequences. Just walking through the area and breathing the air could infect one. The Containment Laboratory. This laboratory has special engineering features that make it possible for laboratory workers to handle hazardous materials without endangering themselves, the community, or the environment. The unique features that distinguish this laboratory from the basic laboratory are the provisions for access control and a specialized ventilation system. The containment laboratory may be an entire building, a single module, or complex of modules within a building. In all cases, a controlled access zone from areas open to the public separates the laboratory.

4. BL4: Practices, safety equipment, and facilities appropriate for work performed with dangerous and exotic agents that pose a high individual risk of life-threatening disease. Exposure to the skin could cause infection. The Maximum Containment Laboratory. This laboratory has special engineering and containment features that allow activities involving infectious agents that are extremely hazardous to the laboratory worker or that may cause serious epidemic disease to be conducted safely. Although the maximum containment laboratory is generally a separate building, it can be constructed as an isolated area within the building. The laboratory's distinguishing characteristic is that it has secondary barriers to prevent hazardous materials from escaping into the environment. Such barriers include sealed openings into the laboratory, airlocks or liquid disinfectant barriers, a clothing-change and shower room contiguous to the laboratory, a double door autoclave, a biowaste treatment system, and a treatment system to decontaminate exhaust air.

Biosphere All the living matter on or in the earth, the oceans and seas, and the atmosphere.

Biostatistics Branch of statistics applied to the analysis of biological phenomena.

Biosynthesis The production, by biological synthesis or degradation, of compounds by a living organism (e.g. amino acid synthesis, nucleotide synthesis).

Biotechnology A process of applying genetic engineering (recombinant DNA), hybrid (monoclonal antibody), hybridization (gene probes), bioelectric, etc. to commercial applications in pharmaceutical, chemical, medical diagnostic device, food, animal and plant industries.

Biotechnology drugs Defined as products based on recombinant DNA, monoclonal antibodies, continuous cell lines, gene therapy, and cellular therapy.

Biotransformation Chemical alteration of an agent (drug) that occurs by virtue of the sojourn of the agent in a biological system. Spontaneous decay of radium would not be considered a biotransformation even if it occurred within the body; chemical alteration of a chemical by enzymatic attack would be considered a biotransformation even if it occurred in a model system, in vitro. Pharmacodynamics involves the chemical effects of a drug on the body; biotransformation involves the chemical effect of the body on a drug! "Biotransformation " should be used in preference to "drug metabolism", and the word "metabolism" should probably be reserved to denote the biotransformation of materials essential to an adequate nutritional state. "Biotransformation" and "detoxication" are not synonyms: the product of a biotransformation may be more, not less, biologically active, or potent, than the starting material.

Biotranslocation The movement of chemicals (drugs) into, through, and out of biological organisms or their parts. In studying biotranslocation one is concerned with the identification and description of such movement, elucidation of the mechanisms by which they occur, and investigation of the factors which control them. Ultimately, the study of biotranslocation involves consideration of how chemicals cross cellular membranes and other biological barriers.

Biowaiver A biowaiver is an exemption granted by the US department of health from conducting human bioequivalence studies when the active ingredient(s) meet certain solubility and permeability criteria in vitro and when the dissolution profile of the dose form meets the requirements for an "immediate" release dose form. Biowaivers are based on the Biopharmaceutics (BCS) classification of the active ingredient. Currently BCS class I and class III compounds are eligible for biowaivers.

Biowaste inactivation The inactivation or "killing" of biological organisms using heat or chemicals. This step is done at the end of the processing to ensure that there are no living organisms remaining in the effluent that is sent to the sanitary sewer system. Heat is usually applied at 130°C (266°F) for mammalian cells. Chemicals used include caustic or acid.

BLA Biologics License Application, a document filed with the U.S. Food and Drug Administration (FDA) as part of the late-stage approval process for biotherapeutic products, such as proteins and antibodies.

Blank A preliminary analysis omitting only the sample to provide an unbiased reference point or baseline for comparison. It is important to minimize extraneous contamination that could be confused with constituents in the sample itself.

Bleomycin Agent widely used for testicular, head and neck as well as some of the pelvic and lung cancers.

Blind experiment A form of experiment in which the participants are, to some degree, kept ignorant of the nature and doses of materials administered as specific parts of the experiment. The purpose of the device is, obviously to prevent a prejudiced interpretation of the drug effects observed, and to prevent a presumed knowledge of effects to be expected from influencing the kinds of effects manifested by a subject. Blind experiments are not limited in use to experiments involving only human subjects. Needless to say, both experimenters and subjects may have general knowledge of the purpose, materials and design of the experiment; their ignorance is limited to the nature of individual drug administrations.

In a "single-blind" experiment, one participant - usually the subject - is left uninformed. In a "double-blind" experiment two participants - usually the subject and observer - are uninformed, and in a "triple-blind" experiment the subject, the observer, and the person responsible for the actual administration of the drug are left unaware of the nature of the material administered.

In clinical experimentation, particularly, the use of blind experimentation is frequently associated with the use of dummy or placebo medication as part of the experimental design, and the use of a "cross-over" experimental design.

Blind study One in which the subject or the investigator (or both) are unaware of what trial product a subject is taking.

Blind weld A "blind weld" is defined as a pipe or tube joint welded automatically in which there is no physical way to inspect the weld either visually or with a borescope.

Blinding Clinical trial technique in which, to eliminate bias in a research study, subjects and/or clinical investigators remain unaware of which investigational product is provided.

Blinded medications Products that appear identical in size, shape, color, flavor, and other attributes to make it very difficult for subjects and investigators to determine which medication is being administered.

Blinding/masking/open label A procedure in which one or more parties to the trial are kept unaware of the treatment assignment(s). Single blinding usually refers to the subject(s) being unaware, and double blinding usually refers to the subject(s), investigator(s), monitor, and, in some cases, data analyst(s) being unaware of the treatment assignment(s). In an open-label trial the identity of treatment is known to all.

Blood borne pathogens Infectious microorganisms that are carried in the blood of infected humans or animals and that can be transmitted through contact with infected blood, body fluids, tissues, or organs. Blood-borne pathogens are implicated in diseases such as malaria, syphilis, brucellosis, tuberculosis, hepatitis B, and AIDS (Acquired Immunodeficiency Syndrome). Workplace transmission of a blood-borne pathogen can occur via accidental inoculation with a contaminated "sharp" exposure through open cuts, skin abrasions, and mucous membranes of eyes and mouth indirect transmission (e.g., touching mouth, eyes, nose or open cuts with contaminated hands).

Blood brain barrier The blood-brain barrier (BBB) is a physiological filter that protects the brain from potentially injurious foreign and endogenous substances in the blood and maintains a constant environment for the brain. It functions as a semi-permeable filter that allows nutrients and some other materials to cross, but excludes many others. Anatomically it consists of capillary endothelial cells and, possibly astrocytes and glial cells that accomplish their physiological roles through a combination of structural—tight junctions between brain capillary endothelial cells and biochemical—

expression of efflux pump proteins and nutrient transporters—means.

Blood clot The conversion of blood from a liquid form to a solid through the process of coagulation.

Blood corpuscle A cell that circulates in the blood.

Blood plasma Blood from which all blood corpuscles, with the exception of platelet cells, have been removed (e.g. by centrifugation) resulting in a clear, straw-colored fluid, which clots as easily as whole blood.

Blood platelets Small, disc-shaped, metabolically active cells circulating in the blood. They are essential in the blood clotting process since they aggregate to form a plug on the injured surface of the blood vessel.

Blood serum The liquid expressed from clotted blood or clotted blood plasma.

Blow (Form) fill, seal Refers to machines that combine formation of a plastic container by blow molding, aseptic filling of a liquid product and sealing of the final package. In the U.S., a major company is ALP, or Automatic Liquid Packaging (Weiler Engineering) and in Europe, Rommilog.

Blowdown The bleeding-off of fixed quantities of accumulated feed water to reduce concentrated impurities. If these impurities are permitted to accumulate, they may pass through the distillation process and contaminate the distillate or foul the distillation system.

BME (Basic medium eagles) One of the most common tissue culture media composed of isotonic salts, carbohydrates and vitamins. When combined with animal serum. BME is a good medium for cell proliferation.

BNP A marker for congestive heart failure.

BOD (Biochemical oxygen demand) The amount of oxygen required to oxidize the dissolved organic matter in a water sample by aerobic (bacterial) decay. A measure of the oxygen depletion that would result from discharging organic impurities into a waterway.

Bolus dosing Instantaneous intravascular injection. If the duration of drug administration is long enough to have more than 5% of your AUC (CL) lost during administration, then you did not have a bolus but an

infusion. Further you would have to collect samples during the administration to quantify this AUC (CL).

Borderline products Products which are close to the boundary between medicines, which need a licence, and others, such as nutritional supplements, cosmetics etc., which do not. Classification depends either on the ingredient or the claim or both.

BPC (Bulk pharmaceutical chemical) A pharmaceutical product derived by chemical synthesis, in bulk form, for later dispensing, formulation or compounding, and filling in a pharmaceutical finishing facility.

Breakthrough Passage of a substance through a bed, filter, or process designed to eliminate it. For ion exchange processes, the first signs are leakage of ions (in mixed beds, usually Silica) and the resultant increase in conductivity. For organic removal beds, usually small, volatile compounds (Trihalomethanes (THMs) are common in activated carbon).

Brand name drug A new prescription drug that holds a patent. The patent gives the company that developed the drug exclusive rights to make and market that drug for a period of time, usually 20 years. When the exclusive rights run out, other drug companies can make and sell generic versions of the drug.

Braze welding A welding process using nonferrous filler metal that has a melting point below that of the base metals, but above 427ºC (800ºF). The filler metal is not distributed in the joint by capillary attraction. This type of welding has been also called Bronze welding, a misnomer.

Brazing A metal joining process wherein coalescence is produced by use of a nonferrous filler metal having a melting point above 427ºC (800ºF), but lower than that of the base metals being joined. The filler metal is distributed between the closely fitted surfaces of the joint by capillary action.

Breakthrough The first appearance in the effluent of an ion-exchange unit of unadsorbed components similar to those that deplete the activity of the resin bed. Breakthrough indicates that the resin is exhausted and needs to be regenerated.

Breath control shields Typically made of acrylic or plastic materials, shields protect product, equipment, or the work from particulate contamination expelled by people.

Broad spectrum Over a wide range. A broad-spectrum disinfectant is effective against a wide range of microorganisms including bacterial spores, mycobacteria, non-lipid and lipid viruses, fungi, and vegetative bacteria.

Bronchitis Bronchitis is an inflammation of the bronchi (lung airways), resulting in persistent cough that produces consideration quantities of sputum (phlegm). Bronchitis is more common in smokers and in areas with high atmospheric pollution.

Bronchodilator drugs Bronchodilators are a group of drugs that widen the airways in the lungs.

Bronchodilators Drugs dilating bronchi used, for example, in bronchial asthma; they belong to the category of anti-asthmatic drugs.

Bronchus Any of the larger air passages that connect the trachea (windpipe) to the lungs. The plural form of "bronchus" as "bronchi."

Broth The liquid culture medium in which fermentation or cell culture takes place.

Browser Computer program that runs on the user's desktop computer and is used to navigate the World Wide Web.

BSE (Bovine spongiform encephalopathy) Sometimes called "Mad Cow Disease". A disease of cattle presumably caused by a virus or other unidentified entity that affects the brain and causes the cow to behave erratically. Prevalent in parts of Europe but not in the United States. BSE is a contaminant that is undesirable in bovine sera. It is not known whether the causative agent can be filtered out since the causative agent itself is not known. In humans, it is believed to cause Creutzfeld-Jacob, a disease affecting the nervous system.

BTU (British thermal unit) The unit used to measure the amount of heat in a substance. One Btu is the heat required to produce a temperature rise of 1°F. in one lb. of water.

Bubble point test A filter leakage test in which the filter is wetted and air pressure is applied and slowly increased until water is expelled from the largest pores and bubbles appear from a submerged tube in a downstream collection vessel. Vigorous bubbling, as opposed to a diffusional airflow or occasional bubbles, is indicative of reaching the bubble point. This visual test can be fairly accurate for low area filters, such as discs. When used to evaluate high area filters, it is subject to limitations in observation, test time, collection conditions, and pressurization rates. The bubble point test is not recommended for integrity testing of filter cartridges.

Buffer A buffer is a compound or mixture of compounds which, added to a solution, helps maintain a certain pH. A buffered solution prevents changes in pH if either acids or bases are added to the solution or if the solution was diluted

Buffer prep Area Section of most biotech facilities devoted to the preparation of controlled bioburden buffer solutions for use in the chromatographic separation area of those facilities.

Bug (ANSI/IEEE) A manifestation of an error in software (a fault).

Bulk handling The transferring of flammable or combustible liquids from tanks or drums into smaller containers for distribution.

Bulk oxygen system An assembly of equipment, such as storage containers, pressure regulators, safety devices, vaporizers, manifolds, and interconnecting piping that has a storage capacity of more than 12,000 cubic feet (340 m^3) of oxygen at normal temperature and pressure, connected in service or ready for service, or more than 25,000 cubic feet (708 m^3) of oxygen, including unconnected reserve on hand at the site.

BUN BUN stands for Blood Urea Nitrogen and is a waste product, which should be removed from the blood by the kidneys. This test measures kidney function.

Bundling Refers to the inclusion of multiple devices or multiple indications for use for a device in a single premarket submission, including products subject to the device and biologics license application (BLA) authorities, for purposes of review and user fee payment. In CBER, the term may also include the designation of separate submissions as one premarket submission for review and user fee payment. Multiple devices may include different models within a generic type of device2 or devices that are of differing generic types.

Busulfan Drug used in treatment of leukaemia.

BVD (Bovine viral diarrhea) Viral contaminant found in bovine sera. Able to be filtered out using 0.1 µm nylon filters.

Bovine Of, relating to, or from a cow: such as Bovine Blood: blood from a cow.

Byte An abbreviation for binary term. A storage unit capable of holding eight bits or the space required for a single letter or number, a single character.

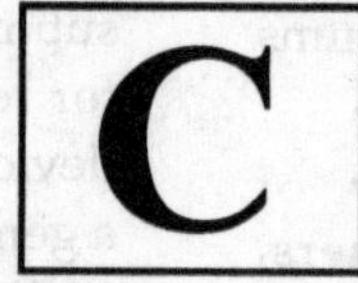

C, Cx The concentration (in units of mass/volume) of a chemical in a body fluid such as blood, plasma, serum, urine, etc.; the specific fluid may be indicated by a subscript, i.e. CU, the concentration of drug in the urine; when no subscript is used, C is commonly taken to be the concentration in the plasma.

C0 The fictive concentration of a drug or chemical in the plasma at the time (in theory) of an instantaneous intravenous injection of a drug that is instantaneously distributed to its volume of distribution. C0 is determined by extrapolating, to zero-time, the plot of log C against t (for apparently "first-order " decline of C) or of C against t (for apparently "zero-order" decline of C).

CA 125 A protein that can be found in the blood and is useful in detecting and evaluating ovarian cancer.

Cache Storage area on a computer's hard drive where the browser stores (for a limited time) Web pages and/or graphic elements.

Caco 2 Human colonic carcinoma; The Caco-2 cell line is widely used in in vitro assays to predict the absorption rate of candidate drug compounds across the intestinal epithelial cell barrier. The assay requires that drug absorption rates (Papp) be determined 21 days after Caco-2 cell seeding to allow for monolayer formation and cell differentiation (localization of active transporters to the apical or basolateral plasma membrane).

Cadmium A metallic element that occurs naturally in tiny amounts in air, water, soil, and food. It is a byproduct of zinc refining, and is used to make batteries, pigments, plastics, alloys, and electroplate. It is also found in cigarette smoke. Exposure to high levels of cadmium may cause certain cancers and other health problems.

Calcitonin A hormone formed by the C cells of the thyroid gland. It helps maintain a healthy level of calcium in the blood. When the calcium level is too high, calcitonin lowers it.

Calcitriol The active form of vitamin D. Calcitriol is formed in the kidneys or made in the laboratory. It is used as a drug to increase calcium levels in the body in order to treat skeletal and tissue-related calcium deficiencies caused by kidney or thyroid disorders.

Calcium A metallic dyad element of a lustrous yellow color, symbol Ca, atomic number 20, atomic weight 40.09, melting point 810°, often found in water usually as dissolved calcium carbonate, chalk ($CaCO_3$). Soluble in water, it causes hardness and subsequent scaling.

Calcium carbonate A mineral taken primarily as a supplement to prevent osteoporosis. It is also being studied for cancer prevention.

Calcium carbonate equivalent The value obtained when salts are calculated in terms of equivalent quantities of calcium carbonate. This is a convenient method of reducing all salts to a common basis for comparison.

ppm $CaCO_3$ = ppm ion X

Equivalent weight of $CaCO_3$———————————————Equivalent weight of ion

Where ion = magnesium, calcium, or other elements that contribute to hardness.

Calibration (ICH API defintion) The demonstration that a particular instrument or device produces results within specified limits by comparison with those produced by a reference or traceable standard over an appropriate range of measurements.

Calibration (PMA CSVC) Demonstration that a particular measuringdevice produces results within specified limits by comparison withthose produced by a reference standard device over an appropriate rangeof measurements. This process results in corrections that may beapplied to optimise accuracy.

Calibration standards A biological matrix that has been fortified with a known amount of test compound. Calibration standards are used to construct calibration curves from which the concentration of the test compound is determined in both the quality control (QC) samples and incurred samples . These samples are treated identically to the collected biological (plasma, feces, etc.) samples. The guidelines for generating a standard curve from calibration standards include:

Standard curve should cover the entire range of expected concentration of the test compound in the incurred samples,

The simplest curve fitting model should be applied such that the model adequately describes the concentration-response relationship,

The Lowest Limit of Quantification (LLOQ) on the calibration curve should have acceptable accuracy and precision.

Calorie Any of several approximately equal units of heat, each measured as the quantity of heat required to raise the temperature of one 1. gram of water by °C from a standard initial temperature, specially from 3.98°C, 14.5°C, or 19.5°C, at a constant pressure of one (1) atmosphere. Also called "gram calorie", "small calorie".

The unit of heat equal to 1/100 the quantity of heat required to raise the temperature of one (1) gram of water from 0°C to 100°C at one (10 atmosphere pressure. Also called "mean calorie".

The unit required to raise the temperature of one (1) Kilogram of water by 1°C at one (1) atmosphere pressure. Also called "kilogram calorie", "large calorie".

Calorimetry Analytical method that measures heat loss or gain resulting from physical or chemical changes in a sample. Differential scanning calorimetry compares the results of heating a sample to those for heating a reference material. For example, a method to measure the temperature at which the sample crystallizes, changes phases, or decomposes.

Camptothecin An anticancer drug that belongs to the family of drugs called topoisomerase inhibitors.

Camptothecin analog An anticancer drug related in structure to camptothecin, a topoisomerase inhibitor. One such drug is aminocamptothecin.

Canabis Products from the plant Cannabis sativa, or marijuana, are the most commonly abused and widely trafficked illicit drugs in the world. The most normally encountered form of cannabis is the dried leaves and flowers of the plant, which have a tobacco-like appearance and are either rolled into cigarettes (joints) or packed into cigars (blunts). Sinsemilla is the same form of the drug prepared from the unpollinated (seedless) female plant and has a higher level of the psychoactive chemical Delta-9-tetrahydrocannabinol (THC). Cannabis resin is the term applied to the dried secretion of the flowering top of the cannabis plant. Also called hashish, the drug can be in the form of a fine powder or compressed into slabs, and is either mixed with tobacco or orally ingested. Cannabis oil, while not as common as the other two forms, is made by extracting the cannabis resin in a manner similar to percolating coffee.

Cancer A term for diseases characterized by abnormal and uncontrolled growth of cells. The resulting mass, a tumor, can invade and destroy surrounding normal tissues. Cancer cells can spread (metastasize) throughout the body via blood and lymph systems. Cancer can originate almost anywhere in the body.

Capitation A reimbursement system in which healthcare providers receive a fixed fee for every patient served, regardless of how many or few services the patient uses. For example, an insurer negotiates to pay a Physician $100.00 a month to care for each of its subscribers, regardless of the amount of services each subscriber uses.

Capsaicin Pungent active principle of red peppers that activates specific sensory ion channels, possibly involved in pain transmission.

Capsid The external protein shell or coat of a virus particle.

Captopril A drug used to treat high blood pressure that is also being studied in the prevention of side effects caused by radiation therapy used in the treatment of cancer. It belongs to the family of drugs called ACE inhibitors.

Carbendazim An anticancer drug that belongs to the family of drugs called antifungal agents.

Carbogen An inhalant of oxygen and carbon dioxide that increases the sensitivity of tumor cells to the effects of radiation therapy.

Carbohydrates A large class of carbon-hydrogen-oxygen compounds that includes the sugars and their polymers (mainly starch, glycogen and cellulose). Most carbohydrates are produced by photosynthesis in plants. They are the major food compounds for both plants and animals. One group of carbohydrates, cellulose, is the primary structural material of plants.

Carbon filter A vessel loaded with activated carbon and used to remove organics, chlorine, tastes, and odors from liquids, operating on the principle of adsorption.

Carbon thickness A measurement of surface organic material. Carbon thickness values typically range from 5 to 20 angstroms (⊕). Significantly contaminated surfaces can show surface carbon thickness of 20 angstroms (⊕) or more.

Carbonate hardness That hardness in water caused by bicarbonates and carbonates of calcium and magnesium. If alkalinity exceeds total hardness, all hardness is carbonate hardness; if hardness exceeds alkalinity, the carbonate hardness equals the alkalinity.

Carboplatin An anticancer drug that belongs to the family of drugs called platinum compounds.

Carboxyamidotriazole An anticancer drug that belongs to the family of drugs called angiogenesis inhibitors.

Carboxypeptidase G2 A bacterial enzyme that is used to neutralize the toxic effects of methotrexate. It belongs to the family of drugs called chemoprotective agents.

Carcinogen A substance that causes the development of cancerous growths in living tissue. A chemical is considered to be a carcinogen if it has been evaluated by the International Agency for Cancer Research (IARC) and found to be a carcinogen or potential carcinogen, or if it is listed in the Annual Report on Carcinogens published by the National Toxicology Program, or if it is regulated by OSHA as a carcinogen.

Carcinogenic Cancer-causing. Many agents that are carcinogenic are mutagens.

Cardiac insufficiency Restricted physical capacity caused by a dysfunction of the myocardial muscle

Cardiac ischemia Ischemia means that a part of the body is receiving a less than adequate supply of blood and oxygen; cardiac ischemia means not enough blood and oxygen are flowing into the heart.

Cardiac toxicity Having an adverse effect (medication-induced) on the heart (also: "cardiotoxicity").

Cardiomyopathy A life-threatening disease in which the heart muscle becomes inflamed, resulting in impaired function.

Cardiovascular Concerning heart and circulation

Carnitine A substance made in the muscles and liver, and also found in certain foods such as meat, poultry, fish, and some dairy products. The body needs carnitine to make energy from fat.

Carotenoid A substance found in yellow and orange fruits and vegetables and in dark green, leafy vegetables. Carotenoids may reduce the risk of developing cancer.

Carrier A person who has a recessive mutated gene, together with its normal allele. Carriers do not usually develop disease but can pass the mutated gene on to their children.

Carry over effect Effects of treatment that persist after treatment has been stopped, sometimes beyond the time of a medication's known biological activity.

Carve out When a service such as pharmacy benefits management is contracted with a separate benefits carrier from the company providing medical benefits.

Carzelesin An anticancer drug that belongs to the family of drugs called alkylating agents.

Case control study A study that compares two groups of people: those with the disease or condition under study (cases) and a very similar group of people who do not have the disease or condition (controls). Researchers study the medical and lifestyle histories of the people in each group to learn what factors may be associated with the disease or condition. For example, one group may have been exposed to a particular substance that the other was not. Also called a retrospective study.

Case report form (CRF) A printed, optical, or electronic document designed to record all of the protocol-required information to be reported to the sponsor on each trial subject.

Case series A group or series of case reports involving patients who were given similar treatment. Reports of case series usually contain detailed information about the individual patients. This includes demographic information (for example, age, gender, ethnic origin) and information on diagnosis, treatment, response to treatment, and follow-up after treatment.

Cash flow Cash Flow is a financial ratio to evaluate a company's profit situation. It will be worked out by building the difference between income and expenditure during a fiscal period

Caspofungin acetate A drug used to prevent or treat infections caused by a fungus (a type of microorganism). It belongs to the family of drugs called antifungal agents.

Catabolism The intracellular phase of metabolism involved in the energy-yielding degradation of nutrient molecules (for example, glucose to CO2 and H2O). Waste products are called catabolites.

Catalase An enzyme that catalyzes the decomposition of hydrogen peroxide and molecular oxygen and water.

Catalyst A compound that increases the rate of a chemical reaction without being consumed or changed. In the biosciences, the term enzyme is used. Enzymes catalyze biological reactions.

Catalytic A chemical reaction happens more quickly without changing the catalyst

Catecholamines The class of neurotransmitters that includes norepinephrine and dopamine.

Categorical data Data evaluated by sorting values (for example, severe, moderate, and mild) into various categories.

Cation A positively charged particle or ion.

Cation exchange resin An Ion exchange resin, which removes positively charged ions (cations) by exchanging them for hydrogen ions.

Cation exchange The displacement of one positively charged particle by another on a cation-exchange material.

Catoplexy Is a condition of sudden muscular weakness or fatigue.

Causality assessment Determining whether there is a reasonable possibility that the drug caused or contributed to an adverse event. It includes assessing temporal relationships, dechallenge/rechallenge information, association (or lack of association) with underlying disease, and the presence (or absence) of a more likely cause.

Cavitation A condition of liquid flow where, after partial vaporization of the liquid, the subsequent collapse of vapor bubbles can produce surface damage.

CBER center for Biologics Evaluation and Research

CC 1088 A drug that is being studied in the treatment of cancer. It is similar but not identical to thalidomide. CC-1088 belongs to the family of drugs called angiogenesis inhibitors.

CC 49 A type of monoclonal antibody used in cancer detection or therapy. Monoclonal antibodies are laboratory-produced substances that can locate and bind to cancer cells.

CC 49 monoclonal antibody A type of monoclonal antibody used in cancer detection or therapy. Monoclonal antibodies are laboratory-produced substances that can locate and bind to cancer cells.

CC 8490 A substance that is being studied in the treatment of brain cancer. It belongs to the family of drugs called benzopyrans.

CC49 streptavidin A substance that is being studied in the treatment of cancer. It is made by combining the monoclonal antibody CC49 with a chemical called streptavidin. It can find tumor cells that have the protein TAG-72 on their surface, including colon, prostate, breast, and ovary cancer cells. After CC49-streptavidin binds to cancer cells, a radioactive compound called yttrium Y 90 DOTA-biotin will find those cells and kill them.

CCI-779 A substance that is being studied in the treatment of cancer. It belongs to the family of drugs called rapamycin analogs. Also called temsirolimus.

CDS Constant delivery system (patch technology)

Cefepime A drug used to treat infection. It belongs to the family of drugs called cephalosporin antibiotics.

Cefixime An antibiotic drug used to treat infection. It belongs to the family of drugs called cephalosporins.

Ceftriaxone A drug used to treat infection. It belongs to the family of drugs called cephalosporin antibiotics.

Ceiling (drug) The maximum biological effect that can be induced in a tissue by a given drug, regardless of how large a dose is administered. The maximum effect produced by a given drug may be less than the maximum response of which the reacting tissue is capable, and less than the maximum response which can be induced by another drug of greater intrinsic activity. "Ceiling" is analogous to the maximum reaction velocity of an enzymatic reaction when the enzyme is saturated with substrate.

Clearance of a chemical is the volume of body fluid from which the chemical is, apparently, completely removed by biotransformation and/or excretion, per unit time. In fact, the chemical is only partially removed from each unit volume of the total volume in which it is dissolved. Since the concentration of the chemical in its volume of distribution is most commonly sampled by analysis of blood or plasma, clearances are most commonly described as the "plasma clearance" or "blood clearance" of a substance.

Coombs Test is used to detect autoantibodies against your own red blood cells (RBCs). Many diseases and drugs (e.g., quinidine, methyldopa, and procainamide) can lead to production of these antibodies. The test is only rarely used to diagnose a medical condition but is essential for use by laboratories such as blood banks. Blood banks use the Coombs' test is to determine whether there is likely to be an adverse reaction to blood that is going to be used for a blood transfusion.

Celecoxib (Celebrex) A nonsteroidal anti-inflammatory drug (NSAID) used to treat osteoarthritis and rheumatoid arthritis. Some research suggests that it might reduce Alzheimer's risk in persons with a family history of dementia.

Cell The fundamental unit of life. The living tissue of almost every organism is composed of these fundamental living units. Unicellular organisms, such as yeast or a bacterium, perform all life functions within the one cell. In a higher organism, a multicellular organism, entire populations of cells may be designated a particular task. The cells of muscle tissue, for example, are specialized for movement.

Cell bank Master Cell Bank: The bank of cells, which contain the original unused mutated cells from which, the Manufacturing Working Cell Bank is taken. This is usually kept under lock with very limited access.

Manufacturing Working Cell Bank: The bank of cells derived from the Master Cell Bank, which are used to seed the fermentation manufacturing process.

Cell based assay The term is used to refer to any of a number of different experiments based on the use of live cells. This is a general definition and can include a variety of assays that measure cell proliferation, toxicity, motility, production of a measurable product, and morphology. Cell-based assays offer a more accurate representation of the real-life model since live cells are used, and also offer the possibility of a dynamic experiment through monitoring the numbers or behavior of the live cells. Thus, they provide a framework to determine the changes an external factor may exert on overall cellular function and viability

Cell culture The in vitro propagation of cells removed from organisms in a laboratory environment that has strict sterility, temperature, and nutrient requirement; also used to refer to any particular individual sample. Usually, cell culture takes place in a bioreactor.

Cell differentiation The process whereby descendants of a common parental cell achieve and maintain specialization of structure and function. Muscle cells become muscle cells and bone cells develop. In humans all the different types of cells differentiate from the simple sperm and egg.

Cell fusion The fusing together of two or more cells to become a single cell. This technique has had important consequences in immunology, developmental biology, and genetics. For example, monoclonal antibodies are produced by fusing a spleen cell (producing an antibody specific for the antigen of interest) with a mouse myeloma cell to produce a hybridoma which has an indefinitely long life because of the myeloma component and which secretes a specific antibody. When a human cell is fused with a mouse cell, the human chromosomes are progressively lost from the resultant hybrid and by correlating the presence of proteins in the hybrid with the presence of particular human chromosomes, genes can be assigned to individual chromosomes.

Cell growth, proliferation based assays Response testing methods that select drugs based upon their ability to stop cell growth or division.

Cell lines When cells from the first culture (taken from the organism) are used to make subsequent cultures, a cell line is established. "Immortal" cell lines can replicate indefinitely.

Cellulose A polymer of six-carbon sugars found in all plant matter, the most abundant biological compound on earth.

Celsius Of or pertaining to a temperature scale that registers the freezing point of water as 0°C and the boiling point as 100°C under normal atmospheric pressure. Also called "centigrade". The designation Celsius has been official since 1948, but centigrade remains in common use.

Center for biologics evaluation and research (CBER) The Bureau of Biologics concerned with biologic drugs, and most importantly, with the new protein and peptide drugs emanating from biotechnology.

Center for drug evaluation and research (CDER) The successor to the Bureau of Drugs concerned with all SVPs (Small Volume Parenterals), LVPs (Large Volume Parenterals), and non-biological drugs.

Centimorgan (cM) A unit of measure of recombination frequency. One centimorgan is equal to a 1% chance that a marker at one genetic locus will be separated from a marker at a second locus due to crossing over in a single generation. In human beings, one centimorgan is equivalent, on average, to one million base pairs.

Central nervous system (CNS) Is the brain, spinal cord and their associated nerves.

Centrifugation Mechanical means of separation based on differences in sedimentation rates due to differences in density between the suspended particles in the liquid.

Centrifuge A centrifuge operates on the principle of centrifugal force, the inertial reaction by which a body tends to move away from a center about which it revolves. This technique is commonly used to separate solids from liquids or liquids of different densities. Centrifugal equipment is divided into two major types, sedimenters and filters:

Centromere A specialized chromosome region to which mitotic or meiotic spindle fibers attach during cell division.

CEP 2563 dihydrochloride A growth factor antagonist that may stop tumor cells from growing.

CEP 701 A substance that is being studied in the treatment of cancer. It belongs to the family of drugs called protein tyrosine kinase inhibitors.

Cephalexin An antibiotic drug that belongs to the family of drugs called cephalosporins.

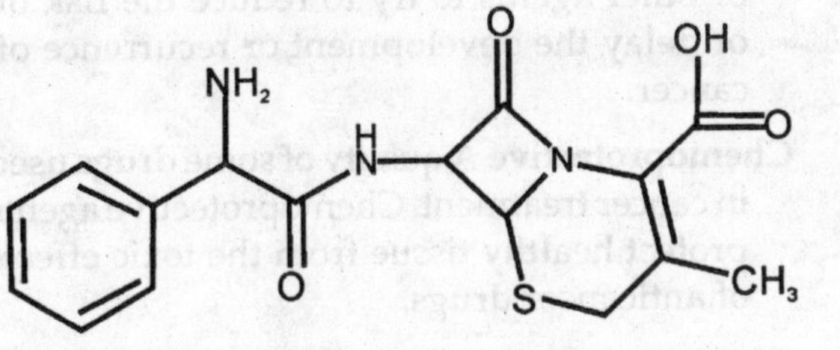

Cephalosporin A drug used to treat bacterial infections. It belongs to the family of drugs called antibiotics.

Cerebrovascular insufficiency An inadequate supply of blood to the brain because of a narrowing of the blood vessels which lead to, or are in various areas of the brain.

Certification (b. ANSI/ASQC A3 1978) Documented testimony by qualified authorities that a systemqualification, calibration, validation or revalidation has beenperformed appropriately and that the results are acceptable.

The procedure and action by a duly authorised body of determining,verifying, and attesting in writing to the qualifications of personnel,processes, procedures, or items in accordance with applicablerequirements.

Certified vendor drawings Drawings prepared by vendors for the fabrication of equipment, specialty components and skid mounted systems. These are certified as fabricated by the vendor and become the official document for the equipment involved.

Cetuximab A type of monoclonal antibody being studied in the diagnosis and treatment of cancer. Monoclonal antibodies are laboratory-produced substances that can locate and bind to cancer cells.

Cevimeline A substance that increases production of saliva and tears. It is being studied as a treatment for dry mouth caused by radiation therapy to the head and neck. It belongs to the family of drugs called cholinergic enhancers.

CFU (Colony forming unit) A measure of the number of bacteria present in the environment or on the surfaces of an aseptic processing room, measured as part of qualification and ongoing monitoring. Also applied to the testing of purified water samples.

CGMPs (current Good manufacturing practices) Current accepted standards of design, operation, practice, and sanitization. The department of health is empowered to inspect drug-manufacturing plants in which drugs are processed, manufactured, packaged, and stored for compliance with these standards.

CGP 48664 A substance that is being studied in the treatment of cancer. It belongs to the family of drugs called S-adenosylmethionine decarboxylase inhibitors.

Change control (PMA CSVC) A formal system by which qualifiedrepresentatives of appropriate disciplines review proposed or actualchanges that might affect a validated status. The intent is todetermine the need for action that would ensure and document that thesystem is maintained in a validated state.

Change note A document specifying the details of an authorised changerequest.

Change over The program by which a processing area is cleared of supplies and components used in the manufacture of a previous product and then readied for production of a new product. This often includes parts change over and/or special cleaning to eliminate cross-contamination.

Change plan A plan defining the details of the authorised changerequest, defining actions, responsibilities and procedures.

Channeling Cleavage, cracking, and furrowing of a resin bed due to resin age, a change in one of the feed solutions, or faulty operational procedures. The solution being treated follows the path of least resistance, runs through these furrows, and fails to contact active resin material in other parts of the bed.

Characterization Precisely deciphering and describing all the characteristics of a drug substance that affect its efficacy and its purity. Or the chemical, physical, and sometimes biological properties that are attributes of a specific drug substance.

Checksum A record of the number of bits transmitted and included with the transmission so that the receiving program can check to see whether the same number of bits arrived. If the counts match, it is assumed that the complete transmission was received.

Chelating agents Organic compounds that can withdraw ions from solution, forming insoluble complexes.

Chemical Caused by combination of agonist with antagonist, with resulting inactivation of the agonist, e.g., dimercaprol and mercuric ion.

Chemical equivalents Those multiple-source drug products which contain essentially identical amounts of the identical active ingredients, in identical dosage forms, and which meet existing physicochemical standards in the official compendia.

Chemoautotrophs Facultative autotrophs that obtain their energy from the oxidation of inorganic compounds.

Chemoimmunotherapy Chemotherapy combined with immunotherapy. Chemotherapy uses different drugs to kill or slow the growth of cancer cells; immunotherapy uses treatments to stimulate or restore the ability of the immune system to fight cancer.

Chemoprevention studies In cancer prevention clinical trials, studies test whether taking certain medicines, vitamins, minerals, or food supplements can prevent cancer. Also called agent studies.

Chemoprevention The use of drugs, vitamins, or other agents to try to reduce the risk of, or delay the development or recurrence of, cancer.

Chemoprotective A quality of some drugs used in cancer treatment. Chemoprotective agents protect healthy tissue from the toxic effects of anticancer drugs.

Chemoresponse assay or test A laboratory test that measures the number of tumor cells that are killed by a cancer drug. The test is done after the tumor cells are removed from the body. A chemosensitivity test may help in choosing the best drug or drugs for the cancer being treated.

Chemosensitivity The susceptibility of tumor cells to the cell-killing effects of chemotherapy drugs.

Chemosensitizer A drug that makes tumor cells more sensitive to the effects of chemotherapy.

Chemostat A growth chamber that keeps a bacterial culture at a specific volume and rate of growth by limiting nutrient medium and removing spent culture.

Chemotherapeutic agent A drug used to treat cancer.

Chemotherapy Drug treatment of parasitic or neoplastic disease in which the drug has a selective effect on the invading cells or organisms.

Chemotherapy Regimen A treatment plan that specifies the dosage, the schedule, and the duration of treatment.

Chemotherapy Treatment with anti-cancer drugs that usually act by interfering with the replication of cancer cell DNA, resulting in cancer cell death. There are several different ways drugs can damage cancer cells, and these different mechanisms often define different classes of chemotherapeutic drugs. Advances in the treatment of cancer over the past 2 decades are due largely to the development and study of chemotherapy.

Chimeric An organism, especially a plant, containing tissues from at least two genetically distinct parents. Type of antibody, partially human and partially mouse.

Chirality The geometric property of a rigid object (or spatial arrangement of points or atoms) of being non- superimposable on its mirror image; such an object has no symmetry elements of the second kind.

Chlorambucil A tablet form of chemotherapy, often used in low grade lymphoma.

Chloramine A chlorine compound formed by reaction with organic amines or ammonia.

Chloride A body salt/electrolyte, it usually follows the same pattern as sodium.

Chlorinated vinyls Thermoplastic chlorinated vinyls include PVC, CPVC, and VDC. PVC and CPVC are very similar materials, the primary difference being the addition of more chlorine to the PVC molecule to synthesize CPVC. This results in a higher glass transition temperature that equates to a higher use temperature for CPVC. The polymerization with chlorine also makes these materials inherently flame resistant. In addition to being resistant to higher temperatures, CPVC is more resistant to process chemicals.

Chlorination Adding chlorine or chlorine compounds to water for disinfection.

Chlorine An element used to kill microorganisms in water. At room temperature and atmospheric pressure a greenish yellow gas.

Chlorine demand Amount of chlorine used up by reacting with oxidizable substances in water before chlorine residual can be measured.

Chloroplasts Relatively large, chlorophyll containing, green organelles responsible for photosynthesis in photosynthetic eukaryotes, such as algae and plant cells. Every chloroplast contains an outer membrane and a large number of inner membranes called thylakoids.

Chlortetracycline The first drug of the tetracycline family, to be introduced (in 1948).

CHO (Chinese hamster ovary) cells In cell culture, the cells of a female hamster's reproductive organs, which historically have proven to be excellent expression systems in analytical studies and for producing pharmaceutical proteins.

Cholagogues Substances inducing a spasm of the gall bladder thus expelling bile to the biliary duct and then to the intestine.

Cholecalciferol A nutrient that helps the body use calcium and phosphorus and make strong bones and teeth. It is found in fatty fish, eggs, and dairy products. The skin can also make cholecalciferol when exposed to sunshine. Not getting enough cholecalciferol can cause a bone disease called rickets. Cholecalciferol is being studied in the prevention and treatment of some types of cancer. Also called vitamin D.

Cholekinetics Substances inducing the gall bladder to empty.

Choleretics Substances supporting bile production and its excretion.

Cholesterol A blood fat related in part to eating animal fats such as eggs, cheese, cream, liver, pork, beef, etc. Increased values may indicate a tendency to have hardening of the arteries. Values of 180 or less are associated with least risk of heart disease.

Cholinergic The parts of the nervous system that use acetylcholine as a neurotransmitter.

Chromatids Copies of a chromosome produced by replication.

Chromatography Procedure by which solutes (e.g., proteins and other chemical products) are selectively separated by a dynamic differential migration process in a system consisting of two or more phases, one of which moves continuously in a given direction and in which the individual substances exhibit different mobilities by reason of differences in adsorption, partition, solubility, vapor pressure, molecular size, or ionic charge density. The individual substances thus obtained can be identified or determined by analytical methods. There are several types of chromatography in use with different operating principles: 1. Adsorption - separates products by their different affinities for the surface of a solid medium, either an inorganic carrier such as silica gel, alumina, or hydroxyapatite, or an organic polymer.

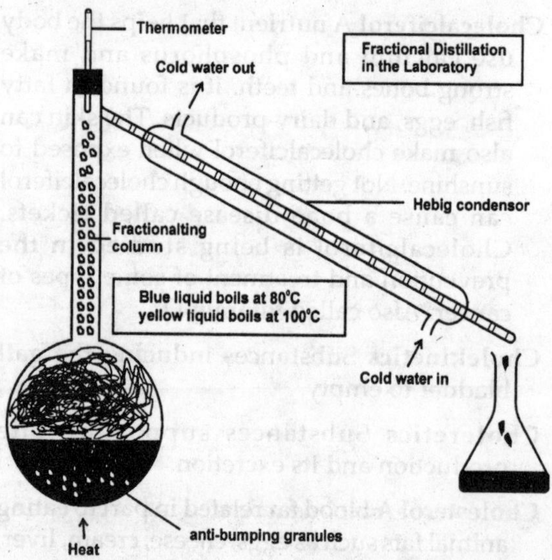

Fig. Chromatography

2. Ion Exchange - uses ion exchange resin to which ionized functional groups have been attached. At an appropriate pH, target proteins acquire a net surface charge that allows them to selectively bind to an ion exchange resin. Other impurities are eluted through the column.

3. Gel Filtration - employs a neutral cross-linked carrier with a defined pore size for molecular fractionation. Molecules larger than the largest pores cannot enter the matrix and pass directly through the column; smaller molecules enter the carrier and are retarded. Gel filtration thus separates on the basis of molecular size, eluting larger molecules first, followed by progressively smaller species.

4. Affinity - relies on the propensity of each biomolecule to have an affinity for another highly specific biomolecule, such as an antibody-antigen relationship. Once bound together, the drug molecules can be detached by altering various chemical attributes in the column.

5. Hydrophobic - separates by molecule polarity and reverse interaction with water.

6. High Pressure Liquid Chromatography (HPLC)-

Chromium enrichment layer thickness In stainless steel, the same as its maximum depth of enrichment, unless a surface iron layer is present in which case the chromium enrichment layer is calculated as the maximum depth of enrichment minus the thickness of the surface iron oxide layer.

Chromophore assisted laser inactivation Antibodies specific for the targeted protein, but not neutralizing, bring a reagent into proximity of the protein, and when activated by a laser, the reagent generates hydroxyl radicals that effectively inactivate the protein.

Chromophore That part of a molecular entity consisting of an atom or group of atoms in which the electronic transition responsible for a given spectral band is approximately located.

That part of a molecular entity consisting of an atom or group of atoms in which the electronic transition responsible for a given spectral band is approximately localized.

Chromosome The self-replicating genetic structure of cells containing the cellular DNA that bears in its nucleotide sequence the linear array of genes. In prokaryotes, chromosomal DNA is circular, and the entire genome is carried on one chromosome. Eukaryotic genomes consist of a number of chromosomes whose DNA is associated with different kind of proteins.

Chronic arrhythmia Any variation from the normal rhythm of the heart (which thereby causes the heart to pump less effectively) that persists over a long period of time.

Chronic obstructive pulmonary disease (COPD) COPD is a chronic respiratory disorder characterised by airflow limitation, accompanied by shortness of breath, cough, wheezing and increased sputum production. Patients are unable to perform their usual daily activities. COPD is mainly associated with smoking, with up to 20% of all smokers developing the disease. COPD progresses with age, leading to disability and early death.

According to the Annual World Health Report of the World Health Organisation (WHO), about 600 million people suffer from COPD, with some three million dying from the disease each year.

CHS 828 A drug that is being studied in the treatment of solid tumors.

CI 1033 A substance that is being studied in the treatment of cancer. It belongs to the family of drugs called tyrosine kinase inhibitors.

CI 958 A substance that is being studied in the treatment of cancer. It belongs to the family of drugs called DNA-intercalating compounds. Also called sedoxantrone trihydrochloride.

CI 980 An anticancer drug that belongs to the family of drugs called mitotic inhibitors. Also called mivobulin isethionate.

CI 994 A substance that is being studied in the treatment of non-small cell lung cancer. Also called N-acetyldinaline.

Cidofovir (Vistide)

Indications: Treatment of CMV infection, including ganciclovir-resistant strains.

Contraindications: Known hypersensitivity, significant renal dysfunction, use of other nephrotoxic medications.

Dosage: Initial therapy: 5 mg/kg IV once a week x 2.

Maintenance therapy (secondary prophylaxis): 5 mg/kg IV once every other week.

Probenecid 2 gm po 3 hr prior, and 1 gm po 2 hr prior and 8 hr after infusion should be administered to prevent nephrotoxicity; 1 liter normal saline is also given prior to cidofovir dosing.

Toxicity: Nephrotoxicity, neutropenia. Probenecid is associated with fever, chills, headache, rash, nausea.

Cilengitide A substance that is being studied as an anticancer and antiangiogenesis drug. Also called EMD 121974.

Cimetidine A drug usually used to treat stomach ulcers and heartburn. It is also commonly used in a regimen to prevent allergic reactions.

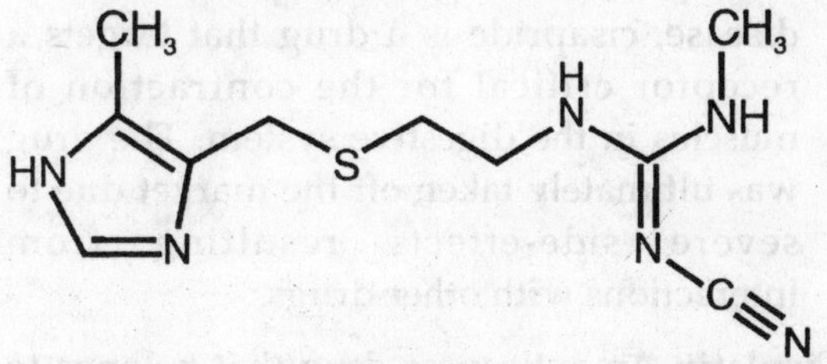

CIP (Clean in place) Internally cleaning a piece of equipment without relocation or disassembly. The equipment is cleaned but not necessarily sterilized. The cleaning is normally done by acid, caustic, or a combination of both, with WFI rinse. The design of a CIP system should considered the operating volume design for the water consumption, chemical and biowaste effluent, and energy required to clean a given circuit or piece of equipment.

Cipro A drug used to treat infections caused by bacteria. It is also being studied in the treatment of bladder cancer. Cipro belongs to the family of drugs called fluoroquinolones. Also called ciprofloxacin.

Ciprofloxacin A drug used to treat infections caused by bacteria. It is also being studied in the treatment of bladder cancer. Ciprofloxacin belongs to the family of drugs called fluoroquinolones. Also called Cipro.

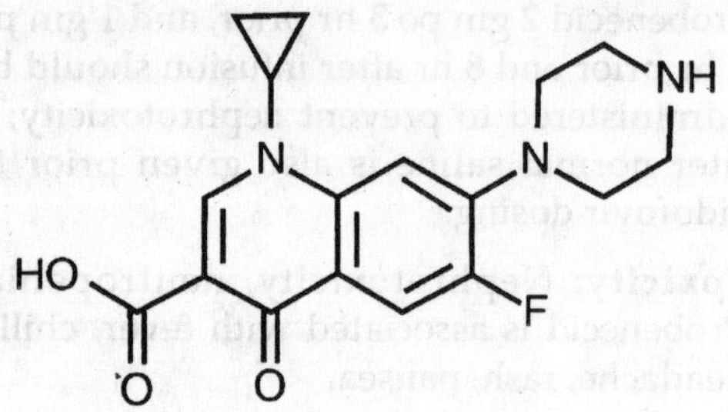

Circadian rhythm Biological timing and rhythmicity that, in human beings, is characterized by cycles of approximately 24 hours. Synonym: biological clock.

Cisapride (Propulsid) Indicated for the treatment of gastroparesis, ileus, chronic constipation, and gastroesophageal reflux disease, cisapride is a drug that targets a receptor critical for the contraction of muscles in the digestive system. The drug was ultimately taken off the market due to severe side-effects resulting from interactions with other drugs.

Cisplatin An anticancer drug that belongs to the family of drugs called platinum compounds.

Citric acid/potassium sodium citrate A drug used in the treatment of metabolic acidosis (a disorder in which the blood is too acidic).

Cl, Clx Clearance - in volume/unit time - of a drug or chemical from a body fluid, usually plasma or blood, by specified route(s) and mechanism(s) of elimination, as indicated by a subscript, e.g., Cl_R, urinary clearance; Cl_H, hepatic clearance, etc. Cl_T, total clearance, indicates clearance by all routes and mechanisms of biotransformation and excretion, operating simultaneously. $Cl_T = k_{el} \cdot V_d$. Following intravenous administration, $Cl_T = D/AUC$; following administration of drug by any route other than the intravenous, $Cl_T = F\,D/AUC$.

Cladribine An anticancer drug that belongs to the family of drugs called antimetabolites.

Claim A formal demand for reimbursement of expenses covered by an insurance policy. Insured individuals may submit claims to health plans for reimbursement.

Clarithromycin An antibiotic drug used in the treatment of infections. It belongs to the family of drugs called macrolides.

Clarithromycin (Biaxin) Indications: Treatment of MAC infection in combination with other agents; prophylaxis of MAC infection.

Contraindications: Known hypersensitivity to macrolide antibiotics.

Dosage: MAC treatment and prophylaxis: 500 mg po bid.

Toxicity: Gastrointestinal intolerance, abnormal liver function tests.

teratogenic in animals.

Class 100 Classification of an aseptic processing area where particle count should not exceed 100 particles (3,530 particles per cubic meter) 0.5μm or larger, per cubic foot of air, and no more than 0.1 CFU (Colony Forming Units) per cubic foot. Target uniform air velocity is 90 fpm plus or minus 20%, HEPA filtered air.

Class 1,000 Classification of an area where particle count should not exceed 1,000 particles (35,300 particles per cubic meter) 0.5μm or larger, per cubic foot of air. Supplied by HEPA filtered air. Class 1,000 is not a pharmaceutical GMP expectation.

Class 10,000 Classification of an area where particle count should not exceed 10,000 particles (353,000 particles per cubic meter) 0.5μm or larger, per cubic foot of air. Minimum of 20 air changes per hour, HEPA filtered air.

Class 100,000 Classification of an area where particle count should not exceed 100,000 particles (3,530,000 particles per cubic meter) 0.5μm or larger, per cubic foot of air, and no more than 2.5 CFU (Colony Forming Units) per cubic foot. Minimum of 20 air changes per hour of HEPA filtered air.

Class 30% ashrae area This area would have 30% efficient filtration. This classification is not specified in ISO 14644-1.

Class 65% ashrae area This area would have 65% efficient filtration. This classification is not specified in ISO 14644-1.

Class 95% ashrae area This area designation refers to the efficiency of the filters based on ASHRAE standard 52-76. These areas would have 95% efficient supply air filtration, unlike classified areas, which would have HEPA filtration. This classification is not specified in ISO 14644-1.

Class name "For naming and describing the classes, SI names and units are preferred; however, English (U.S. customary) units may be used".

Classical pharmaceuticals Small-molecule, nonbiotech drugs produced by chemical synthesis.

Classification The level (or the process of specifying or determining the level) of airborne particulate cleanliness applicable to a cleanroom or clean zone, expressed in terms of an ISO Class N, which represents maximum allowable concentrations (in particles per cubic meter of air) for considered sizes of particles.

Classified space A space in which the number of airborne particles is limited. This is accomplished by the strict use of HVAC systems. Areas are classified as Class 10, Class 100, Class 1,000, Class 10,000, and Class 100,000. In pharmaceutical production, only classes 100, 10,000, and 100,000 are used.

Clean air device Stand-alone equipment for treating and distributing clean air to achieve defined environmental conditions.

Clean air projector Fan and filter unit used to locally clean room air and deliver it to a desired location. Often called a fan/filter unit.

Clean area An area where particulate and microbial levels are specified (e.g., Filling Room - Class 10,000 "In Operation")

Clean database (or file) One from which errors have been eliminated and in which measurements and other values are provided in the same units.

Clean space A room or volume controlled to meet a certain airborne particulate limit (Class or Grade). In pharmaceutical facilities, clean spaces are usually classified and controlled only for aseptic processing facilities, but may also be defined for certain biotech processes. Final non-sterile bulk facilities, oral product, most topical product manufacturing facilities, and warehouses are normally not classified as clean spaces.

Clean steam Steam free from boiler additives that may be purified, filtered, or separated. When condensed, clean steam meets the specification for WFI. Usually utilized to sterilize process equipment.

Clean zone ISO 14644-1 defines it as "a dedicated space in which the concentration of airborne particles is controlled, and which is constructed and used in a manner to minimize the introduction, generation, and retention of particles inside the zone and in which other relevant parameters, e.g. temperature, humidity, and pressure, are controlled as necessary". Additionally, ISO 14644-1 states, "this zone may be open or enclosed and may or may not be located within a cleanroom".

Cleanroom A specially constructed space environmentally controlled with respect to airborne particles (size and count), temperature, humidity, air pressure, airflow patterns, air motion, and lighting. ISO 14644-1 defines it as "a room in which the concentration of airborne particles is controlled, and which is constructed and used in a manner to minimize the introduction, generation, and retention of particles inside the room, and in which other relevant parameters, e.g. temperature, humidity, and pressure, are controlled as necessary."

Cleanroom classification The maximum number of particles greater than or equal to 0.5μm in diameter that may be present in a cubic foot of room air.

Clearance The clearance of a chemical is the volume of body fluid from which the chemical is, apparently, completely removed by biotransformation and/or excretion, per unit time. In fact, the chemical is only partially removed from each unit volume of the total volume in which it is dissolved. Since the concentration of the chemical in its volume of distribution is most commonly sampled by analysis of blood or plasma, clearances are most commonly described as the "plasma clearance" or " blood clearance" of a substance.

A single compartment system, total clearance, by all routes (ClT), is estimated as the product of the elimination constant and the volume of distribution, in liters: ClT = kel · Vd the dimensions of ClT are, of course, volume/time.

Cleavage The splitting up of a complex molecule into two or more simpler molecules. The series of cell divisions occurring in the ovum immediately following its fertilization.

client A program that makes a service request of another program (the server) that fulfills the request. Web browsers (such as Netscape Navigator and Microsoft Explorer) are clients that request HTML files from Web servers.

Clindamycin Indications: Treatment of toxoplasmic encephalitis (for patients unable to tolerate sulfadiazine) in combination with pyrimethamine.

Contraindications: Known hypersensitivity.

Dosage: Initial therapy: 900 mg IV q8h for initial therapy or 300-450 mg po q6h.

Maintenance therapy (secondary prophylaxis): 300-450 mg po q6h.

Toxicity: Diarrhea, nausea, rash.

Clindamycin/Primaquine Indications: Treatment of PCP in patients unable to tolerate TMP-SMX.

Contraindications: Known hypersensitivity; glucose 6-phosphate dehydrogenase (G6PD) deficiency is contraindication to primaquine use.

Dosage: Clindamycin 600 mg IV q6-8h (or 300-450 mg po qid) and primaquine 15 mg base po qd x three weeks.

Toxicity: Clindamycin: diarrhea, nausea, rash. Primaquine: nausea, dyspepsia, hemolytic anemia (G6PD deficiency).

Pregnancy categories B (clindamycin) and C (primaquine).

Clinical Refers to physical signs and symptoms directly observable in the human body.

Clinical development The phase of drug development in which investigational new drugs (INDs) are tested on humans under the control of clinicians. Clinical development is necessary to obtain approval to market new drugs.

Clinical endpoint A characteristic or variable that reflects how a patient feels, functions, or survives. Clinical endpoints are distinct measurements or analyses of disease characteristics reflecting the effect of a therapeutic intervention in a clinical trial or study.

Clinical equivalents Those chemical equivalents which, when administered in the same amounts, will provide essentially the same therapeutic effect as measured by the control of a symptom or a disease.

Clinical hold The temporary cessation of a clinical trial by department of health if the agency is concerned about a drug or study protocol. The trial may resume when the problem is solved.

Clinical informatics Capturing, Managing and Measuring Clinical Data Quality to Ensure Accurate Statistical Analysis and Optimum Outcomes , Progress on Standards and Interoperability, Adapting Clinical Trial Operations in Tandem with EDC Technologies and Implementation,

The application of informatics approaches to the clinical- evaluation phase of drug development. These approaches can include clinical- trial simulations to improve trial design and patient selection, as well as electronic capturing and storing of clinical data and protocols. The goal is to reduce expenses and time to market.

Clinical pharmacology The branch of pharmacology that deals directly with the effectiveness and safety of drugs in humans.

Clinical pharmacometabolomics The segregation of patient populations using small molecule biomarkers in clinical trials, adverse drug reaction, and drug efficacy evaluation.

Clinical practice guidelines Guidelines developed to help health care professionals and patients make decisions about screening, prevention, or treatment of a specific health condition.

Clinical research Involving or concerned with the direct observation and treatment of living patients vs. theoretical science. Evaluating the safety and effectiveness of new drugs or therapies by monitoring their effects on people.

Clinical research associate (CRA) Person employed by a sponsor, or by a contract research organization acting on a sponsor's behalf, who monitors the progress of investigator sites participating in a clinical study. At some sites (primarily in academic settings), clinical research coordinators are called CRAs.

Clinical research coordinator (CRC) Person who handles most of the administrative responsibilities of a clinical trial, acts as liaison between investigative site and sponsor, and reviews all data and records before a monitor's visit. Synonyms: trial coordinator, study coordinator, research coordinator, clinical coordinator, research nurse, protocol nurse.

Clinical significance Change in a subject's clinical condition regarded as important whether or not due to the test article. Some statistically significant changes (in blood tests, for example) have no clinical significance. The criterion or criteria for clinical significance should be stated in the protocol.

Clinical study A type of research study that tests how well new medical approaches work in people. These studies test new methods of screening, prevention, diagnosis, or treatment of a disease. Also called a clinical trial.

Clinical therapeutic index Some indices of relative safety or relative effectiveness cannot be defined explicitly and uniquely, although it is presumed that the same quantifiable and precise criteria of efficacy and safety will be used in comparing drugs of similar kinds. The Food and Drug Administration has considered the following definition of an improved Clinical Therapeutic Index to be used in comparing different drug combinations or formulations; the assumption is retained that an improved or " better" drug has a higher Clinical Therapeutic Index " 1. increased safety (or patient acceptance) at an accepted level of efficacy within the recommended dosage range, or

2. increased efficacy at equivalent levels of safety (or patient acceptance) within the recommended dosage range."

Clinical trial A scientific means of evaluating the effectiveness and safety of a treatment, drug, or device in one or more human subjects including surgery, chemotherapy, or radiotherapy. There are different phases of a clinical trial

Phase I Trial: The first step in testing a new treatment in humans. These studies test the best way to give a new treatment (for example, by mouth, intravenous infusion, or injection) and the best dose. The dose is usually increased a little at a time in order to find the highest dose that does not cause harmful side effects. Because little is known about the possible risks and benefits of the treatments being tested, phase I trials usually include only a small number of patients who have not been helped by other treatments.

Phase II Trial: A study to test if a new treatment has an anticancer effect (for example, shrinks a tumor or improves blood test results) and if it works against a certain type of cancer.

Phase III Trial: A study to compare the results of people taking a new treatment with the results of people taking the standard treatment (for example, which group has better survival rates or fewer side effects). In most cases, studies move into phase III only after a treatment seems to work in phases I and II. Phase III trials may include hundreds of people.

Phase IV Trial: After a treatment has been approved and is being marketed, it is studied in a phase IV trial to evaluate side effects that were not apparent in the phase III trial. Thousands of people are involved in a phase IV trial.

Clinical trial exemption (CTX) A scheme that allows sponsors to apply for approval for each clinical study in turn, submitting supporting data to the Medicines Control Agency (MCA), which approves or rejects the application (generally within 35 working days). Approval means that the company is exempt from the requirement to hold a clinical trial certificate (CTC).

Clinical trial materials Complete set of supplies provided to an investigator by the trial sponsor.

Clinical trial simulation A relatively new effort to devise in silico simulations of human physiology and genetic variation to help identify which compounds will eventually fail in the drug development process.

Clinical trial/study Any investigation in human subjects intended to discover or verify the clinical, pharmacological, and/or other pharmacodynamic effects of an investigational product(s), and/or to identify any adverse reactions to an investigational product(s), and/or to study absorption, distribution, metabolism, and excretion of an investigational product(s) with the object of ascertaining its safety and/ or efficacy. The terms clinical trial and clinical study are synonymous.

Clinical trial/study report A written description of a trial/study of any therapeutic, prophylactic, or diagnostic agent conducted in human subjects, in which the clinical and statistical description, presentations, and analyses are fully integrated into a single report.

Clodronate A drug used in the treatment of hypercalcemia (abnormally high levels of calcium in the blood) and cancer that has spread to the bone (bone metastases). It may decrease pain, the risk of fractures, and the development of new bone metastases.

Clofarabine A substance that is being studied in the treatment of cancer. It belongs to the family of drugs called nucleoside analogs.

Clone A group of individuals produced from one individual through asexual processes that do not involve the interchange or combination of genetic material. As a result, members of a clone have identical genetic compositions. Protozoa and bacteria, for example, frequently reproduce asexually by a process called binary fission. In binary fission, a single-celled organism undergoes cell division and the result is two cells with identical genetic composition. Next, these two identical cells undergo division and the result is four cells with identical genetic composition. These identical offspring are all members of a clone.

Cloning Using specialized DNA technology to produce multiple, exact copies of a single gene or other segment of DNA to obtain enough material for further study. This process is used by researchers in the Human Genome Project, and is referred to as cloning DNA. The resulting cloned (copied) collections of DNA molecules are called clone libraries. A second type of cloning exploits the natural process of cell division to make many copies of an entire cell. The genetic makeup of these cloned cells, called a cell line, is identical to the original cell. A third type of cloning produces complete, genetically identical animals such as the famous Scottish sheep, Dolly.

Cloning vector DNA molecule originating from a virus, a plasmid, or the cell of a higher organism into which another DNA fragment of appropriate size can be integrated without loss of the vectors capacity for self-replication; vectors introduce foreign DNA into host cells, where it can be reproduced in large quantities. Examples are plasmids, cosmids, and yeast artificial chromosomes; vectors are often recombinant molecules containing DNA sequences from several sources.

Closed formulary A prescription benefits plan that has a closed-formulary design generally will not cover the cost of certain drugs unless a member's physician authorizes a medical exception.

Closed formulary plan – in this type of plan, pharmacy benefits do not cover medications on the Formulary Exclusions List unless the member's doctor obtains a medical exception.

Closed system System sterilized-in-place or sterilized while closed prior to use, is pressure or vacuum tight to some predefined leak rate, can be utilized for its intended purpose without breach to the integrity of the system, can be adapted for fluid transfers in or out while maintaining asepsis, and is connectable to other closed systems while maintaining integrity of all closed systems. (From PDA TR-28 for sterile product manufacture)

Clostridium A genus of bacteria, most are obligate anaerobes and form endospores.

Clotrimazole Indications: Treatment of mucosal candidiasis.

Contraindications: Known hypersensitivity.

Dosage: Oral candidiasis: 10 mg lozenge dissolved in the mouth 5 times a day; vaginal candidiasis: 100 mg tablet per vagina bid x 3 days.

Toxicity: Nausea, abnormal liver function tests.

Cmax, Cmin The maximum or "peak" concentration (Cmax) of a drug observed after its administration; the minimum or "trough" concentration (Cmin) of a drug observed after its administration and just prior to the administration of a subsequent dose. For drugs eliminated by first-order kinetics from a single-compartment system, Cmax, after n equal doses given at equal intervals is given by C0(1 - fn)/(1 - f) = Cmax, and Cmin = Cmax - C0.

The time following drug administration at which the peak concentration of Cmax occurs, tp (for any route of administration but the intravenous), is given by tp = (ln ka - ln kel)/(ka - kel). (Remember that ln is the natural logarithm, to the base e, rather than the common logarithm or logarithm to the base 10; ln X=2.303 log X.).

CMC (Chemistry, manufacturing, and controls) The section on a BLA (Biologics License Application) or IND (Investigational New Drug) describing the composition, manufacture, and specifications of a drug product and its ingredients.

CMF Standard drug reigmen used in the treatment of breast cancer

CNS Central Nervous System.

CNS prophylaxis Chemotherapy or radiation therapy given to the central nervous system (CNS) as a preventive treatment. It is given to kill cancer cells that may be in the brain and spinal cord, even though no cancer has been detected there. Also called CNS sanctuary therapy.

CNS sanctuary therapy Central nervous system sanctuary therapy. Chemotherapy or radiation therapy given to the central nervous system (CNS) as a preventive treatment. It is given to kill cancer cells that may be in the brain and spinal cord, even though no cancer has been detected there. Also called CNS

Co codamol Analgesic for mild or moderate pain.

Co dydramol Analgesic for mild or moderate pain.

Co proxamol (Distalgesic) Analgesic to deal with mild or moderate pain.

Co2 Buffer system assists in the transport of carbon dioxide from the tissue to the lungs.

Coagulation Adding insoluble compounds to water to neutralize the electrical charge on colloids, causing them to coalesce to form larger particles that can be removed by settling.

Coaguligand A VTA (Vascular Targeting Agent) that utilizes a human coagulation protein to induce tumor blood vessel clotting.

Cobalamin A vitamin that is needed to make red blood cells and DNA (the genetic material in cells) and to keep nerve cells healthy. It is found in eggs, meat, poultry, shellfish, milk, and milk products. Cobalamin, along with folate, may be given to help reduce side effects in cancer patients being treated with drugs called antimetabolites. Also called vitamin B12.

Cobalamine A vitamin that is needed to make red blood cells and DNA, (the genetic material in cells), and to keep nerve cells healthy. It is found in eggs, meat, poultry, shellfish, milk, and milk products. Cobalamine, along with folate, may be given to help reduce side effects in cancer patients being treated with drugs called antimetabolites. Also called vitamin B12.

Coccus A bacterium of round, spheroidal, or ovoid form, including micrococcus, staphylococcus, streptococcus, and pneumococcus.

COD (Chemical oxygen demand) The amount of oxygen needed to completely oxidize all oxidizable organic and inorganic substances in water.

Codeine Drug for stronger pain relief; best used in conjunction with a laxative.

Coding In clinical trials, the process of assigning data to categories for analysis. Adverse events, for example, may be coded using MedDRA.

Coding sequence The region of a gene (DNA) that encodes the amino acid sequence of a protein.

Coenzyme A non-polypeptide molecule required for the action of certain enzymes; often contains a vitamin as a component.

Cofactor Small molecular weight, heat stable inorganic or organic substance required for the action of an enzyme.

Cognome, human The **Human Cognome Project** seeks to reverse- engineer the human brain, paralleling in many ways the Human Genome Project and its success in deciphering the human genome. Analytical techniques used in the Human Cognome Project include: studying brain biology and chemistry in wet lab experiments, studying brain structure using frozen tissue sample scanning and imaging, studying brain activity and function using active brain imaging, (which is improving both spatial and temporal resolutions in successive technology generations), studying brain development though the field of morphogenesis, studying brain disease, injury and dysfunction through the fields of brain pathology, neurology and psychopharmacology, and studying psychology relative to brain structure and function through neuropsychology,

Cohort Group of subjects in a clinical trial followed up at regular, predetermined intervals.

Coinsurance Is the portion you pay for most covered expenses, in addition to the deductible and any copayment. For example, if the Plan pays 80% of covered expenses, the 20% of covered expenses you have to pay is your coinsurance.

Coliform bacteria A group of bacteria found in mammalian intestines and soil, used as a measure of fecal pollution in water. They are easy to identify and count in the laboratory because of their ability to ferment lactose.

Collagen An albuminoid present in connective tissue, bone (ossein), and cartilage (chondrin), notable for its high content of the imino acids proline and hydroproxilone. On boiling with water it is converted into gelatin.

Collateral targeting The therapeutic strategy of targeting structures and cell types other than cancer cells common to all solid tumors as a means to attack a solid tumor.

Colloid A translucent, yellowish material of the consistency of glue, less fluid than mucoid or mucinoid, found in the cells and tissues in a state of colloid degeneration or colloid carcinoma.

A substance, such as gelatin or cytoplasm that because of the size of its molecules, is slowly diffusible rather than soluble in water and is incapable of passing through an animal membrane.

Colonoscopy Examination of the large intestine using a colonoscopy introduced through the anus and guided up the colon.

Colony A growth of microorganisms on a solid medium. The growth is visible without magnification.

Combination chemotherapy Use of two or more anti-cancer drugs. This approach can enhance the effectiveness of treatment. Combinations of drugs are used to target many types of cancerous cells and prevent or slow the development of resistant cells. A tumor may respond to more than one drug's mechanism of action; therefore a combination of drugs can provide better results.

Combination products Include 1. A product comprised of two or more regulated components, i.e., drug/device, biologic/device, drug/biologic, or drug/device/biologic, that are physically, chemically, or otherwise combined or mixed and produced as a single entity;

2. Two or more separate products packaged together in a single package or as a unit and comprised of drug and device products, device and biological products, or biological and drug products;

3. A drug, device, or biological product packaged separately that according to its investigational plan or proposed labeling is intended for use only with an approved individually specified drug, device, or biological product where both are required to achieve the intended use, indication, or effect and where upon approval of the proposed product the labeling of the approved product would need to be changed, e.g., to reflect a change in intended use, dosage form, strength, route of administration, or significant change in dose; or

4. Any investigational drug, device, or biological product packaged separately that according to its proposed labeling is for use only with another individually specified investigational drug, device, or biological product where both are required to achieve the intended use, indication, or effect.

Combinatorial chemistry Automated technology that allows chemists to synthesize (manufacture) small quantities of different compounds that share a similar chemical structure.

Combined modality therapy The use of two or more modes of treatment - surgery, radiotherapy, chemotherapy, immunotherapy - in combination, alternately or together, to achieve optimum results against disease.

Combustible dust Any finely divided solid material that is 420µ or 0.017 inches or less in diameter, or any material capable of passing through an US No. 40 standard sieve that when dispersed in air in the proper proportions, could be ignited by a flame, spark or other source of ignition.

Combustible liquid A liquid having a closed cup flash point at or above 100°F (37.8°C). Combustible liquids do not include compressed gases or cryogenic fluids. Combustible liquids are subdivided as follows: 1. Class II - Liquids having a closed cup flash point at or above 100°F (37.8°C) and below 140°F (60°C)

2. Class III-A - liquids having a closed cup flash point at or above 140°F (60°C) and below 200°F (93.3°C)

Class III-B - liquids having a closed cup flash point at or above 200°F (93.3°C).

Commissioning The documented process, verifying that equipment and systems are installed according to specifications, placing the equipment and systems into active service and verifying its proper operation. Commissioning is done for good business, but can include many Qualification activities.

Communications standards It is clear that shared understanding of the basic data elements within pharmacogenomics is a critical building block upon which to build an information infrastructure. Methods for communicating these data are therefore equally as important. The two main areas that require progress are the definition of shared syntax (how information is structured in a data file) and semantics (how the information should be interpreted by others).

Comparability The ability of a system to deliver data that can be compared in standard units of measurement and by standard statistical techniques with the data delivered by other systems. While not a critical component of accuracy, comparability of data generated by a system is critical to evaluating its accuracy and usefulness.

Comparative study One in which the investigative drug is compared against another product, either active drug or placebo.

Comparator (Product) An investigational or marketed product (i.e., active control), or placebo, used as a reference in a clinical trial.

Compartment(s) The space or spaces in the body, which a drug appears to occupy after it has been absorbed. Pharmacokinetic compartments are mathematical constructs and need not correspond to the fluid volumes of the body which are defined physiologically and anatomically, i.e., the intravascular, extracellular and intracellular volumes.

Some drugs make the body "behave" as if it consisted of only a single pharmacokinetic compartment. Tissue and plasma concentrations of the drug rapidly and simultaneously reach equilibrium in all the tissues to which the drug is distributed. A plot of plasma concentration against time after intravenous administration can be rectified into only a single straight line of negative slope, which can intersect the ordinate at only one point; only one volume of distribution can be calculated. Hence, the existence of only one compartment or volume of distribution can be inferred.

Some drugs make the body appear to consist of two or more pharmacokinetic compartments, since tissue/plasma equilibrium is achieved at different times in different tissues or groups of tissues. A plot of plasma concentration against time after intravenous administration can, at best, be resolved into a series of connected straight-line segments with progressively decreasing slopes. Each of these segments may be extrapolated to intersect the ordinate, and one may infer the existence of as many pharmacokinetic compartments, of volumes of distribution, for the drug as there are intersections or segments.

Compartments in which equilibrium is achieved relatively late are referred to as "deep" compartments; compartments in which equilibrium is achieved early - and from which drug is redistributed to other sites - are referred to as "shallow" or "superficial" compartments.

Compendial Official; purported to comply with USP or NF.

Competent authority (CA) The regulatory body charged with monitoring compliance with the national statutes and regulations of European Member States.

Compiler (ANSI/IEEE) A program used to translate a higher orderlanguage into its re-locatable or absolute machine code equivalent.

Complementary DNA (cDNA) DNA that is synthesized from a messenger RNA template; the single-stranded form is often used as a probe in physical mapping.

Compliance (in relation to trials) Adherence to all the trial-related requirements, good clinical practice (GCP) and ethical requirements, and the applicable regulatory requirements.

Compounding The bringing together of excipient and solvent components into a homogeneous mix of active ingredients.

Compressed gas A material, or mixture of materials that are either liquefied, nonliquefied, or in solution having a boiling point of 68°F (20°C) or less at 14.7 psia (101.3 kPa) of pressure. The exceptions to this rule are those gases that have no health or physical hazard properties. These gases are not considered compressed until the pressure in their packaging exceeds 41 psia (282.5 kPa) at 68°F (20°C).

Computational chemistry Computer-assisted techniques that enable chemists to understand and design compound structures in the context of a biological target.

Computer controlled system Computer system plus its controlled function.

Computer hardware (PMA CSVC) Any physical element used in a computersystem.

Computer related system Computerized system plus its operating environment.

Computer system (PMA CSVC) A group of hardware components andassociated software designed and assembled to perform a specificfunction or group of functions. Added Configuration: The documented physical and functional characteristicsof a particular item or system. A change converts one configurationinto a new one.

Concavity (welding) A condition in which the surface of a welded joint is depressed relative to the surface of the tube or pipe. Concavity is measured as a maximum distance from the outside or the inside diameter surface of a welded joint along a line perpendicular to a line joining the weld toes.

Concentration polarization The phenomenon in ultrafiltration (UF) in which solutes form a dense, polarized layer next to the membrane surface eventually blocking further flow. UF systems counteract this by continuously flushing the solute away from the membrane surface.

Concurrent process validation Establishing documented evidence that a process does what it purports to do based on information generated during actual implementation of the process.

Condensate Distillate just after it has been cooled from steam into the liquid state.

Condenser The heat exchanger used in distillation to cool steam in order to convert it from the vapor to the liquid state.

Conductivity The reciprocal of resistivity (C=1/R). A measure of the ability to conduct an electric current. Since ionized impurities increase the conductivity of water, it is also an accurate measure of ionic purity. Conductivity is normally expressed in micromhos/cm (μmho/cm) or microsiemens/cm (μS/cm). To measure it, current is passed between two electrodes a fixed distance apart.

Confidentiality Prevention of disclosure, to other than authorized individuals, of a sponsor's proprietary information or of a subject's identity and personal data.

Configurable software Commercial, off-the-shelf software that can be configured to specific user applications without altering the basic program.

Configuration management (ANSI/IEEE) The process of identifying anddefining the configuration items in a system, controlling the releaseand change of these items throughout the system life cycle, recordingand reporting the status of configuration items and change requests,and verifying the completeness and correctness of configurationitems.

Conformation The characteristic three-dimensional shape (tertiary structure) of a macromolecule.

Conformers Molecules with the same molecular structure (same number of atoms and same atoms are bonded within the molecule) but with a different 3-Dimension representation due to twisting of various internal bonds.

Conformity assessment The process by which compliance with the ERs is assessed.

Conjugated protein A protein containing a metal or an organic prosthetic group or both. Hemoglobin is a conjugated protein.

Consent decree The result of a serious violation of regulations and related safety and quality standards. A company must agree to a series of measures aimed at bringing its manufacturing standards in compliance with regulations. Until agreed-upon conditions are met, a company may be forbidden to distribute its products in interstate commerce, except for those products deemed essential for the public health.

Consent form (CF) Document used during the consent process that is the basis for explaining to potential subjects the risks and potential benefits of a study and the rights and responsibilities of the parties involved.

Conserved sequence A base sequence in a DNA molecule (or an amino acid sequence in a protein) that has remained essentially unchanged throughout evolution.

Construction qualification Documented evidence to show that thoseconstructional aspects of a facility which can affect product qualityhave been constructed in accordance with the approved specification.

Consumer safety officer department of health official who coordinates the review process of various applications.

Contact dermatitis Contact dermatitis is an inflammation of the skin or a rash caused by contact with various substances of a chemical, animal or vegetable nature. The reaction may be an immunologic response or a direct toxic effect of the substance. Among the more common causes of a contact dermatitis reaction are detergents left on washed clothes, nickel (in watch straps, bracelets and necklaces, and the fastenings on underclothes), chemicals in rubber gloves and condoms, certain cosmetics, plants such as poison ivy, and topical medications.

Containment The action of confining within a defined space a microbiological agent or other entity that is being cultured, stored, manipulated, transported, or destroyed in order to prevent or limit its contact with people and/or the environment. Methods to achieve containment include physical and biological barriers and inactivation using physical or chemical means. 1. Primary Containment. Addresses the protection of personnel and the immediate laboratory environment from exposure to infectious agents. It involves the use of closed containers or safety biological cabinets along with secure operating procedures.

2. Secondary Containment. A system of containment that prevents the escape of infectious agents into the environment external to the laboratory. It involves the use of rooms with specially designed air handling, the existence of airlocks and/or sterilizers for the exit of materials and secure operating procedures. In many cases it may add to the effectiveness of primary containment.

Contig Group of cloned (copied) pieces of DNA representing overlapping regions of a particular chromosome.

Contig map A map depicting the relative order of a linked library of small overlapping clones representing a complete chromosomal segment.

Continuous fermentation A process in which sterile medium is added without interruption to the fermentation system with a balancing withdrawal (or "harvesting") of broth for product extraction. The length of fermentation can be measured in weeks or months. Commercial applications of continuous fermentation are limited in number, with ethanol production by yeast the most important example.

Contract A written, dated, and signed agreement between two or more involved parties that sets out any arrangements on delegation and distribution of tasks and obligations and, if appropriate, on financial matters. The protocol may serve as the basis of a contract.

Contract manufacturer A company holding an agreement requiring the performance of some aspect of API manufacturing

Contract research organization (CRO) A person or an organization (commercial, academic, or other) contracted by the sponsor to perform one or more of a sponsor's trial-related duties and functions.

Contributing employer Is the AFTRA Health and Retirement Funds and any employer who is required and permitted under the Trust Agreement to contribute to the AFTRA Health Fund under the terms of a collective bargaining agreement with AFTRA or a written agreement with the Fund.

Control area A building or portion of a building within which the exempted amounts of hazardous materials may be stored, dispensed, handled, or used.

Control group The group of subjects in a controlled study that receives no treatment, receives a standard treatment, or receives a placebo.

Control parameter range Range of values for a given control parameterthat lies between its two outer limits or control levels.

Control parameters Those operating variables that can be assignedvalues that are used as control levels.

Control serum Serum used as a standard for clinical chemistry lab tests. Most often produced from outdated whole blood plasma. Most often turbid and difficult to filter.

Controlled area An area constructed and operated in such a manner that some attempt is made to control the introduction of potential contamination, and the consequences of accidental release of living organisms. The level of control exercised should reflect the nature of the organism employed in the process. At a minimum, the area should be maintained at a pressure negative to the immediate external environment and allow for the efficient removal of small quantities of airborne contaminants.

Controlled study A study in which a test article is compared with a treatment that has known effects. The control group may receive no treatment, standard treatment, or placebo.

Conventional drugs New compounds made up by chemical synthesis or fermentation. These are termed by the department of health as NCEs (New Chemical Entities). The department of health rates conventional drugs with important therapeutic gain as 1-A drugs, for priority review. For example, AIDS drugs are conventional drugs approved for AIDS or AIDS-associated conditions.

Conventional flow cleanroom A room supplied with filtered air with no specified requirement for uniform airflow patterns or velocity. Airflow patterns are usually turbulent.

Converted data Any original data that has been entered into a user-developed application (spreadsheet, database, report, etc.) for manipulation, evaluation, or review.

Convexity A condition in which the surface of a welded joint is extended relative to the surface of the tube or pipe. Convexity is measured as a maximum distance from the outside or inside diameter surface of a welded joint along a line perpendicular to a line joining the weld toes.

Coordinating center Headquarters for a multisite trial that collects all data.

Coordinating committee A committee that a sponsor may organize to coordinate the conduct of a multicenter trial.

Coordinating investigator An investigator assigned the responsibility for the coordination of investigators at different centers participating in a multicenter trial.

Copay The copay or copayment is the amount that the insured member must pay for a prescription. The copay amount may be different for a brand drug versus a generic drug.

Copayment Is the portion you pay before you pay your deductible and coinsurance.

Corn steep liquor An ingredient in the culture medium for producing penicillin. A natural nitrogenous material that is a by-product of the corn milling industry.

Coronary heart disease Reduction of blood flow in the heart caused by the narrowing or blocking of the coronary vessels.

Correlation The relationship of one variable to another, not to be confused with causation. (statistics).

Corrosive A chemical that causes visible destruction or irreversible alterations in living tissue by chemical action at the site of contact. A chemical is considered corrosive if, when tested on the intact skin of albino rabbits, it destroys or changes irreversibly the structure of the tissue at the site of contact following an exposure period of four hours. This term shall not refer to action on inanimate surfaces.

Corrosive liquid A liquid which when in contact with living tissue, will cause destruction or irreversible alteration of such tissue by chemical action. Examples include acidic, alkaline, or caustic materials.

Corticoids Substances similar to the hormone of the adrenal glands called cortisone; corticoids are differentiated into two groups – mineralocorticoids and glucocorticoids applied both locally and systemically, mainly as anti-phlogistics, immunosuppressives, anti-asthmathics or in the treatment of an allergy.

Corticosteroid drugs Corticosteroids are a group of anti-inflammatory drugs similar to the natural corticosteroid hormones produced by the cortex of the adrenal glands. Among the disorders that often improve with corticosteroid treatment include asthma, allergic rhinitis, eczema and rheumatoid arthritis.

Cosmid Artificially constructed cloning vector containing the cos gene of phage lambda. Cosmids can be packaged in lambda p0hage particles for infection into E. coli: this permits cloning of larger DNA fragments (up to 45kb) that can be introduced into bacterial hosts in plasmid vectors.

Cost containment The process by which companies implement new programs or modify existing programs to continuously monitor costs so as to better manage the costs to their business. In the case of pharmacy benefits, this usually refers to providing similar acting drugs at lower costs. For example, switching to Allegra® from Claritin.

Cough Suppressants Drugs suppressing cough administered to reduce a dry, irritating cough.

Covered earnings Are those payments made to you by a contributing employer for work under a collective bargaining agreement that provides for contributions to the AFTRA Health Fund.

Covered expenses Are the costs of services or supplies for which the Fund will pay all or a portion. The description of each program will set forth those expenses it covers.

Covered roster artist Is an individual (whether or not part of a group) bound by an exclusive recording agreement with the record label (signed to the sideletter agreement) as of the last day of the immediately preceding semi-annual Schedule C period.

COX (COX-2) Cyclooxygenase enzyme (Cyclooxygenase enzyme, subtype 2).

CP (Cyclic polarization) An electrochemical test (ASTM G61) for metals that measures the point at which pitting corrosion begins. CP uses an electrolytic cell to directly measure the corrosion rate. By using the test piece as the working electrode, initiation of localized corrosion is shown by the potential at which the current density increases rapidly. This point is called the "pitting potential". The lower the current density at this point, the more resistance to pitting corrosion. The current density is measured in micro-amps per square centimeter.

Cream A word with many meanings that, in medicine and pharmacy, refers to a water-soluble preparation applied to the skin. An ointment differs from a cream in that it has an oil base.

Creatinine Creatinine is a waste product, which should be removed from the blood by the kidneys. This test measures kidney function.

Critical A material, process step, or process condition, test requirement, or any other relevant parameter is considered critical when non-compliance with predetermined criteria directly influences the quality attributes of the API (Active Pharmaceutical Ingredient) in a detrimental manner.

Critical area An area where (sterile) product or contact surface is exposed, normally Class 100 (e.g., Point of Fill).

Critical device A device that directly ensures that a GMP Critical Parameter is maintained within predetermined limits (e.g., terminal HEPA filter, point of use filter). A malfunction of such a device would place product quality directly at risk.

Critical instrument An instrument that measures a GMP Critical Parameter, used to monitor and document that parameter.

Critical parameter A GMP or product quality parameter (e.g., differential pressure, unidirectional airflow pattern) that must be maintained within predefined limits to ensure product SISPQ (Strength, Identity, Safety, Purity, or Quality).

Critical point The combination of pressure and temperature at which the gas and liquid phases of a substance become indistinguishable.

Critical process parameter A process-related variable which, whenout-of-control, can potentially cause an adverse effect onfitness-for-use of an end product.

Critical process step For sterile products, this normally is an activity where product or product contact parts are exposed to the surrounding environment.

Critical step(s) The point or points in the process which, if not carried out properly or if contaminated, will not allow drug substances to be made such that they will meet their intended characterizations and impurity profiles.

Critical surface The part of the working surface to be protected from particulate contamination. It is within the Critical Zone.

Critical system A structural, mechanical, or electrical system that can impact the processing parameters and attributes of the finished product or regulatory study. Critical systems may include utilities, process equipment, and systems.

CRO Contract Research Organization.

Cross contamination The measurable and detrimental contamination of a material or product with another material or product.

Cross linking An oxidation reaction in which undesirable bonds form between nucleic acids (RNA and DNA) or between proteins (bit into an apple and watch it do yellow over time, this is protein cross linking).

Cross over experiment A form of experiment in which each subject receives the test preparation at least once, and every test preparation is administered to every subject. At successive experimental sessions each preparation is "crossed-over" from one subject to another. The purpose of the cross-over experiment is to permit the effects of every preparation to be studied in every subject, and to permit the data for each preparation to be similarly and equally affected by the peculiarities of each subject. In a well-designed cross-over experiment, if it is at all possible, the sequence in which the test preparations are administered is not the same for all subjects, in order to avoid bias in the experiment as a result of changes in the behavior of the subjects that are a function of time rather than of drug administration, or a function of drug interactions. At least, the cross-over design permits detecting such biases when they occur. The preparations under test in a cross-over experiment may - ideally, should - include one or more doses, of an experimental or "unknown" drug, one or more doses of a dummy or placebo medication ("negative control drugs"), and one or more doses of a standard drug, the actions of which are expected to be similar to those of the "unknown" ("positive control drug"). Even for the investigator with the best knowledge and intentions, the economics and logistics of experimentation may prevent carrying out a complete and perfect cross-over experiment.

Cross tolerance Tolerance to a drug that generalizes to drugs that are chemically related of that produce similar affects. For example, a patient who is tolerant to heroin will also exhibit cross-tolerance to morphine.

Cross validation Is a comparison of validation parameters when two or more bioanalytical methods are used to generate data within the same study, e.g., when sample analysis are conducted at more than one site, a cross validation with calibration standards and a sub-set of incurred samples should be conducted at each site to establish interlaboratory reliability.

Crossing over The breaking during meiosis of one maternal and one paternal chromosome, the exchanging of corresponding sections of DNA, and the rejoining of the chromosomes. This process can result in an exchange of alleles between chromosomes.

Crossover trial In crossover trials, each subject receives both treatments being compared or the treatment and control. Such trials are used for patients who have a stable, usually chronic, condition during both treatment periods.

Cryogenic liquid A fluid that has a normal boiling point below -150°F (-101.1°C).

Cryothermy Also called cryoablation, the technique uses very cold temperatures through a probe (called a cryoprobe) to create lesions. It is a technique commonly used during arrhythmia surgery to replace the incisions made during the Maze Procedure, and has a success rate of about 80%.

Cryptography The mathematical science of deliberately scrambling and unscrambling information. Information is protected by being transformed (encrypted) into an unreadable format, called cipher text. Only those who posses a secret key can decypher (or decrypt) that message into plain text.

CS Colorimetric solution A954.

Css The concentration of a drug or chemical in a body fluid - usually plasma - at the time a "steady state" has been achieved, and rates of drug administration and drug elimination are equal. Css is a value approached as a limit and is achieved, theoretically, following the last of an infinite number of equal doses given at equal intervals. The maximum value under such conditions (Css,max) is given by Css,max = C0/(1 -f), for a drug eliminated by first-order kinetics from a single compartment system. The ratio Css,max/C0 indicates the extent to which drug accumulates under the conditions of a particular dose regimen of, theoretically, an infinitely long duration; the corresponding ratio 1/(1 - f) is sometimes called the Accumulation Ratio, R. Css is also the limit achieved, theoretically, at the "end" of an infusion of infinite duration, at a constant rate.

CT 2103 A protein that can be linked to a chemotherapy drug to deliver the drug directly to the tumor with fewer side effects. It is being studied in the treatment of cancer. Also called polyglutamate paclitaxel.

CT 2106 A form of the anticancer drug camptothecin that may have fewer side effects and work better than camptothecin. It is being studied in the treatment of cancer. It belongs to the family of drugs called DNA topoisomerase inhibitors. Also called polyglutamate camptothecin.

CT 2584 A substance that is being studied in the treatment of cancer. It may prevent the growth of blood vessels from surrounding tissue into a solid tumor.

CT index A measure of drug "potency" calculated from data appropriate to the construction of a Time-Concentration curve; the product of the concentration (C) of an agent applied to a biological system to produce a specific effect and the duration (T) of application required to produce the effect.

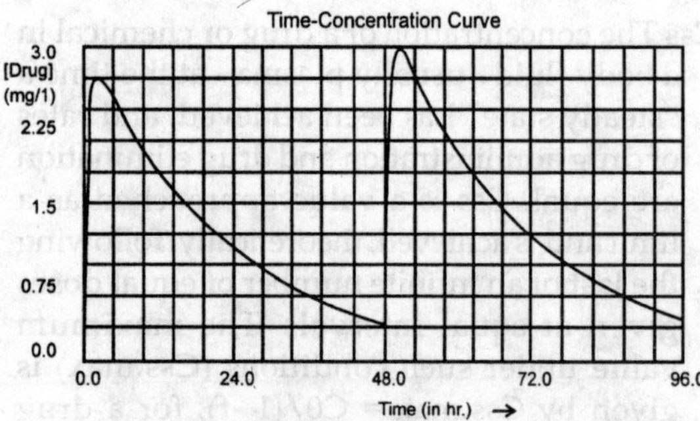

Fig. CT index

The index is calculated on the assumption that the time-concentration curve is precisely and symmetrically hyperbolic and convex to the origin, and that the products of the coordinates for all points on the line are constant. The time-concentration curve of an agent with high potentiality for producing a specified effect lies closer to the axis than the curve for an agent of lesser potential; the CT index for the agent of greater potential is smaller than the index for the agent of lesser potential, i.e., the smaller the CT index, the more "potent" the compound. CT indices have found their greatest application in toxicology, in assessing the potential for effect of noxious vapors, etc.

Culture medium Any nutrient system for the artificial cultivation of bacteria or other cells; usually a complex mixture of organic and inorganic materials.

current Good Manufacturing Practices (cGMP's)

Curative or specific therapy Treatment directed toward eradication of one or more of the agencies etiologic to the patient's condition. Antimicrobial drugs such as penicillin have specific or curative effects.

Curriculum vitae (cv) Document that outlines a person's educational and professional history.

Custodial care Means all services and supplies, including room and board, provided primarily to assist a covered individual in the activities of daily living, regardless of the practitioner or provider by whom they are prescribed, recommended or performed.

Customer The pharmaceutical customer or user organisation contractinga supplier to provide a product. In the context of this document it issynonymous with User.

Cut An enzymatic break that occurs in both strands of a DNA molecule opposite one another by restriction enzymes.

Cycle A predetermined schedule for chemotherapy administration. Some cycles of chemotherapy repeat every 3 weeks, while others repeat every 4 or even 8 weeks. Each cycle consists of a group of drugs given on particular days according to a specific treatment plan.

Cyclic nucleotide phosphodiesterase (PDE) Enzymes which take cyclic nucleotides (cAMP, cGMP) and convert them to simple nucleotides. cAMP is an important secondary messenger. Stimulation of Beta receptors produces cAMP. Clinically PDE is important because drugs that can block PDE can prolong the effects of cAMP. PDE inhibitors are used in the treatment of CHF.

Cyclophosphamide Chemotherapy drug used in treatment of breast cancer .

Cycloplegia Paralysis or loss of function of the ciliary muscle; this results in loss of accommodation (ability to focus).

CYP CYP is shorthand for cytochrome P450, a family of heme-containing terminal oxygenases that are active in a range of metabolic and biosynthetic pathways. They are involved in the metabolism (breakdown) of both endogenous and exogenous (xenobiotic) substrates, includingdrugs and environmental chemicals, and in the synthesis of metabolome components such as leukotrienes, prostacyclins, HETEs, retinoic acids, steroids and bile acids. They are divided into families of structurally related proteins based on their gene sequence. Families are designated by a number, their subfamilies by a letter and their species-specific subfamily by a second number. Thus, CYP 3A4 is a human CYP that is a member of the CYP 3 family and CYP 3A subfamily. The study of CYPs is complicated by the fact that the metabolic products and pathways of individual CYPs overlap and their relative levels of expression differ among species, making interspecies extrapolation of xenobiotic metabolism extremely problematic. However, the availability of recombinant CYPs has made the study of metabolic pathways mediated by individual CYPs more feasible, but with some loss of the physiological and pharmacological relevance of studying the CYPs acting in concert in their natural membrane environment. Within a species, some CYPs are expressed exclusively, or nearly so, in particular tissues, while others are expressed in multiple tissues but at very different levels.

Do you want to mention their subcellular localization in the endoplasmic reticulum (microsomal fraction), their importance in Phase I drug metabolism, their involvement in drug-drug interactions via inhibition and induction, intestinal drug metabolism, and/ or the many and varied model systems that ASLP can bring to bear on these issues?

Cyproterone Anti-androgen agent widely used in the treatment of prostate cancer.

Cystic fibrosis An inherited disease in which thick mucus clogs the lungs and blocks the ducts of the pancreas.

Cytochrome P450 enzymes The most important and well- studied group of drug-metabolizing enzymes, the cytochrome P450 enzymes (found in the liver) are responsible for the metabolism of a large number of pharmaceutical compounds. These enzymes function to detoxify xenobiotics (foreign molecules in the body, including drugs). The various genetic polymorphisms in cytochrome P450 can result in increased enzymatic activity, decreased enzymatic activity, or complete loss of enzyme activity. These changes can, in turn, lead to increased (or decreased) activation of pro- drugs, or to increased (or decreased) metabolism and excretion of drugs.

Cytochrome P-450 oxidase (CYP) CYP is a class of enzymes that function to alter molecules so that they become more water soluble. These enzymes are most predominant in the liver but can also be found in the intestines, lung and other organs. CYP is not only involved in drug metabolism but other important physiologic functions, including the synthesis of certain hormones.

Cytokine A protein that acts as a chemical messenger to stimulate cell migration, usually toward where the protein is released.

Interlukins, lymphokines, and interferons are the most common.

Cytolysis The dissolution of cells particularly by destruction of their cell membrane.

Cytopathic Damaging to cells.

Cytoplasm The protoplasmic contents of the cell outside the nucleus in which the cell's organelles are suspended.

Cytoplasmic and nuclear receptors Proteins in the cytoplasm or nucleus that specifically bind signaling molecules and trigger changes which influence the behavior of cells. The major groups are the steroid hormone receptors (RECEPTORS, STEROID), which usually are found in the cytoplasm, and the thyroid hormone receptors (RECEPTORS, THYROID HORMONE), which usually are found in the nucleus. Receptors, unlike enzymes, generally do not catalyze chemical changes in their ligands.

Cytosine (C) A pyrimidine occurring as a fundamental unit or base of nucleic acids.

Cytostatic agents Therapeutics that inhibit cell division and growth. This term can refer to machinery, such as those that would freeze cells.

Cytostatics Drugs used in the treatment of malign tumours.

Cytotoxic A toxin or antibody that has a special toxic effect on cells (cell-killing).

Cytotoxic Chemotherapy Anti-cancer drugs that kill cells, especially cancer cells.

Cytotoxicity The ability of a substance or compound to cause a cytotoxic effect.

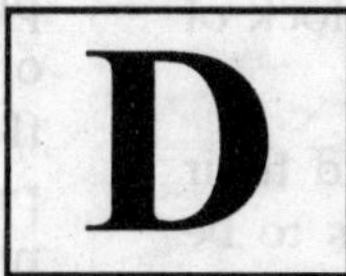

D Value The time under a stated set of exposure conditions (temperature in an autoclave) required to reduce a microbial population by a factor of 90% (e.g. from 10,000 to 1,000).

D5W (5 D/W) One of the most prevalent of LVPs . Five percent dextrose in water. Presence of dextrose presents significant filtration problems. Usually requires activated charcoal pretreatment.

Daclximab A monoclonal antibody that is being studied in the treatment of adult T-cell leukemia and in the treatment of cytopenia (low blood cell count). Also called daclizumab.

Daclizumab A monoclonal antibody that is being studied in the treatment of adult T-cell leukemia and in the treatment of cytopenia (low blood cell count). Also called daclximab.

Dalton The unit of molecular weight, equal to the weight of a hydrogen atom.

Danazol A synthetic hormone that belongs to the family of drugs called androgens and is used to treat endometriosis. It is being evaluated in the treatment of endometrial cancer.

Dapsone Indications Treatment of PCP (mild to moderate infection) in combination with trimethoprim; prophylaxis of PCP in patients unable to tolerate TMP-SMX; primary prophylaxis of toxoplasmosis in combination with pyrimethamine.

Contraindications: Known hypersensitivity, G6PD deficiency.

Dosage: PCP treatment: dapsone 100 mg qd and trimethoprim 15 mg/kg/day x three weeks.

PCP prophylaxis: 100 mg po qd; toxoplasmosis prophylaxis: add pyrimethamine 50 mg weekly with folinic acid 25 mg.

Toxicity: Rash, fever, gastrointestinal intolerance, neutropenia, methemoglobinemia.

Darbepoetin alfa A substance made in the laboratory that stimulates the bone marrow to produce red blood cells. It belongs to the family of drugs called antianemics.

Data and safety monitoring board (DSMB) Researchers – ideally independent of the trials they monitor – who periodically review data from blinded, placebo-controlled trials. A DSMB can stop a trial if toxicities are found or if treatment is proved beneficial.

Data base A collection of data, typically organized for easy search and retrieval.

Data encryption standard (DES) A widely used method of data encryption using a private (secret) key that the U.S. government judged so difficult to break that it was restricted for export to other countries. Each message uses one of 72 quadrillion or more possible encryption keys that are chosen at random. The sender and receiver must both know and use the same private key. DES applies a 56-bit key to each 64-bit block of data.

Data integrity The validity of data and their relationships. For electronic records to be trustworthy and reliable, the links between raw data, metadata, and results must not be compromised or broken. Without data integrity, it is not possible to regenerate a previous result reliably.

Data migration The process of translating data from one system to another when a company replaces the current computing systems with a new one.

Data monitoring Process by which case report forms are examined for completeness, consistency, and accuracy.

Database Data stored in computer form for retrieval, processing, and/or analysis.

Database mining A highly automated process that compares the recorded sequence for each identified gene to all known genes; results are stored in an annotated database.

DCS Distributed Control System.

DDC (direct digital control) A collection of control units (analog and discrete) connected into a data highway, usually with a host or alarming/recording computer attached.

DDD Daily dose definition – an artificially established administration unit used, for example, for monitoring the consumption of drugs.

De minimis release The release of viable microbiological agents or eukaryotic cells that does not result in the establishment of disease in healthy people, plants, or animals; or in uncontrolled proliferation of any microbiological agents or eukaryotic cells.

De novo structure A de novo structure, or de novo derivative, is a molecule that has actually been altered slightly rather than just contorted.

Dead leg An area of entrapment in a vessel or piping run that could lead to contamination of the product. In a piping system, a non-flowing pocket, tee, or extension from a primary piping run that exceeds a defined number of pipe diameters from the ID of the primary pipe. Denoted by the term L/D or L/A, where L is equal to the leg extension perpendicular to the normal flow pattern or direction, A is the annular gap width, and D is equal to the ID (or inside dimension) of the extension or leg. In some existing standards, the dimension L is measured from the centerline of the primary pipe. For bioprocessing systems, an L/D of 2:1 is achievable with today's component technology for most valving and piping configurations.

Dead source code (K.G. Chapman) 1. Superseded code from earlier versions. Avoided by using qualitysoftware development standards; .

2. Residue from system modification. Avoided by effective configurationchange controls; .

3. Rarely used code that appears dead such as: - modules in some largeconfigurable programs; - certain diagnostic programs that are intendedto be inactive until needed.Removal of code in category 3 leads to serious potential futureproblems. "Idle code" can be "parked" in libraries until needed.

Debugging (IEEE) The process of locating, analysing, and correctingsuspected faults.

Declaration of helsinki A set of recommendations or basic principles that guide medical doctors in the conduct of biomedical research involving human subjects. It was originally adopted by the 18th World Medical Assembly (Helsinki, Finland, 1964.

Decontamination A process that reduces contaminating substances to a defined acceptance level.

Deductible Is that initial part of each year's covered expenses under a particular program for which you are responsible and for which you will not be reimbursed by the Fund.

Deferoxamine An iron-chelating agent that removes iron from tumors by inhibiting DNA synthesis and causing cancer cell death. It is used in conjunction with other anticancer agents in pediatric neuroblastoma therapy.

Defibrotide A substance that is being studied in the prevention of veno-occlusive disease, a rare complication of high-dose chemotherapy and stem cell transplantation in which small veins in the liver become blocked.

Deflagration An exothermic reaction, such as the extremely rapid oxidation of a combustible dust or flammable vapor in air, in which the reaction progresses through the unburned material at a rate less than the velocity of sound. A deflagration can have an explosive effect.

Degrading Deterioration of a surface finish so that pieces of the finish (or substrate) material large enough to be visible to the unaided eye, dislodge without any direct physical contact and fall from the surface of the material.

Deionization Removing dissolved ions from solution by passing the solution through a bed of ion exchange resin, consisting of polymer beads that exchange hydrogen ions for cations and hydroxyl ions for anions in solution. The ionic impurities remain bound to the resins and the hydrogen and hydroxyl ions combine with each other to form water.

Delavirdine (Rescriptor)

Indications: Treatment of HIV infection in combination with other agents.

Contraindications: Known hypersensitivity.

Dosage: 400 mg po tid. Two tablets must be dissolved in 3 or more ounces of water to produce a slurry. Antacids and ddI should not be taken one hour before or after the dose. There are many potential drug interactions, some of which require dosage modification

Toxicity: Rash is common and does not require discontinuation of the drug unless accompanied by fever, mucous membrane involvement, or other systemic manifestations. Stevens-Johnson syndrome has been reported infrequently.

Delayed rectifier potassium channel (IKr) A cardiac protein that is important in synchronizing individual cardiac cells critical to normal heart function.

Deletion map A description of a specific chromosome that uses defined mutations - specific deleted areas in the genome - as "biochemical signposts", or markers for specific areas.

Dementia Severe impairment of mental functioning.

Demineralization Sometimes used interchangeably with deionization, it refers to the removal of minerals and mineral salts using ion exchange. Water softening is a common form of demineralization.

Demographic data Characteristics of subjects or study populations, which include such information as age, sex, family history of the disease or condition for which they are being treated, and other characteristics relevant to the study in which they are participating.

Denaturation The loss of the native structure of a macromolecule resulting, from heat treatment, extreme pH changes, chemical treatment, etc. It is accompanied by loss of biological activity. For example, proteins may be denatured by heat, pH extremes, or addition of agents such as urea or guanidinium hydrochloride.

Dendrites The fine network of branches that extend from the body of a nerve, receiving impulses and carrying them into the center of the cell.

Dent A typical stainless steel interior surface anomaly that refers to a large, smooth-bottomed depression whose diameter or width is greater than its depth and which will not produce an indication.

Dependence A somatic state which develops after chronic administration of certain drugs; this state is characterized by the necessity to continue administration of the drug in order to avoid the appearance of uncomfortable or dangerous (withdrawal) symptoms. Withdrawal symptoms, when they occur, may be relieved by the administration of the drug upon which the body was "dependent."

Dermatological drugs Drugs used locally in dermatology.

DES Diethylstilbestrol (dye-ETH-ul-stil-BES-trol). A synthetic form of the hormone estrogen that was prescribed to pregnant women between about 1940 and 1971 because it was thought to prevent miscarriages. DES may increase the risk of uterine, ovarian, or breast cancer in women who took it. DES also has been linked to an increased risk of clear cell carcinoma of the vagina or cervix in daughters exposed to DES before birth.

Desalination The removal of dissolved salts from brine to produce potable water.

Desensitization A decline in the response to repeated or sustained application of an agonist that is a consequence of changes at the level of the receptor.

Desiccant Chemical salt used to dehumidify air, to control moisture in materials contacting that air.

Desiccators Closed containers, usually made of glass or plastic, with an airtight seal used for drying materials.

Design condition The specified range or accuracy of a controlled variable used by the designer to determine performance requirements of an engineered system.

Design qualification (DQ) Formal and systematic verification that therequirements defined during specification are completely covered by thesucceeding specification or implementation.

Design specification (a. GAMP forum, b.IEEE)

A. This is a completedefinition of the equipment or system in sufficient detail to enable itto be built. This links to Installation Qualification which checks thatthe correct equipment or system is supplied, to the required standardsand that it is installed correctly.

b. The specification that documents the design of a system or systemcomponent to satisfy specified requirements.

Designer drugs Are substances whose molecular structure has been modified in order to optimise their effect on the one hand, and in order to by-pass laws and regulations governing the control of substances on the other hand. Once designer drugs have been outlawed by the competent authorities they are called controlled substances (2 C-1).

Deslorelin A substance that is being studied in the treatment of cancer as a way to block sex hormones made by the ovaries or testicles. It belongs to the family of drugs called gonadotropin-releasing hormone analogs.

Detonation An exothermic reaction characterized by the presence of a shock wave in a material that establishes and maintains the reaction. The reaction zone progresses through the material at a rate greater than the velocity of sound. The principal heating mechanism is one of shock compression. Detonations have an explosive effect.

Deuteromycetes Molds that cannot reproduce by sexual means. Some pathogenic fungi such as Trichophyton, which causes athlete's foot, belong to this family.

Development The process by which a compound discovered in research is progressed through human clinical trials prior to approval to market

Dexamethasone A synthetic steroid (similar to steroid hormones produced naturally in the adrenal gland). Dexamethasone is used to treat leukemia and lymphoma and may be used to treat some of the problems caused by other cancers and their treatment.

Dexmethylphenidate A substance that is being studied in the treatment of fatigue and nervous system side effects caused by chemotherapy. It belongs to the family of drugs called central nervous system stimulants.

Dexrazoxane A drug used to protect the heart from the toxic effects of anthracycline drugs such as doxorubicin. It belongs to the family of drugs called chemoprotective agents.

DHL vaccine A tri-valent vaccine. Also, the most common veterinary vaccine that has a combination of viral and bacterial vaccines. Used for distemper, hepatitis (canine), and leptospira.

DHT (dihydrotestosterone) A conversion of testosterone that is considered to be an aging-bio-marker. Among its affects are the appearance of body-hair, the loss of scalp hair and the onset of prostate gland problems.

Diabetes A disease in which the body cannot process or use glucose efficiently. In persons with diabetes, insulin, a hormone produced in the pancreas and essential for glucose use in the body, is not produced or the body does not respond well to the insulin that is produced.

Diagnomics Molecular diagnostic testing that give clinicians information about patients that can be used in making medical decisions.

Diagnosis The identification of a disease or condition through analysis and examination by a physician.

Diagnostic A substance or group of substances used to identify a disease by analyzing the cause and symptoms.

Dialysis The separation of low-molecular weight compounds from high molecular weight components by diffusion through a semipermeable membrane. Frequently utilized to remove salts, introduce salts, remove biological effectors such as nicotinamide adenine dinucleotides, nucleotides phosphates, etc. from polymeric molecules such as protein, DNA, RNA, etc. Commonly used membranes have a molecular weight cutoff around 10,000 but other membrane pore sizes are available.

Diamorphine hydrochloride Opiate used in severe pain. Extremely valuable.

Diatom Any minute, unicellular or colonial algae of the class Bacillariophyceae having siliceous cells walls consisting of two overlapping symmetrical parts.

Diatomaceous earth, diatomite, kiselguhr (DE) Fine silicaceous powder used as a filter aid.

Diclofenac (Voltarol) Anti-inflammatory agent used for moderate pain.

Didanosine (ddI, Videx) Indications: Treatment of HIV infection in combination with other agents.

Contraindications: Known hypersensitivity, history of pancreatitis or significant peripheral neuropathy.

Dosage: Enteric-coated formulation (Videx EC) has been approved by the department of health for once daily dosing and can be given without regard to meals. Dose is 400 mg po qd for weight > 60 kg and 250 mg po qd for weight < 60 kg.

Also available in tablets and buffered powder. Tablets: > 60 kg —> 400 mg po qd or 200 mg po bid; < 60 kg —> 250 mg po qd or 125 mg po bid. Tablets must be chewed or dissolved in water. Buffered Powder: > 60 kg —> 250 mg po bid ;< 60 kg —> 167 mg po bid.

All formulations must be taken on an empty stomach (> 30 minutes before a meal or > 2 hours after a meal).

Coadministration of hydroxyurea 500 mg po bid may enhance the effectiveness of ddI by increasing intracellular level of drug.

Toxicity: Peripheral neuropathy, acute pancreatitis, gastrointestinal intolerance, abnormal liver function tests.

Diethylstilbestrol The earliest synthetic (man-made) form of the hormone estrogen.

CH_2CH_3
HO— —OH
CH_3CH_2

4, 4–(1,2–deityyl–1,2)bisphenol
deitylstilbestrol
DES

Diffusion The random thermal motion of particles, which causes them to flow from a region of higher concentration to one of lower concentration until they are uniformly distributed.

Digestion The enzymatic hydrolysis of major nutrients in the gastrointestinal system to yield their building-block components.

Digestive system The digestive system is the group of organs that breaks down food into chemical components that the body can absorb and use for energy and for building and repairing cells and tissues.

Digital A series of on and off pulses arranged to convey information.

Digital certificate An attachment to an electronic message used for security purposes. The most common use of a digital certificate is to verify that a user sending a message is who he or she claims to be and to provide the receiver with the means to encode a reply.

Digital representation Biometric parameters such as a fingerprint or retinal pattern are turned into data that a computer understands: the digital representation of the biometric. The pattern in the biometric divides it into a grid of boxes, and a zero or a one, depending on whether the box is filled in, marks each box.

Digital signature An electronic signature based upon cryptographic methods of originator authentication, computed by using a set of rules and a set of parameters such that the identity of the signer and the integrity of the data can be verified.

Dihydrocodeine (DF118) Drug for stronger pain relief (codeine derivative); best used in conjunction with a laxative, as very constipating.

Dilated cardiomyopathy The most common of the three forms of cardiomyopathy in which the damaged heart muscle stretches out of shape. The enlarged heart loses its ability to pump blood effectively, leading to blood clots and, ultimately, heart failure.

Dilution factor The ratio of solvent to solute by volume.

Dilution Lowering the concentration of a solution by adding more solvent.

Diploid A full set of genetic material, consisting of paired chromosomes one chromosome from each parental set. Most animal cells except the gametes have a diploid set of chromosomes. The diploid human genome has 46 chromosomes.

Diplophase A phase in the life cycle of an organism where the organism has two copies of each gene. The organism is said to be diploid.

Direct access Permission to examine, analyze, verify, and reproduce any records and reports that are important to evaluation of a clinical trial. Any party (e.g., domestic and foreign regulatory authorities, sponsors, monitors, and auditors) with direct access should take all reasonable precautions within the constraints of the applicable regulatory requirement(s) to maintain the confidentiality of subjects' identities and sponsor's proprietary information.

Direct impact system An engineering system that may have a direct impact on product quality.

Disaster Any event (i.e. fire, earthquake, power failure etc.), which could have a detrimental effect upon an automated system or its associated information.

Discoloration (welding) Any change in surface color from that of the base metal. Usually associated with oxidation occurring on the weld and heat affected zone (HAZ) on the outside diameter and inside diameter of the weld joint as a result of heating the metal during the welding. Colors may range from pale bluish-gray to deep blue, and from pale straw color to a black crusty coating.

Disease Illness, sickness: an interruption, cessation or disorder of body functions systems or organs.

Disease management program A program, available under certain benefits plans, that offers support to members with certain long-term illnesses such as diabetes, asthma, coronary artery disease and low back pain. Disease management programs often may include educational materials and, in some circumstances, may offer other assistance to help the member monitor his or her condition and treatment.

Disease resistant individuals Another interesting group [of phenotypes for pharmacogenomics] includes those who have no disease yet have high risk factors. A classic example are individuals who exposed themselves to multiple risk factors for HIV - unprotected intercourse with multiple partners, intravenous drug use, etc. - and who either did not get the disease, or when they did get it, it progressed very slowly. Interestingly, a gene target was identified in this group - the CCRX deletions. There are many other disease-resistant groups in medicine. ... In general, disease- resistant groups provide a way of identifying given targets that are pre-validated in human subjects.

Disinfection Process by which viable microbiological agents or eukaryotic cells are reduced to a level unlikely to produce disease in healthy people, plants, or animals. These processes may use chemical agents, heat, ultraviolet light, etc. to destroy most (but not necessarily all) of the harmful or objectionable microorganisms, pathogens, and potential pathogens. Disinfection does not necessarily result in sterilization. 1. "High level disinfection" inactivates fungi, viruses, and bacteria. High-level chemical disinfectants maybe ineffective against bacterial spores if they are present in large numbers. Extended exposure times may be required.

2. "Intermediate level disinfection" destroys fungi, some viruses (lipid and most non-lipid medium-size and small viruses), mycobacteria, and bacteria.

3. "Low level disinfection" kills vegetative forms of bacteria, some fungi, and some medium-size and lipid-containing viruses. Low-level disinfectants do not reliably kill bacterial spores, mycobacteria, or small or non-lipid viruses.

Disintegration Breaking up of a tablet in water or in simulated gastric and/or simulated intestinal fluid to the point that the particles pass through a fine screen.

Disintegration time The time required for a tablet to break up into granules of specified size (or smaller), under carefully specified test conditions. The conditions of the laboratory test, in vitro, are set to simulate those that occur in vivo. Factors such as the kind and amount of tablet binders and the degree of compression used in compacting the tablet ingredients help determine disintegration time. The active ingredients in a disintegrated tablet are not necessarily found to be in solution and available for absorption. A long disintegration time is incompatible with rapid drug absorption; a short disintegration time, by itself, does not ensure rapid absorption.

Dispensing The pouring or transferring of any material from a container, tank or similar vessel, whereby vapors, dusts, fumes, mists or gases may be liberated to the atmosphere.

Dissimilation The breakdown of food material to yield energy and building blocks for cellular synthesis.

Dissolution Generally, dissolving; but specifically, a USP test which determines how rapidly the active ingredients of a dosage form dissolve. The test is generally done with six tablets in containers with very specifically defined dimensions, stirring mechanisms, etc.

Dissolution time The time required for a given amount (or fraction) of drug to be released into solution from a solid dosage form. Dissolution time is measured in vitro, under conditions which simulate those which occur in vivo, in experiments in which the amount of drug in solution is determined as a function of time. Needless to say, the availability of a drug in solution - rather than as part of insoluble particulate matter - is a necessary preliminary to the drug's absorption.

Epinephrine reversal describes the response seen to epinephrine (EPI) in the presence of an alpha-blocker. The normal response to EPI alone is an increase in BP and HR. However in the presence of an alpha-blocker, EPI can now only activate the beta-receptors to cause a fall in BP with an increase in HR.

Dissolved solids The amount of nonvolatile matter dissolved in a water sample, usually expressed in parts per million (PPM) by weight.

Distillation The process of separating water from impurities by heating until it changes into vapor and then cooling the vapor to condense it into purified water.

Distribution Distribution is the process by which a drug reversibly leaves the blood stream and enter extracellular fluid and/oe the cells of tissue.

Distribution is the reversible transfer of xenobiotics from one location in the body to another location.

Diuretics Drugs increasing the production and secretion of urine, they are often used as anti-hypertensives to "dehydrate" during a general oedema, for example, in heart failure, kidney or liver diseases.

DMAE (demethylaminoethanol) Is found in small amounts in the brain and is known for its brain enhancing affects.

DNA (deoxyribonucleic acid) The molecule of which the genetic material is composed. It consists of two chains joined together as a double helix. Each chain is composed of a polymer of nucleotides (consisting of a nitrogenous base, a deoxyribosesugar ring, and a phosphate group) joined together by phosphodiester bonds between the 5'-phosphate of one nucleotide and the 3'-hydroxyl of the next. The two chains run in opposite directions and are held together by hydrogen bonds between the bases in equivalent positions in the two chains. There are various forms of double helical DNA. They are: 1. B-DNA (first described by Crick and Watson) is a right-handed helix with 10.6 base pairs per turn and is probably the main form of cellular DNA.

2. A-DNA is also a right-handed helix but is somewhat skewed and contains about 11 base pairs per turn. It is the form taken By DNA-RNA hybrid double helixes.

3. Z-DNA is a left-handed helix with 11 base pairs per turn. It is favored by regions rich in guanine cutosine base pairs and probably occurs infrequently in cellular DNA.

DNA array Spots of DNA arranged on a slide support such as glass or silicon "DNA chip" (or microarray), used for screening, sequencing, genetic mapping, and so on.

DNA replication The use of existing DNA as a template for the synthesis of new DNA strands. In humans and other eukaryotes, replication occurs in the cell nucleus.

DNA sequence The relative order of base pairs, whether in a fragment of DNA, a gene, a chromosome, or an entire genome.

DNA vaccines Recombinant DNA vectors encoding antigens administered for the prevention or treatment of disease. The host cells take up the DNA, express the antigen, and present it to the immune system in a manner similar to that which would occur during natural infection. This induces humoral and cellular immune responses against the encoded antigens. The vector is called naked DNA because there is no need for complex formulations or delivery agents; the plasmid is injected in saline or other buffers.

DNA vector A DNA vehicle for transferring generic information from one cell to another.

Documentation Written or pictorial information describing, defining, specifying, and/or reporting of certifying activities, requirements, procedures or results.

DNAse (Deoxyribonuclease) An enzyme that degrades DNA.

Dobutamine therapy An intravenous form of inotropic therapy that is administered by an infusion pump to monitor the dosage of medicine.

Documentation All records, in any form (including, but not limited to, written, electronic, magnetic, and optical records; and scans, x-rays, and electrocardiograms) that describe or record the methods, conduct, and/or results of a trial, the factors affecting a trial, and the actions taken.

Domain A discrete portion of a protein with its own function. The combination of domains in a single protein determines its overall function.

Domain antibodies The smallest known antigen- binding fragments of antibodies, ranging from 11 kDa to 15 kDa. ... owing to their small size and inherent stability, can be formatted into larger molecules to create drugs with prolonged serum half- lives or other pharmacological activities

Domain name The way a particular Web server is identified on the Internet. For example, www.tripod.com names the World Wide Web (www) server for Tripod (tripod), which is a commercial (com) entity.

Dominant allele A gene that is expressed, regardless of whether its counterpart allele on the other chromosome is dominant or recessive. Autosomal dominant disorders are produced by a single mutated dominant allele, even though its corresponding allele is normal.

Domperidone Anti-nausea drug.

Donepezil A drug used in the treatment of Alzheimer's disease. It belongs to the family of drugs called cholinesterase inhibitors. It is being studied in the treatment of side effects caused by radiation therapy to the brain.

DOP (dioctyl phthalate) A mono-dispersed test aerosol of sub-micron particles, generated to challenge (evaluate integrity) of HEPA filters for HVAC.

Dopamine A neurotransmitter critical to fine motor co-ordination, immune function, motivation, insulin regulation, physical energy, thinking, short term memory, emotions such as sexual desire and autonomic nervous system balance.

Dopaminergic The parts of the nervous system which use dopamine as a neurotransmitter.

Dose The quantity of drug, or dosage form, administered to a subject at a given time; for example, the usual dose of aspirin for relief of pain in an adult is 300-600 milligrams. Dose may be expressed in terms appropriate to a specific dosage form, i.e., one teaspoonful of a liquid medication, rather than the weight of drug in the teaspoonful. Dose may be described as an absolute dose (the total amount administered to a subject) or as a relative dose (relative to some property of the subject as body weight or surface area, mg/kg, or mg/m 2).

Dosage form The physical state in which a drug is dispensed for use. For example: a frequent dosage form of procaine is a sterile solution of procaine. The most frequent dosage form of aspirin is a tablet.

Dosage group A group of subjects in a clinical trial receiving the same dosage (amount) of a drug being tested.

Dosage regimen (a) The number of doses per given time period; (b) the time that elapses between doses (for example, every six hours) or the time that the doses are to be given (for example, at 8 a.m. and 4 p.m. daily); or (c) the amount of a medicine (the number of capsules, for example) to be given at each specific dosing time.

Dose effect curve A characteristic, even the sine qua non, of a true drug effect is that a larger dose produces a greater effect than does a smaller dose, up to the limit to which the cells affected can respond. While characteristic of a drug effect, this relationship is not unique to active drugs, since increasing doses of placebos (q.v.) can, under certain conditions, result in increasing effects. Distinguishing between " true" and "inactive" drugs requires more than demonstration of a relationship between "dose" and effect.

The curve relating effect (as the dependent variable) to dose (as the independent variable) for a drug-cell system is the "dose-effect curve" for the system. For a unique system, i.e., one involving a single drug and a single effect, such curves have three characteristics, regardless of whether effects are measured as continuous (measurement) or discontinuous (quantal, all-or-none) variates:

The curves are continuous, i.e. there are no gaps in the curve, and effect is a continuous function of dose. Some effect corresponds to every dose above the threshold dose (q.v.), and every dose has a corresponding effect; there is no inherent invalidity in interpolating doses or effects from a dose-effect curve.

The curves are "monotonic". The curve may have a positive slope, or a negative slope, but not both if the system under study is unique. The slope of the curve may show varying degrees of positivity (negativity), but the sign of the slope stays the same throughout the range of testable doses. When monotonicity of a dose-effect curve does not obtain, one may infer that the system under study is not unique or singular: either more than one active agent or more than one effect is under study.

The curves approach some maximum value as an asymptote, and the asymptote is a measure of the intrinsic activity (q.v.) of the drug in the system.

Dosing Dosing means determining the quantity per dose of a substance/substances to achieve its/their optimum efficacy, safety and high-level of comfort for the patient; moreover, for making a drug effective and safe, it is necessary to follow precisely the dosing prescribed by the physician; drug dosing is often unique while depending on the nature and severity of a specific disease, the overall condition and age of the patient; a special modification of dosing is applied for children, elderly patients and patients suffering from hepatic or renal diseases.

Double blind A type of scientific experiment in which neither the subjects nor the researchers know who is receiving an active substance and who is receiving a placebo. Researchers who do not know which subjects received the active substance then usually evaluate the data generated from the experiment. This type of experiment helps to eliminate personal bias from research.

Double blind crossover This is a study where at one point in the experiment all of the subjects switch from an active substance to a placebo or vice versa.

Double blind test Used in Clinical Trials, this is a method to ensure that any one party cannot improperly influence the test. The product (either in a single strength dosage or in multiple dosages) and the placebo are packaged and given a code name known to only the initiating party. These are then sent to another party who gives the coded packages yet another code name or number, and makes a matrix of the previous name/number to the new name/number. This is then sent to the physician who administers these to the patient. At the end of the test, the physician provides records of which patient received which code name/number product. This is then cross-referenced to the intermediate matrix to determine the original code name/number. The results of the treatment are then correlated to determine the efficacy of the drug.

The structure of DNA as proposed by Watson and Crick. It consists of two right-handed helical polynucleotide chains coiled around the same axis. The two chains are anti-parallel with their 3rd to 5th internucleotide phosphodiester bonds running in opposite directions. Under most conditions, the coiling of the chains is such that if the ends are held still, as in circular DNA or in a large chromosome, the chains cannot be separated except by cleavage of one of the strands.

Double blind study A study in which neither the subject(s) nor the investigator(s) know what treatment a subject is receiving.

Doxercalciferol A substance that is being studied in the prevention of recurrent prostate cancer. It belongs to the family of drugs called vitamin D analogs.

Doxorubicin (Adriamycin) Chemotherapy drug, with a wide spectrum of activity. Toxic to the heart in high dosage. A part of the CHOP chemotherapy regimen used to treat NHL.

OH O OH O ''OH MeO O OH O O NH$_2$ HO

Doxycycline Brand name: Vibramycin. A synthetic broad-spectrum antibiotic derived from tetracycline . Doxycycline is used for many different types of infections, including respiratory tract infections due to Hemophilus influenzae, Streptococcus pneumoniae, or Mycoplasma pneumoniae. It is also used for the treatment of nongonococcal urethritis (due to Ureaplasma), Rocky Mountain spotted fever, typhus, chancroid, cholera , brucellosis, syphilis, and acne .

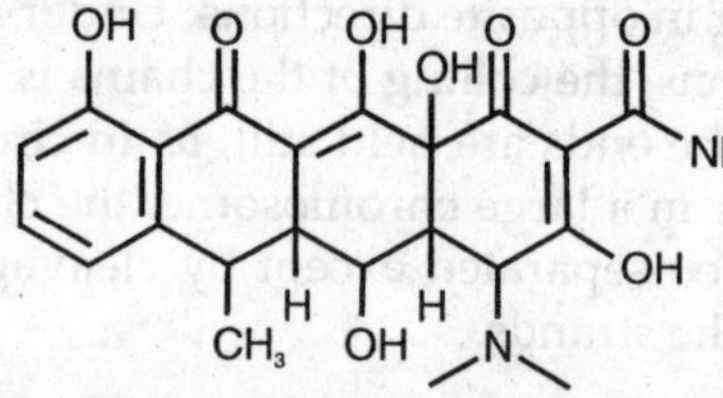

Dronabinol (Marinol) Indications: Appetite stimulant for treatment of AIDS wasting syndrome.

Contraindications: Known hypersensitivity, significant cognitive dysfunction.

Dosage: 2.5 mg po bid.

Toxicity: Neuropsychiatric symptoms, gastrointestinal intolerance.

Dronabinol A synthetic pill form of delta-9-tetrahydrocannabinol (THC), an active ingredient in marijuana that is used to treat nausea and vomiting associated with cancer chemotherapy.

Drug A chemical used in the diagnosis, treatment, or prevention of disease. More generally, a chemical, which, in a solution of sufficient concentration, will modify the behavior of cells exposed to the solution. Drugs produce only quantitative changes in the behavior of cells; i.e., drugs increase or decrease the magnitude, frequency, of duration of the normal activities of cells. Drugs used in therapy never produce qualitative changes in cell behavior short of producing death of the cell, e.g., a nerve cell cannot be made to contract or a muscle cell cannot be made to secrete saliva by use of a drug. The degree to which this point of view will be modified by the discovery and development of agents which act on cells at a genetic level remains to be seen.

Drug abuse Use or misuse of a drug under conditions, or to an extent, considered "more destructive than constructive for society and the individual." More specifically, the use of drugs for their effects chiefly on the central nervous system, to an extent and/or at a frequency and/or for a duration of time that is inimical to the welfare of the user and/or the total of social groups in which she/he lives. The abuse potential of a drug depends on its capacity to induce compulsive drug-seeking behavior in the user, its capacity to induce acute and chronic toxic effects (and to permit occurrence of associated diseases), and upon social attitudes toward the drug, its use, and its effects.

Drug active substance Basic active substance which is the bearer of the drug effects is usually indicated as a sub-heading of the drug trade name; apart from active substances, the drug usually also contains additives processed in the drug form.

Drug administration Drug application; there are several types of drug administration, such as sublingual where a drug is put under the tongue and left to dissolve, oral (the drug is swallowed), parenteral – most frequently injections (depending on the point of application we differentiate them into, for example, muscular – intramuscular, venous – intravenous, subcutaneous), topical, where drugs are applied on a certain area, while the most frequently used drugs are those affecting the skin (dermal drugs), followed by solutions for ear, nose and eyes, suppositories, vaginal tablets; the type of drug administration depends amongst other things on whether the active substance is required to deliver local or systemic effect; the correct drug administration is important for achieving the required drug effect and that is why sometimes various aids are used for administration, for example, in inhalation of anti-asthmatics.

Drug administration contraindication This is any circumstance or condition of the patient under which administration of a specific drug is inconvenient, not recommended or impossible; contraindication can be absolute or relative while absolute contraindication is a situation where drug administration is totally inconvenient, as drug administration of such a contraindication can result in a situation threatening the patient's life; relative contraindication of the drug is a situation where drug administration is not recommended, but if the physician assesses the drug as being advantageous for the patient in terms of his/her health condition and availability of other drugs, the drug can be administered to control a disease; in general, the attending physician must always assess the significance or benefit of a specific drug administration on an individual basis; the majority of drugs feature their contraindications, while frequent contraindication is, for example, represented by known allergy to the active substance or additive and many drugs are contraindicated in pregnancy or lactation; the opposite of indication.

Drug allergy Drug allergy is a hypersensitivity condition of the body against a certain drug manifesting most frequently in various skin reactions, bronchiostenosis and oedema, while the most severe form of allergy is anaphylactic shock, which is an acute life-threatening allergic reaction connected with oedema of the respiratory tract. Drugs which may induce an allergic reaction contain, for example, certain antibiotics, acetylsalicylic acid or local anaesthetics.

Drug application Specifies how the preparation should be used.

Drug approval glossary Adaptive clinical trials: A process for improving the efficiency of clinical trials based on interim analyses of clinical data, potentially leading to reductions in overall sample size, shorter project duration, improved quality of results, and reduced costs.

The pressure to speed up trials reduce their costs and get new products to the market place will only increase. Flexible methods for design and monitoring will be key factors for responding to this pressure. The combination of electronic data capture technology, group sequential technology, and adaptive technology will provide an integrated solution to the logistical and statistical complexities of monitoring trials in flexible ways without biasing their conclusions.

Drug benefit A benefit normally included with a medical plan that allows prescription medicine to be obtained using a benefit card. The member normally pays only a small copayment or coinsurance amount for each prescription obtained.

Drug dependence A somatic state which develops after chronic administration of certain drugs; this state is characterized by the necessity to continue administration of the drug in order to avoid the appearance of uncomfortable or dangerous (withdrawal) symptoms. Withdrawal symptoms, when they occur, may be relieved by the administration of the drug upon which the body was "dependent". Recommended as a term to be substituted for such words as "addiction" and "habituation " since it is frequently difficult to classify specific agents as being only addictive, habituating, or non-addicting or non-habituating. e.g., drug dependence of the barbiturate type.

Drug development process

Discovery: Identification of a biological, genetic or protein target linked to a particular disease, and subsequent lead identification of a potential drug that interacts with the target to help cure the disease or halt its progression.

Pre-clinical: Comprehensive in vitro (lab dish) and animal testing of the drug candidate to establish its target specificity, toxicity in various doses and pharmacokinetics.

Clinical Phase I: Human trials conducted to demonstrate the safety and effectiveness or (efficacy) of an experimental drug or procedure. Tests are conducted with paid volunteers to establish dosage, side effects and pharmacokinetics.

Clinical Phase II: Trials with small numbers of patients conducted to identify drug performance characteristics (optimal dosing, administration, key indication).

Clinical Phase III: Pivotal trials conducted with larger patient populations to establish efficacy and provide additional safety information.

Drug form Drug form is the complete form of medical preparations in which, except for the prescribed dose of an active substance additives are added thus getting the drug form suitable for its administration while masking its adverse appearance, taste or odour connected with the drug administration, the drug onset of efficacy is postponed, the drug effect is extended, etc. Drug form is represented, for example, by tablets (various types of tablets including vaginal, chewing and others), capsules, injections, ointments, suppositories, solutions and a number of others; a single active substance can be administered in various drug forms. A drug form may have a significant impact on the active substance characteristics. For each drug form to fulfil its role, certain administration rules are required which are included on the leaflet and the patient is informed about them by his or her physician or pharmacist.

Drug group indication Identifies a drug group – the group of drugs determined for treatment of a specific impairment; usually a specific name in Latin is used.

Drug half life The amount of time it takes for one-half of an administered drug to be metabolized and eliminated through biological processes.

Drug interactions Incidents that occur in the body when a medication is affected by another medication.

Drug metabolism The process by which the body converts a drug into a more water soluble product so that it may be easily excreted. In this process, a drug is acted on by an enzyme or enzyme pathway. The biological substance produced from metabolic processes is termed a "metabolite."

Drug metabolizing enzymes DME genes The biochemical and transcriptional mechanisms by which drugs and xenobiotics affect the expression of the Phase I (cytochrome P450) and Phase II (e.g, glutathione S-transferase) drug metabolizing enzymes (DMEs). These important proteins are responsible for metabolizing endogenous compounds such as steroids, prostaglandins, and leukotrienes, as well as drugs and environmental pollutants. A notable characteristic of some DME genes is their ability to be transcriptionally upregulated by treatment with chemical inducers such as phenobarbital (PB).

Drug optimization A method to improve the efficacy of a drug.

Drug product A finished dosage form, for example, tablet, capsule, solution, etc., that contains one or more APIs (Active Pharmaceutical Ingredients) generally, but not necessarily, in association with inactive ingredients. The term also includes a finished dosage form, which does not contain an API but is intended to be used as a placebo.

Drug receptors Proteins that bind specific drugs with high affinity and trigger intracellular changes influencing the behavior of cells. Drug receptors are generally thought to be receptors for some endogenous substance not otherwise specified.

Drug regimen The approved directions for when and how to take a specific medication.

Drug registration Drug registration means permission granted by the relevant state authority (State Institute of Drug Control in the Czech Republic) to use and distribute a certain drug in the Czech Republic; on the basis of the registration proceedings each drug is given a registration number and registration itself is valid for 5 years. Then it must be renewed. The main aim of registration is to ensure that the patients get only safe, effective drugs of high quality.

Drug resistance The failure of cancer cells, viruses, or bacteria to respond to a drug used to kill or weaken them. The cells, viruses, or bacteria may be resistant to the drug at the beginning of treatment, or may become resistant after being exposed to the drug.

Drug response Comparison of pharmacogenomics studies will be difficult until a more standard definition of "response" and of various phenotypes can be agreed upon.

Drug response phenotype SNPs are also useful in pharmacogenomics for matching an individual's genotype with a drug- response phenotype. It is possible, in this context, to identify individuals who cannot adequately metabolize the drug and must be dosed accordingly, or those with a compromised drug target, who could not benefit from the drug. The discovery of such a relationship will require measuring hundreds of SNPs in or near candidate genes in several thousands of individuals. Validation will require detecting very few SNPs in several hundred to several thousand individuals. These relationships can be used either for clinical trials or diagnostically to determine therapy. Each clinical trial will involve measuring few SNPs in the low thousands of individuals.

Drug safety Improving products' effective clinical safety will increase the industry's fundamental value proposition to patients, healthcare providers, payors and regulators. Topics include: Implementing programs that yield the greatest possible ROI in terms of both increasing the probability of timely approval and mitigating safety risks. Aligning resources to design and execute a proactive risk management plan. Integrating drug safety knowledge longitudinally across a compound's lifecycle. Optimizing the allocation of an organization's scarce and increasingly costly drug safety assessment resources. Understanding regulatory authorities' evolving drug safety risk management expectations and how they should be applied in practice. Differentiating the value and rigor of assessment methods and tools—including Phase IV trials, observational studies, patient and drug registries, and database mining. Utilizing quantitative approaches for surveillance and signal detection in pharmacovigilance.

Drug selectivity The propensity of a drug to affect one receptor population in preference to others. ie. propranolol is a non-selective beta-blocker (blocks all beta-receptors equally), whereas metoprolol is a beta1-selective blocker in that it has a greater preference (affinity) for beta1- over beta2-receptors. Selectivity is generally a desirable property in a drug as it can minimize potential side-effects ie. potential of propranolol causing bronchospasm. Selectivity is not to be confused with "potency"; a potent drug may be non-selective or a selective drug may not be very potent.

Drug storage conditions The correct storage of the drug is important in order to maintain its efficacy and safety; the majority of drugs should be stored at a temperature of up to 25°C, protected against light and humidity. However, certain substances require special storage, for example at a lower temperature, i.e. they should be kept in the refrigerator (for example some hormones, ointments and vaccines); all drugs should be kept out of the reach of children; drugs which are not stored under the recommended conditions might degrade even prior to the expiration date.

Drug target A gene or gene product (protein) against small molecule drugs will be screened and developed

Drug tolerance A condition that occurs when the body gets used to a medicine so that either more medicine is needed or different medicine is needed.

Drug toxicity Adverse effects caused by a drug that may occur with overdose of the drug, accumulation in the body over time or the inability of the person's body to eliminate the drug.

Drug trade name Name (made up identification) under which the preparation enters the market and under which it is approved by the State Institute of Drug Control .

Drug using The effects of drugs may be influenced by a series of external and internal factors, therefore, a successful treatment requires the correct use of drugs. For example it is necessary to follow the recommendations given by the physician or pharmacist on drug administration relating to food intake (fasting means 30 minutes before meals or 2 hours after meals) and even having a drink after drug administration should not be underestimated (for the majority of drugs it is recommended to drink water or mild lukewarm tea; the optimum quantity in adults is considered to be 250 ml of drink. With certain drugs it is recommended to use milk as a drink, but on the contrary, with some drugs milk is not suitable at all; you should be careful regarding acid drinks, fruit juices, coffee, dark tea and of course alcohol). In some cases the time of day that the drug is administered can play an important role (some drugs are to be administered in the morning, while others before going to bed). Certain drugs should be used regularly for a certain period of time, some for a person's whole life, while others are used only when problems occur. When using certain drugs it is advisable to avoid sunshine, etc.

Dry air Air from which all water vapor and contaminants have been removed. Its composition by volume is: 1. Nitrogen 78.08%

2. Oxygen 20.95%

3. Argon 0.93%

4. Carbon Dioxide 0.03

5. Other gases 0.00003.

Dry heat sterilization Sterilization utilizing a heating oven or continuous tunnel (gas or electric heated), as opposed to steam sterilization in an autoclave, usually used for glassware and metal parts. In depyrogenation temperatures of 250°C result in sterilization and the inactivation of endotoxin present on the surface of the equipment.

Dry orgasm Sexual climax without the release of semen from the penis.

DTC Direct to consumer advertising Ads targeted directly to people who might take a drug urging them to ask their doctor about the drug.

DTGM fusion protein An anticancer drug formed by the combination of diphtheria toxin and a colony-stimulating factor (GM-CSF). The colony-stimulating factor is attracted to cancer cells, and the diphtheria toxin kills the cells.

Dummy "A counterfeit object;" a form of treatment - as in an experimental investigation of drug effects - which is intended to have no effects, to be biologically inert. The dummy treatment should mimic in every way (dosage form, route of administration, etc.) the purportedly active ingredient upon which the effectiveness of the active treatment is expected to depend. In contrast to a dummy, a placebo is expected to have an effect through the agency of "suggestion" or other psychological mechanisms, even though the effects of placebos may be psychological or physical. Dummies may, of course, have the effects of placebos, but it is useful to be aware of the difference expected to exist between the two.

According to Gaddum, dummies have two functions: 1. to distinguish between drug effects in a subject and other effects, such as those of suggestion: obviously, an experiment might properly incorporate both a dummy and a placebo.

2. to obtain an unbiased assessment of the result of a pharmacologic experiment.

Durability The ability to withstand the rigors of the environment without degrading or requiring repair.

Dust Dusting Deterioration of the finish at the surface so it is easily loosened from the surface by light physical contact (such as wiping one's hand across the surface), mechanically induced air movements or naturally occurring air movements.

Dye Dyes are additives used for colour treatment of the drug appearance, followed by differentiation of the similar shaped drugs containing various active substances, and if needed, to differentiate drugs of various concentrations of the same active substance.

Dynamic conditions Environmental conditions of a manufacturing room occupied by the normal number of workers appropriately garbed and with production equipment in operation. However, dynamic conditions for some dusty operations, such as aseptic powder filling, may be measured in the absence of product.

Dynamic HTML Collective term for a combination of new tags and options, style sheets, and programming that lets you create Web pages in Hypertext Mark-up Language (HTML) that are more responsive to user interaction than previous versions of HTML.

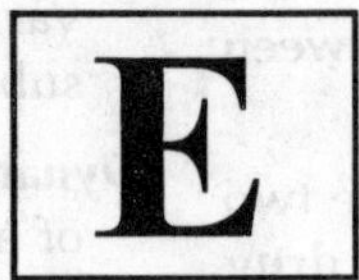

E coli (escherichia coli) A fast growing, Gram-negative bacteria commonly found in the body with a comparatively simple structure. The genetic make up of E. coli is the best known of any organism, having been widely studied during the development of genetic engineering. It has been used extensively as the host cell for novel proteins made by rDNA technology.

EBCT (electron beam computerized tomography or "Ultrafast CT") EBCT is a very fast form of computerized tomography (popularly known as CT scan or "CAT scan") that measures calcium deposits in the coronary arteries; the measurement is reported as a "calcium score."

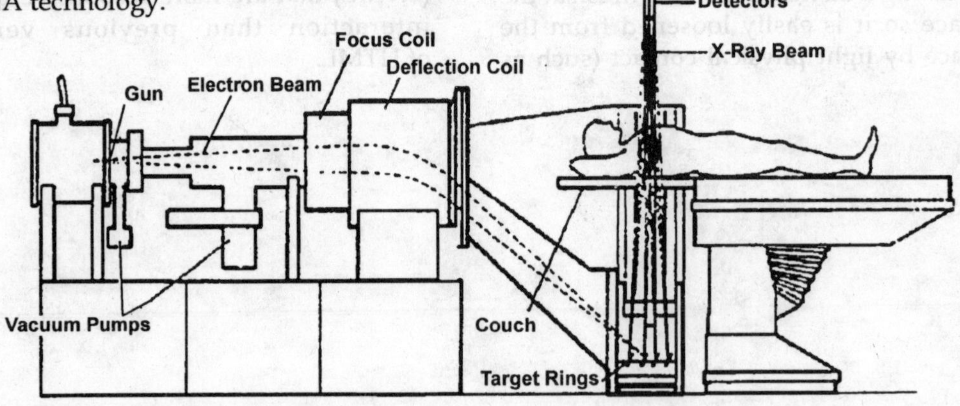

Fig. EBCT

EC50 The concentration of an agonist that produces 50% of the maximal possible effect of that agonist. Other percentage values (EC10, EC20, etc.) may be specified. Concentration is preferably expressed in molar units, but the mass concentration (g/l) may be used if the molecular weight of the substance is unknown.

Ecology The study of the interrelationships between organisms and their environment.

Economy The ability of a system to deliver data of high information content at a low overall cost per item of data; economy does not, of course, contribute to " accuracy" but is an important determinant of the practical usefulness of a system or method.

Eculizumab A monoclonal antibody that is being studied in the prevention of red blood cell destruction in patients with paroxysmal nocturnal hemoglobinuria (a red blood cell disorder).

Eczema An inflammation of the skin, usually causing itching and sometimes accompanied by crusting, scaling or blisters. A type of eczema often made worse by allergen exposure is termed "atopic dermatitis".

ED50 1. In a quantal assay, the median effective dose.

2. In a graded (non-quantal) assay, the dose of a drug that produces 50% of the maximal response to that drug. It is preferable, where possible, to express potency in terms of EC50 but ED50 is appropriate for in vivo measurements and for those in vitro experiments where the absolute concentration is uncertain. If the maximum response is unknown, it is acceptable to express the effectiveness of a drug in terms of the dose that produces a particular level of response, for example a certain change in blood pressure or heart rate. In such a case, the appropriate units must be included (e.g. ED20mm) to avoid confusion.

Edge of failure A control parameter value that, if exceeded, meansadverse effect on state of control and/or fitness for use of theproduct.

Edotecarin A substance that is being studied in the treatment of cancer. It belongs to the family of drugs called topoisomerase I inhibitors. Also called J-107088.

Edrecolomab A type of monoclonal antibody used in cancer detection or therapy. Monoclonal antibodies are laboratory-produced substances that can locate and bind to cancer cells.

Efavirenz (Sustiva) Indications: Treatment of HIV infection in combination with other agents.

Contraindications: Known hypersensitivity.

Dosage: 600 mg po qhs. Avoid taking with high fat meals. There are many potential drug interactions, some of which require dosage modification

Toxicity: Rash is common and does not require discontinuation of the drug unless accompanied by fever, mucous membrane involvement, or other systemic manifestations. Other side effects include vivid dreams and nightmares, neurocognitive dysfunction, hyperlipidemia, abnormal liver function tests.

Teratogenic in non-human primates. Women taking efavirenz should use two forms of contraception.

H N O O Cl CF_3

Effective permeability Similar in principle to apparent permeability (Papp) effective permeability (Peff) is calculated based on the disappearance of a compound from one side of a biological barrier (slope of the disappearance vs. time profile) whereas Papp is calculated based on the appearance of a compound on the opposite side of a biological barrier. In an ideal case, Peff = Papp. However in the case of intestinal transport of a prodrug that is converted rapidly to the active moiety inside intestinal epithelial cells, Peff is much greater than Papp because the prodrug disappears from the intestinal lumen but does not appear on the serosal side.

Effective Adequate and well-controlled investigations, including clinical investigations, by experts qualified by scientific training and experience to evaluate the effectiveness of the drug involved."

Effectiveness The desired measure of a drug's influence on a disease condition as proved by substantial evidence from adequate and well-controlled investigations.

Efficacy Broadly, efficacy refers to the capacity of a drug to produce an alteration in a target cell/organ after binding to its receptor. A competitive antagonist, that occupies a binding site without producing any alteration in the receptor, is considered to have an efficacy of zero.

Efficacy is generally independent of potency/affinity, and is related to the maximum effect that a particular drug is capable of producing.

As originally formulated by Stephenson (1956), binding of an agonist A to its receptor R is considered to result in a "stimulus" S=ε A x P AR where ε A is the efficacy of A and PAR is the proportion of the receptors occupied. The effect of the drug on the cell or tissue is given by Effect = f (S), where f is an unspecified monotonic function that is dependent upon the nature of the receptor and its interaction with the cell or tissue. Efficacy is both agonist and tissue-dependent.

Efficacy is related to Intrinsic Activity, which was originally defined by Furchgott (1966) as e=ε/R T , i.e. as the efficacy per receptor. In practice, the two terms are sometimes loosely used synonymously.

Effluent The output or discharge from a process, such as a wastewater treatment process.

Elastin An albuminoid, or scleroprotein present especially in yellow elastic fibrous tissue.

Elastomer Long chain co-polymers or terpolymers (two or three different monomers in one chain) that contain adequate crosslinks among individual chains. Fluorinated elastomers are more stable than hydrocarbon or silicon elastomers because C-F bonds are approximately 30% stronger than C-H bonds. There are five major department of health compliant elastomers used in the pharmaceutical and biopharmaceutical industries: EPDM (ethylene-propylene-diene rubber), fluororelastomers (FKM), platinum-cured silicon (pt-Si), and finally Kalrez parts using compounds KLR-6221 and KLR-6230, which are perfluoroelastomers.

Elastomeric material A material that can be stretched or compressed repeatedly and, upon immediate release of stress, will return to its approximate original size.

Electrical area classifications Facilities, or portions of facilities are classified electrically according to the type of material present and its flammability and/or explosive potential. Each area classification carries with it specific requirements for the construction requirements found within that space to guard against sparking. The Class of an area refers to the type of material; the Division of the area refers to whether that material is normally found in that area or not. Electrical classifications are covered by the National Electrical Code (NEC) adopted by the National Fire Protection Association (NFPA) as Volume 6 of the National Fire Codes. They are: 1. Class I, Division 1: A Class I, Division 1 location 1. is that in which ignitable concentrations of flammable gases/vapors can exist under normal operating conditions; or

2. in which ignitable concentrations of such gases/vapors may exist frequently because of repair, maintenance operations or because of leakage; or

3. in which breakdown or faulty operation of equipment or process may release ignitable concentrations of flammable gases/vapors, and might also cause simultaneous failure of electric equipment.

2. Class I, Division 2: A Class I, Division 2 location (1) is that in which volatile flammable liquids or flammable gases are handled, processed, or used, but in which the liquids, vapors, or gases will normally be confined within closed containers or closed systems from which they can escape only in case of accidental rupture or breakdown of such containers or systems, or in case of abnormal operation of equipment; or 2. in which ignitable concentrations of gases or vapors are normally prevented by positive mechanical ventilation, and which might become hazardous through failure or abnormal operation of the ventilating equipment; or

3. that is adjacent to a class I, Division 1 location, and to which ignitable concentrations of gases or vapors might occasionally be communicated unless such communication is prevented by adequate positive-pressure ventilation from a source of clean air, and effective safeguards against ventilation failure are provided.

3. Class II, Division 1: A Class II, Division 1 location 1. is that in which combustible dust is in the air under normal operating conditions in quantities sufficient to produce explosive or ignitable mixtures; or 2. where mechanical failure or abnormal operation of machinery or equipment might cause such explosive or ignitable mixtures to be produced, and might also provide a source of ignition through simultaneous failure of electric equipment, operation of protection device, or from other causes; or 3. in which combustible dusts of an electrically conductive nature may be present in hazardous quantities.

4. Class II, Division 2: A Class II, Division 2 location 1. is that in which combustible dust is not normally in the air in quantities sufficient to produce explosive or ignitable mixtures, and dust accumulations are normally insufficient to interfere with the normal operation of electrical equipment or other apparatus but combustible dust may be in suspension in the air as a result of infrequent malfunctioning of handling or processing equipment and where combustible dust accumulations on, in, or in the vicinity of the electrical equipment may be sufficient to interfere with the safe dissipation of heat from electrical equipment or may be ignitable by abnormal operation or failure of electrical equipment.

5. Class III, Division 1: A Class III, Division 1 location is that in which easily ignitable fibers or materials producing combustible filings are handled, manufactured, or used.

6. Class III, Division 2: Class III, Division 2 location is that in which easily ignitable fibers are stored or handled.

Electrical cardioversion A procedure used to restore a chronic irregular heart rhythm.

While the patient is under sedation, a special machine delivers an electrical current or currents to the heart through "paddles" applied to the chest. This shock briefly interrupts the electrical activity of the heart which allows the normal heart rhythm to be restored.

It is often used as an emergency procedure to correct a fast heart rhythm that is causing low blood pressure, chest pain, or heart failure, and in non-urgent situations to convert atrial fibrillation to normal heart rhythm.

Electrical code Electrical Groups Electrical groupings are based on the characteristics of the materials involved. These include the following: 1. Class I, Group A: Atmospheres containing acetylene.

2. Class I, Group B: Atmospheres containing hydrogen, fuel and combustible process gases containing more than 30 percent hydrogen by volume, or gases or vapors of equivalent hazard such as butadiene, ethylene oxide, propylene oxide, and acrolein.

3. Class I, Group C: Atmospheres such as ethyl ether, ethylene, or gases or vapors of equivalent hazard.

4. Class I, Group D: Atmospheres such as acetone, ammonia, benzene, butane, cyclopropane, ethanol, gasoline, hexane, methanol, methane, natural gas, naphtha, propane, or gases or vapors of equivalent hazard.

5. Class II, Group E: Atmospheres containing combustible metal dusts, including aluminum, magnesium and their commercial alloys, or other combustible dusts whose particle size, abrasiveness, and conductivity present similar hazards in the use of electrical equipment.

6. Class II, Group F: Atmospheres containing combustible carbonaceous dusts, including carbon black, charcoal, coal, or coke dusts that have more that 8 percent entrapped volatiles, or dusts that have been sensitized by other materials so that they present an explosion hazard.

7. Class II, Group G: Atmospheres containing combustibles dusts not included in Group E or F, including flour, grain, wood, plastic, and chemicals.

Electrodialysis (ED) A membrane separation method used for the separation of charged molecules from a solution by application of a direct current. The membranes contain ion-exchange groups and have a fixed electrical charge. This method is very effective in the concentration of electrolytes and proteins.

Electrolyte A chemical compound which when dissolved or ionized in water allows it to conduct electric current.

Electron microscopy (EM) A technique for visualizing material that uses beams of electrons instead of light rays and that permits greater magnification than is possible with an optical microscope. Electron microscopes have been used to examine the structure of viruses and bacteria, to identify and classify pollen grains, etc.

Electronic approval An input command requiring restricted entry madeunder a level of higher authorisation, which signifies an act ofapproval.

Electronic identification (eID) An electronic measure that can besubstituted for a hand-written signature or initials for the purpose ofsignifying approval, authorisation or verification of specific dataentries.

Electronic record Any combination of text, graphics, data, audio, pictorial, or other information representation in digital form that is created, modified, maintained, archived, retrieved, or distributed by a computer system.

Electronic signature or e-sig According to department of health, an electronic signature is a computer data compilation of any symbol or series of symbols executed, adopted, or authorized by an individual to be the legally binding equivalent of the individual's handwritten signature.

Electronic verification An input command that enables a designateduser, or the computerised system itself, to electronically signifyverification or endorsement of a specific step, transaction or dataentry. Source of the electronic verification may be made visible orinvisible to users of the data.

Electrophoresis The migration of electrically charged proteins, colloids, molecules, or other particles when dissolved or suspended in an electrolyte through which an electric current is passed. The most important use of electrophoresis is in the analysis of blood proteins. Since the proportion of these proteins varies widely in different diseases, electrophoresis can be used for diagnostic purposes. Electrophoresis is used to study bacteria and viruses, nucleic acids, and some types of smaller molecules, including amino acids.

Electropolishing Also known as "chemical machining" and "reverse plating", electropolishing is an electrochemical process far superior to any available mechanical process for the removal of minute surface imperfections in stainless steel. It levels and brightens the material surface by anodic dissolution in an electrolyte flowing solution with an imposed electrical current. When the proper combination of electrolyte current & temperature is attained, the high points of surface irregularities, or high current density areas, are selectively removed at a greater rate than the remainder of the surface, resulting in improved surface smoothness. During electropolishing, the polarized surface film is subjected to the combined effects of gassing (oxygen) that occurs with electromechanical metal removal, saturation of the surface with dissolved metal, and the agitation and temperature of the electrolyte.

Electrostatic fluidized bed A container holding powder coating material which is aerated from below so as to form an air-supported expanded cloud of such material which is electrically charged with a charge opposite to the charge of the object to be coated. Such object is transported through the container immediately above the charged and aerated materials in order to be coated.

Eligibility period Describes the time during which potential members of a health insurance plan can enroll. Also can be a period under a major medical policy when reimbursable expenses can be accrued. Eligibility requirements are guidelines outlined by insurance companies to determine which individuals can be covered under a group insurance plan.

ELISA (Enzyme linked immunosorbent assay) A test to measure the concentration of antigens or antibodies.

Ellinghausen's medium A complex medium for growing Leptospira . Contains numerous salts, nutrients, and BSA (Bovine Serum Albumin).

Elute To separate one solute from another by washing. Elution may include the removal by means of a suitable solvent of one material (absorbed material) from another (adsorbent) that is insoluble in that solvent.

Embedded system A system, usually microprocessor or PLC based, whosesole purpose is to control a particular piece of automated equipment.This is contrasted with a standalone computer system.

Embriology The study of the early stages in the development of an organism. In these stages a single highly specialized cell, the egg, is transformed into a complex, many-celled organism resembling its parents.

Enantiomer One of a pair of molecular entities that are mirror images of each other and non-superimposable.

Endemic A disease present in a community or among a group of people; used to describe a disease prevailing continually in a region.

Endergonic reaction A chemical reaction with a positive standard free energy change, an "uphill" reaction.

Endocrine glands The glands that secrete their products (hormones) into the blood that then carries them to their specific target organs. Endocrine glands are the pituitary, thyroids, adrenals, pancreas, ovaries (in females), and testes (in males). Endocrine glands are found in some invertebrates as well as in vertebrates.

Endocrine hormones The products secreted by the endocrine glands. These help control long-term processes, such as growth, lactation, sex cycles, and metabolic adjustment. The endocrine system and the nervous system are interdependent and are often referred to collectively as the neuroendocrine system. For example, the juvenile hormone, found in insects and annelids, affects sexual maturation. There is currently great interest in the possible use of such hormones in the control of destructive insects.

Endocrine system Is a term for a group of glands, specifically the pituitary, thyroid, thymus, pancreas, adrenal, testes and ovaries.

Endonuclease An enzyme that cleaves its nucleic acid substrate at internal sites (other than the terminal bonds) in the nucleotide sequence.

Endorphins Endogenous opiates having morphine-like effects consisting of small polypeptides such as enkephalin and leu-enkephalin and longer polypeptides such as alpha-, ß-, and gamma-endorphins. They bind to opiate receptors in the brain. Endorphins induce analgesia when injected intraventricularly but not when administered peripherally, presumably because of their inability to cross the blood/brain barrier. The amino acid sequence of the endorphins is short enough to allow the gene sequences coding for them to be synthesized.

Endospore A highly heat and chemical resistant dormant inclusion (spore) occurring within the substance of certain genera of bacteria, mainly Bacillus and Clostridium.

Endothelial cells A layer of flat cells that line the tumor blood vessel structure.

Endotoxin A poisonous complex molecule (lipopolysaccharide) that forms an integral part of the bacterial (gram-negative bacteria) cell wall and is only released when the integrity of the wall is disturbed. Certain organisms may release endotoxins (e.g. E. coli) during biosynthesis of a recombinant DNA product, thus necessitating purification steps to ensure their removal. In water treatment, it most often refers to pyrogens.

Endpoint An indicator measured in a subject or biological sample to assess the safety, efficacy, or other objective of a trial.

Enhanced documentation Collection of Engineering, Quality Control, and Regulatory Affairs documents, which will be required for the operation, validation, maintenance, and regulatory compliance of a pharmaceutical plant.

Enrollment The number of members in a Health Maintenance Organization (HMO). Also the process by which an HMO signs up individuals or groups as subscribers.

Enteral nutritional support A liquid nutritional supplement is administered directly to the gastrointestinal tract through a feeding tube.

Enthalpy A thermodynamic property that indicates the total energy in a sample of dry air and water vapor, measured in Btu/lb dry air. Dry air at zero degrees Fahrenheit and atmospheric pressure is designated as zero enthalpy.

Enzyme Any of numerous proteins or conjugated proteins produced by living organisms and functioning as complex biochemical catalysts. They not only promote reactions but also function as regulators making sure the organism does not produce too much or too little of any chemical substance. Although all enzymes are proteins, many contain additional non-protein components essential for catalytic activity. Such enzymes are termed haloenzymes. The protein part of this enzyme is termed an apoenzyme and the non-amino acid part is termed a coenzyme.

Enzyme kinetics Most of the chemical reactions which occur in living systems, if left to their own devices, would occur at rates which are very slow, some immeasurably slow. Catalysts are required to make these reactions go at rates that are useful to the cell. In biological systems the catalysts are enzymes

Enzyme product The resulting molecule or molecules after a substrate reacts with an enzyme.

Enzyme substrate The molecule with which an enzyme interacts. Typically, the enzyme-substrate relationship is very specific, analogous to a lock and key. An enzyme will not act on just any substrate, only the one for which it is designed.

Epidemic A disease attacking many people in a community simultaneously; distinguished from endemic, since the disease is not continuously present but has been introduced from outside.

Epilepsy Symptoms may include impairment of motor response and disturbed consciousness

Epinephrine Epinephrine is a naturally occurring hormone, also called adrenaline. It is one of two chemicals (the other is norepinephrine) released by the adrenal gland. Epinephrine increases the speed and force of heart beats and thereby the work that can be done by the heart. It dilates the airways to improve breathing and narrows blood vessels in the skin and intestine so that an increased flow of blood reaches the muscles and allows them to cope with the demands of exercise. Epinephrine has been produced synthetically as a drug since 1900. It remains the drug of choice for treatment of anaphylaxis.

OH, HO, H, N, HO

Epithelium The layer(s) of cells between an organism or its tissues or organs and their environment (skin cells, inner linings of lungs or digestive organs, outer linings of kidneys, etc.).

Epitope Any part of a molecule that acts as an antigenic determinant. A macromolecule can contain many different epitopes each capable of stimulating production of a different specific antibody. The specific interaction between proteins is determined by only limited parts of the proteins involved. In general the epitope (interaction site) of a protein is composed of 7-30 amino acids. ... If an epitope is formed by a continuous stretch of amino acids sequence it is called a linear epitope. In about one third of all proteins the epitope is linear. However, in the majority of cases the epitope is composed of amino acids that are close in space, but can be located on different loops of the amino acid sequence. These epitopes are referred to as discontinuous epitopes.

EPO (Erythropoietin) A glycoprotein hormone that stimulates the production of red blood cells. It is a commercialized product of recombinant DNA technology.

EPO906 A substance that is being studied as a treatment for cancer. It belongs to the family of drugs called epothilones. Also called epothilone B.

Epoetin alfa A substance that is made in the laboratory that stimulates the bone marrow to make red blood cells. It belongs to the family of drugs called antianemics. It is also called recombinant human erythropoietin.

Epoetin beta A substance that is made in the laboratory and that stimulates the bone marrow to make red blood cells. It belongs to the family of drugs called antianemics. It is also called recombinant human erythropoietin.

Epoxy These materials are based on the reactive oxirane group, which are characterized by the attachment of one oxygen atom to two different adjacent carbon atoms. Standard epoxy resins are the reaction product of bisphenol A and epichlorohydrin. Curing of epoxy resins generally occurs at ambient temperatures and is achieved by the chemical reaction of the epoxy with a second reactant such as amines, polyamines, amine products, or other reactants. Cure can occur at higher temperatures when reacted with anhydrides, carboxylic acids, phenol or novolac (phenol-formadehyde) thermoplastic resins. These reactants are sometimes referred to as catalysts, which is a misnomer.

Equine Of, pertaining to, or characteristic of a horse, such as equine hormones.

Equipment suitability The established capacity of process equipment and ancillary systems to operate consistently within established limits and tolerances.

Equipoise A state in which an investigator is uncertain about which arm of a clinical trial would be therapeutically superior for a patient. An investigator who has a treatment preference or finds out that one arm of a comparative trial offers a clinically therapeutic advantage should disclose this information to subjects participating in the trial.

Equipotent Equally potent, or equally capable of producing a pharmacologic effect of a specified intensity. The masses of the drugs required to produce this degree of effect may be compared, quantitatively, to yield estimates of " potency" of the drugs. Obviously, if two drugs are not both capable of producing an effect of a given intensity, they cannot be compared with respect to potency; i.e., drugs with different intrinsic activities or ceiling effects cannot be compared with respect to potency in doses close to those producing the ceiling effect of the drug with the greater intrinsic activity.

Equity ratio The equity ratio will be worked out by comparing the equity to the balance sheet total. It describes the rate of the economical and financial stability of the company.

Equivalence In 1969, a federal Task Force on Prescription Drugs recommended that the words "generic equivalents" no longer be used in describing and comparing drug preparations. The Task Force recommended that an appropriate nomenclature should take into account three kinds of equivalence of drug preparations:

Erectile dysfunction Impairment of erectility, impotence

Erythrocyte The red blood cell consisting largely of hemoglobin and carrying nearly all the oxygen contained in the blood. Erythrocytes are biconcave discs that are manufactured in the bone marrow.

Erythromycin An antibiotic used to improve stomach emptying. It works by increasing the contractions that move food through the stomach. It may also be used to treat certain infections caused by bacteria, such as bronchitis; diphtheria; Legionnaires' disease; pertussis (whooping cough); pneumonia; rheumatic fever; venereal disease (VD); and ear, intestine, lung, urinary tract, and skin infections. Side effects include nausea, vomiting, and abdominal cramps.

Erythropoietin (Procrit) Indications: Treatment of HIV- or ZDV-associated anemia (HCT < 30) in patients with serum erythropoietin levels < 500 milliunits/ml.

Contraindications: Known hypersensitivity to mammalian cell derived products or human albumin, uncontrolled hypertension.

Dosage: 40,000 units SC once a week; response usually seen between 2 and 6 weeks.

Toxicity: Headache, nausea, arthralgia, hypertension, seizures.

Teratogenic in animals.

ESCA Electron spectroscopy for chemical analysis

Escrow Ancient legal term also applied to the deposit of source codedocumentation by the software developer with an independent thirdparty, called the Escrow Agent. The agent holds the source codedocumentation upon the terms and conditions set out in the Escrowagreement. These terms allow him to release it to specified users ofthe software in certain circumstances. These circums- tances are usuallythe bankruptcy, or liquidation of the software developer. More recentlyit is used to allow code documentation used in regulated industries tobe made available to reviewing regulators, without allowing generalaccess that would carry commercial risks.

ESOP (Executive Stock Option Program) In the executive stock option programs managers and employees are issued with share options enabling them to share in the company's success.

Essential amino Acids Amino acids that cannot be synthesized by human and other vertebrates and must be obtained from the diet.

Essential documents Documents with individually and collectively permit evaluation of the conduct of a study and the quality of the data produced. **Essential fatty acids** The group of polyunsaturated fatty acids of plants required in the human diet.

Estrogen Estrogen is a female hormone produced by the ovaries. Estrogen deficiency can lead to osteoporosis .

Etanercept A drug that is commonly used to treat arthritis. It is also being studied in the treatment of cancer, and as a treatment for loss of appetite and weight loss in cancer patients. It belongs to the family of drugs called tumor necrosis factor (TNF) antagonists.

Ethambutol (Myambutol) Indications: Treatment of MAC infection in combination with other agents; treatment of TB in combination with other agents.

Contraindications: Known hypersensitivity, history of optic neuritis.

Dosage: 25 mg/kg/day po for one to two months, followed by 15 mg/kg/day.

Toxicity: Optic neuritis, rash, gastrointestinal intolerance, hepatotoxicity.

teratogenic in animals.

Ethical pharmaceutical A controlled substance for the diagnosis or treatment of disease.

Ethylene oxide (ETO) A toxic compound used in gaseous form as a sterilizing agent, usually as a 10% mixture with carbon dioxide or 12% mixture with freon (referred as 12-88). Sterilization using ETO leaves residual chemicals such as ethylene chlorohydrin and ethylene glycol.

Etidronate A drug that belongs to the family of drugs called bisphosphonates. Bisphosphonates are used as treatment for hypercalcemia (abnormally high levels of calcium in the blood) and for cancer that has spread to the bone (bone metastases).

Etiologic agent A disease-causing organism or toxin.

Etoposide An anticancer drug that belongs to the families of drugs called podophyllotoxin derivatives and topoisomerase inhibitors.

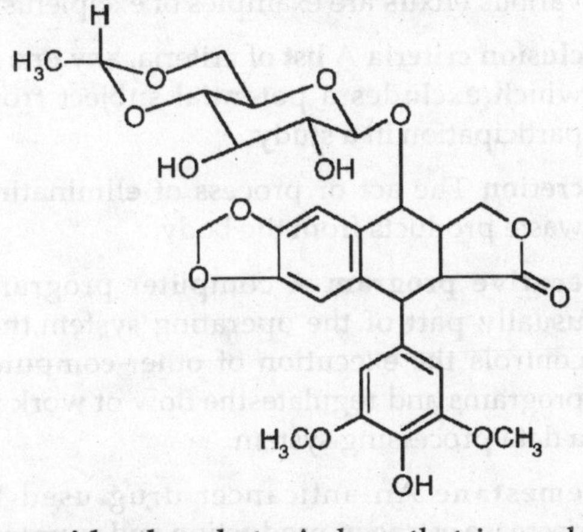

Etoposide phosphate A drug that is used to treat testicular and small cell lung cancers, and is being studied in the treatment of other cancers. It belongs to the families of drugs called podophyllotoxin derivatives and topoisomerase inhibitors.

Eugeroic A unique class of drugs that have stimulatory properties.

Eukaryote An organism that carries its genetic material physically constrained within a nuclear membrane, separate from the cytoplasm. All animal and plant cells except bacteria, viruses, and bluegreen algae are eukaryotic. Eukaryotes are five to ten times larger than prokaryotes in diameter.

European medicines agency (EMEA) Regulatory authority for drugs in Europe

Eutectic Of, pertaining to, or formed at the lowest possible temperature of solidification for any mixture of specified constituents. A common term used to describe metal alloys.

Evaporator Apparatus used in distillation to heat a liquid and create a phase change from the liquid to the vapor state. A steam boiler is an evaporator.

Excipient A more or less inert substance added in a prescription drug compound as a diluent or vehicle or to give form or consistency when the remedy is given in a pill form; simple syrup, aromatic powder, honey, and various elixirs are examples of excipients.

Exclusion criteria A list of criteria, any one of which excludes a potential subject from participation in a study.

Excretion The act or process of eliminating waste products from the body.

Executive program A computer program, usually part of the operating system,that controls the execution of other computer programs and regulatesthe flow of work in a data processing system.

Exemestane An anticancer drug used to decrease estrogen production and suppress the growth of estrogen-dependent tumors.

Exergonic reaction Referring to a chemical reaction that takes place with release of negative standard energy to its surroundings, a "downhill" reaction.

Exfiltration Leakage of air out of a room through cracks in doors and pass-throughs through material transfer openings, etc. due to a difference in room pressures.

Exhaustion Occurs when absorbents, such as activated carbon or ion exchange resins, have depleted their capacity by using up all active sites. Ion exchange resins may be regenerated to reverse the process.

Exisulind A drug that is being studied in the treatment and prevention of cancer. It has been shown to cause apoptosis (cell death) in cancerous and precancerous cells by acting through a group of cellular enzymes called cGMP phosphodiesterases.

Exocytosis Vesicular release of transmitter ie. NE storage vesicle migrates to and fuses with the plasma membrane to release NE (and other compounds within the vesicle ie. DBH) into the synaptic cleft. Non-exocytotic release includes the displacement of NE by amphetamine or tyramine, which can then leak across the plasma membrane in the synaptic cleft.

Exogenous DNA DNA originating outside an organism.

Exon The proteincoding DNA sequence of an eukaryotic gene.

Exonuclease An enzyme that cleaves nucleotides sequentially from free ends of a linear nucleic acid substrate.

Exotic organism A biological agent where either the corresponding disease does not exist in a given country or geographical area, or where the disease is the subject of prophylactic measures or an eradication program undertaken in the given country or geographical area.

Exotoxins Proteins produced by bacteria that are able to diffuse into a medium through the bacterial cell membrane and cell wall. They are generally more potent and specific in their actions than endotoxins.

Expectorans Drugs facilitating expectoration of accumulated mucus produced in the respiratory tract (mainly in bronchi).

Expectorant A medication that helps bring up mucus and other material from the lungs, bronchi, and trachea. An example of as expectorant is guaifenesin which promotes drainage of mucus from the lungs by thinning the mucus and also lubricates the irritated respiratory tract. Sometimes the term "expectorant" is incorrectly extended to any cough medicine. From the Latin expectorare, to expel from the chest, from ex-, out of + pectus, chest.

Experimental procedure means:

a. any medical procedure, equipment, treatment or course of treatment, or drug or medicine that is under investigation and the use of which is limited to research;

b. techniques that are restricted to use at centers which are capable of carrying out disciplined clinical efforts and scientific studies;

c. procedures which are not proven in an objective way to have therapeutic value or benefit; and

d. any procedure or treatment whose effectiveness is medically questionable.

Expiration ("expiration date") Identifies the shelf life, this number is also included in the internal packaging (blister, vial....), after a specified date the preparation must not be used. Usually it is indicated as a month and year (for example 06/2004).

Expiration date A date, determined by stability tests, after which the product may not meet the USP requirements. Expiration dates are generally limited to no more than 3 years after production, but longer stability periods are allowed for some very stable materials such as sulfur or sodium chloride.

Explanatory trial Term used to describe a clinical study designed to demonstrate the efficacy of a product.

Explanatory trials Explanatory questions ask whether a carefully selected group of patients can benefit from a treatment and, if so, by what biological mechanism. Explanatory trials define a population of roughly equivalent risk by imposing strict eligibility criteria, and test a precise hypothesis about the treatment's biological mode of action. The treatment's effect is assessed through endpoints based on the biological mode of action, so follow-up is generally short and the endpoints are usually laboratory measurements, not clinical outcomes. The protocol gives rigid rules for patient management and study drug discontinuation, and any deviation from the protocol must be carefully described, because it may affect the interpretation of the trial.

Explosion resistance A type of construction used to house solvents in sufficiently large quantities, to qualify the space electrically as an explosion potential area. Typically the internal walls, ceiling, and floor are constructed of material strong enough to withstand a specified intensity of explosion, and at least one wall has explosion relief devices that direct the explosion outwardly. In a single story arrangement, or if the explosion resistant area is on the top floor, the roof may also have devices that can be used to relieve the explosion.

Explosive A chemical that causes a sudden, almost instantaneous release of pressure, gas and heat when subjected to sudden shock, pressure, or high temperatures, or a material or chemical, other than a blasting agent, that is commonly used or intended for the purpose of producing an explosive effect.

Exposed or open process The drug substance is exposed to the room environment during processing.

Express To translate the genetic information stored in the DNA into protein.

Expression The process by which the information in a gene is used to create proteins.

Expression pharmacogenomics Applies genome/ proteome scale differential expression technologies to both in vivo and in vitro models of drug response to identify candidate markers correlative with and predictive of drug toxicity and efficacy. It is anticipated to streamline drug development by triaging towards lead compounds and clinical candidates that maximize efficacy while minimizing safety risks.

Expression profiling A method for comparing genes that are expressed (present and active) in healthy tissue with those expressed in diseased tissue. It can help to identify proteins associated with the disease, narrowing the search for appropriate drug targets.

Expression system A host organism combined with a genetic vector (such as virus or circular DNA molecule called a plasmid) that is loaded with a gene of interest. The expression system provides the genetic context in which a gene will function in the cell - that is, the gene will be expressed as a protein.

External consistency The consistency of a procedure between sets of data.

External quality audit A systematic and independent examination todetermine whether quality activities and related results comply to adocumented Quality System and whether this documented Quality System isimplemented effectively and is suitable to achieve the contractualrequirements placed by the customer.

Extractables Undesirable foreign substances that are leached or dissolved by water or process streams from the materials of construction used in filters, storage vessels, distribution piping, and other wetted surfaces.

Extrinsic asthma Extrinsic asthma is asthma that is triggered by an allergic reaction, usually something that is inhaled.

Ex-vivo A Latin term meaning, 'Outside of the living body'.

F

F The fraction of a dose which is absorbed and enters the systemic circulation following administration of a drug by any route other than the intravenous route; the availability of drug to tissues of the body, generally. When the total clearance and the dose of drug administered are known, F can be determined from the relationship: (AUC x CIT)/D = F. When identical doses of a drug have been given by the intravenous and by some other route (x), and the AUCs have been determined, the bioavailability of the drug after administration by route X can be determined: F=AUCx/AUCiv. The amount of free drug recovered in the urine (AU) after administration of identical doses given intravenously and by route X can also be used to determine bioavailability: F=AU,x/AU,iv

Face velocity The velocity obtained by dividing the air quantity by the component face area (NEBB).

Facility flexibility A qualitative measure of the number of different products that can be produced in a facility or area of a facility.

Facility user The end user of a facility, often called the Owner, represented by operating, maintenance, and quality control personnel.

Factor IX (Hemophilia factor) In the clotting of blood, also known as Christmas factor (Biggs and Macfarlane). Deficiency of factor IX causes hemophilia B or Christmas disease that resembles hemophilia A, and is an inherited defect that leads to a severe hemorrhagic disorder. Factor IX is required for the formation of intrinsic blood thromboplastin and affects the amount formed (rather than the rate).

After Gabriel Daniel Fahrenheit (1686-1736). Of or pertaining to a temperature scale that registers the freezing point of water as 32°F. and the boiling point as 212°F. under standard atmospheric pressure (29.921 inches of mercury). Fahrenheit temperatures are related to Centigrade temperatures by the equation F = 1.8C + 32 .

Factor VIII (Hemophilia factor) Also known as antihemophilic factor or AHF (Brinkhous) in the clotting of blood, Factor VIII is a labile protein of the blood-clotting system that assists in the conversion of Factor IX into plasma factor X (Stuart factor). Deficiency of factor VIII is associated with classic hemophilia A, a hereditary, sex-linked, hemorrhagic tendency that occurs almost exclusively in men; clotting time is prolonged, less thromboplastin is formed, and the conversion of prothrombin is diminished.

Famciclovir (Famvir) Indications: Treatment and prophylaxis of HSV and VZV infections.

Contraindications: Known hypersensitivity.

Dosage: HSV treatment: 125 mg po bid x 5-7 days; secondary prophylaxis: 125-250 mg po bid.

VZV treatment: 500 mg po tid x 7 days. Secondary prophylaxis generally is not indicated.

Toxicity: Headache, nausea.

Family qualifying year Refers to eligibility for coverage under the Senior Citizen or Early Retiree Program. A Qualifying year is a year during which an individual had covered earnings at least equal to the greater of $2,000 or the amount required as of the last day of such Base Year to qualify for a year of eligibility under the AFTRA Family Health Plan.

FAS Financial Accounting Standard

Faslodex A drug that blocks estrogen activity in the body and is used in the treatment of estrogen-dependent tumors such as breast cancer. It belongs to the family of drugs called antiestrogens.

Fed batch fermentation The most common operating mode for rDNA fermentation. After an initial partial charge of media to the fermenter and seed transfer, sterile media is added at measured rates during the balance of the fermentation cycle. Cell mass and broth are withdrawn only at the end of the cycle.

Fee for service The traditional method for financing healthcare in which a provider is paid for each service rendered. Fee-for-service is the system of payment used by conventional indemnity health plans.

Feedback loop A central concept in industrial controls in which the value of a process variable is compared with the desired value (setpoint), and any discrepancy (error) is converted into a modified output signal.

Feedwater The water entering a treatment process.

Fermentation The process of growing microorganisms within an enclosed tank (fermenter) under controlled conditions of aeration, agitation, temperature, and pH. The different types organisms used as a basis for fermentation are: 1. Bacteria (E. coli)

2. Yeasts

3. Molds

4. Chinese Hamster Ovary (CHO) cells

5. Kidney cells

6. Vaccines to viruses.

Fermenter A tank or vessel used for carrying out fermentation. There are various choices of fermenters, depending on whether cells are suspended in the medium or attached to some type of support: 1. In suspension reactors

2. Attached growth reactors

3. Stirred-tank reactors

4. Airlift fermenters

5. Packed bed reactors

6. Two-chamber reactors

7. Hollow-fiber reactors.

Ferumoxtran 10 A substance that is being studied as a way of improving magnetic resonance imaging (MRI) in diagnosing cancer and finding lymph nodes to which cancer has spread. Ferumoxtran-10 is made of nanoparticles (ultrasmall pieces) of iron oxide coated with dextran (a type of sugar). It is injected into the blood of the patient and the particles collect in lymph nodes, liver, spleen, or brain tissue where they can be seen using MRI. Ferumoxtran-10 later breaks down and passes from the body in urine.

Ferumoxytol A nanoparticle form of iron made in the laboratory that is being studied for use in iron replacement therapy, and as a contrast agent for magnetic resonance imaging. Contrast agents are substances that are injected into the body and taken up by certain tissues, making the tissues easier to see in imaging scans.

Fetal calf serum The liquid portion remaining after natural coagulation of blood drawn from the heart of an unborn calf. Because of the absence of gamma globulin, fetal calf serum is a good tissue culture serum.

Fever Also known as pyrexia, a human body temperature above the normal 98.6°F (37°C).

Fiber Any particulate contaminant having an aspect (length to width) ratio of 10 or more. ISO 14644-1.

Fibrin A plasma protein that, in its aggregated state, is the major component of a blood clot. It is produced from fibrinogen, a soluble precursor, by the action of the proteolytic enzyme, thrombin.

Fibrinogen In the clotting of blood it is known as Factor I. The plasma protein that becomes converted to a clot at the end of the coagulation process. Present in plasma; absent in serum.

Fibrinolytics Drugs used to dissolve thrombus.

File transfer protocol (FTP) A standard protocol for exchanging files between computers on the Internet. Used to transfer Web page files to the computer that acts as a server for everyone on the Internet. Also commonly used to download programs and other files to your computer from other servers. FTP is usually one of the programs that come with TCP/IP.

Filgrastim SD/01 A drug used to increase numbers of white blood cells in patients who are receiving chemotherapy. It belongs to the family of drugs called colony-stimulating factors. Also called pegfilgrastim and Neulasta.

Fill and finish (parenteral drugs) Preparation of parenteral drugs, either LVPs or SVPs, demands the highest level of contamination control, because the human body's normal defenses against infection are bypassed when parenteral medications are introduced either intramuscularly (I.M.) or intravenously (I.V.) directly into the body. The processing of raw materials into finished dosage forms must comply at all times with cGMPs and must be able to support process validation. Mechanical design should include HVAC Classifications considered essential to attain global regulatory acceptance. The desire for increased levels of sterility assurance has led the department of health to promote the use of terminal sterilization for aseptically filled products. The department of health has stated that terminal sterilization processing is the method of choice unless the manufacturer can show that it is detrimental to the product. Terminal sterilization may be accomplished using autoclaves that apply overpressure to balance the pressures that are developed across the inside and outside of the containers. Because of product sensitivities, biologics, and blood products are not appropriate applications for terminal sterilization.

Filters Filtering centrifuges accommodate a range of liquid-solid separations. The two batch types, basket and peeler centrifuges, can separate almost any liquid-solid slurry. For continuous operation, there are pusher and conical centrifuges. a) Pusher - with a horizontal axis, the pusher centrifuge operates at a constant fixed speed. It has a perforated bowl, generally with a bar-type screen. One end of the bowl is open while the opposite end is closed with a reciprocating diaphragm, or disc, which rotates with the bowl. b) Conical - the standard conical centrifuge consists of a cone with a small closed end and a large open end to which is attached a coarsely woven drainage screen, topped with a filter screen or perforated plate. A compartmentalized casing surrounds the bowl. There are two variations of the basic conical centrifuge: the tilting conical centrifuge and the conveyor conical type.

Filtration Removal of suspended matter from a fluid by passing it through a porous matrix that prevents particles from getting through, usually by entrapment on or in the filter matrix.

Final bulk product The final drug product after chemical or biological processing and purification, ready for concentration, drying, and filling into containers prior to dispensing and final filling.

Final report Complete, comprehensive description of a completed trial that describes the experimental materials and statistical design. It also presents and evaluates the trial results and statistical analyses.

Finished product A medicinal product that has undergone all stages of production, including packaging in its final container.

Firmware A combination of hardware and software with the programming written directly into read-only memory (ROM).

First in humans study The first Phase 1 study in which the test product is administered to human beings.

First order kinetics According to the law of mass action, the velocity of a chemical reaction is proportional to the product of the active masses (concentrations) of the reactants. In a monomolecular reaction, i.e., one in which only a single molecular species reacts, the velocity of the reaction is proportional to the concentration of the unreacted substance (C). The change in concentration (dC) over a time interval (dT) is the velocity of the reaction (dC/dT) and is proportional to C. For infinitely small changes of concentration over infinitely small periods of time, the reaction velocity can be written in the form of a differential equation: $-dC/dt=kC$. Here, dC/dt is the reaction velocity, C is concentration, and k is the constant of proportionality, or monomolecular velocity constant, which uniquely characterizes the reaction. The minus sign indicates that the velocity decreases with the passage of time, as the concentration of unreacted substance decreases; a plot of C against time would yield a curve of progressively decreasing slope.

The mechanisms, the kinetics, described by the differential equation are termed first order kinetics because - although the exponent is not written - concentration (C) is raised to only the first power (C^1).

The differential equation above may be integrated and rearranged to yield: $\ln (C/C_0)= kt$, where ln indicates use of the natural logarithm, to the base e; C_0 is the concentration of unreacted substance at the beginning of an observation period; t is the duration of the observation period; and k is the familiar proportionality or velocity constant. The units of k are independent of the units in which C is expressed; indeed, since a logarithm is dimensionless, and t has the dimension of time, the integrated equation balances, dimensionally, because k has the dimension of reciprocal time, t^{-1}. Notice that for observation periods of equal length, the ratio C/C_0 is always the same; after equal intervals, the final concentration is a constant fraction of the starting concentration, or, in equal time intervals, constant fractions of the starting concentration are lost, even though absolute decreases in concentration become progressively less as time passes and C becomes smaller and smaller.

Let $t_{1/2}$ represent the length of time required for C_0 to be halved, so that $C=0.5\ C_0$. Then, substituting in the integrated equation above, $\ln 0.5 = -kt_{1/2}$, or, since -0.693 is the natural logarithm of 0.5: $-0.693 = kt_{1/2}$. Multiplying both sides of the equation by -1 yields $0.693 = kt_{1/2}$ or $0.693/k = t_{1/2}$: the natural logarithm of 2 (0.693) divided by the monomolecular velocity constant yields the time required for the concentration to be halved, the " half-life " or "half-time" of the reaction.

Since ln (C/C0) may be rewritten (lnC - lnC0), the integrated equation may be rewritten and given the form of a linear equation: ln C = ln C0 - kt. The existence of a monomolecular reaction can be established by plotting ln C, for unreacted material, against t and finding the relationship to be linear; the slope of the line is the original proportionality or velocity constant, and the intercept of the line with the ordinate is the natural logarithm of the original concentration of unreacted material. Since natural logarithms have a fixed relationship to common logarithms, i.e., logarithms to the base 10 (lnX =2.303 log X), one may write: 2.303 log C =2.303 log C - kt. When common logarithms of C are plotted against t, a first order reaction yields a straight line with a slope of k/2.303, and an intercept that is the common logarithm of C0.

When two molecular species react with each other (a bimolecular reaction), but one of the substances is present in a concentration greatly in excess of the concentration of the other and/or does not change in concentration during the reaction, the velocity of the reaction at any time is really determined only by the concentration of the other substance. Such a pseudo-monomolecular reaction, because the velocity is determined by the concentration of only one of the two reactants, still follows first order kinetics.

Following administration of a drug, it may be eliminated from the body only after "reacting " with tissue components which are present in high concentrations and which are not used up to any degree during the drug's stay in the body. Such eliminative processes mimic pseudo-monomolecular reactions, and the drug is eliminated from the body according to first order kinetics,. The apparent velocity constant determined for such a process is called the elimination rate constant, kel, and the elimination half-life can be computed as 0.693/kel.

First pass effect All drugs that are absorbed from the intestine enter the hepatic portal vein and pass through the liver before they are distributed systemically. Some drugs (ie. propranolol) have a high degree of removal from the circulation on their first passage through the liver.

First-line treatment The initial treatment of a disease .

FISH (Fluorescent in situ hybridization) A physical mapping approach that uses fluorescein tags to detect hybridization of probes with metaphase chromosomes and with the less condensed somatic interface chromatin.

Fissile material A radioisotope that could undergo a nuclear fission reaction and is usually found at reactor sites or as part of a nuclear weapon.

Flaggelae Thin, helical filaments attached to the surface of bacterial and eukaryotic (e.g. sperm, protozoa) cells. They are motile structures containing microtubules (composed of proteins called tubulin) that enable cells possessing them to move.

Flagyl A drug that is used to treat infection and is being studied in the treatment of cancer. It belongs to the families of drugs called antibacterials, antiprotozoals, and anthelmintics. Also called metronidazole.

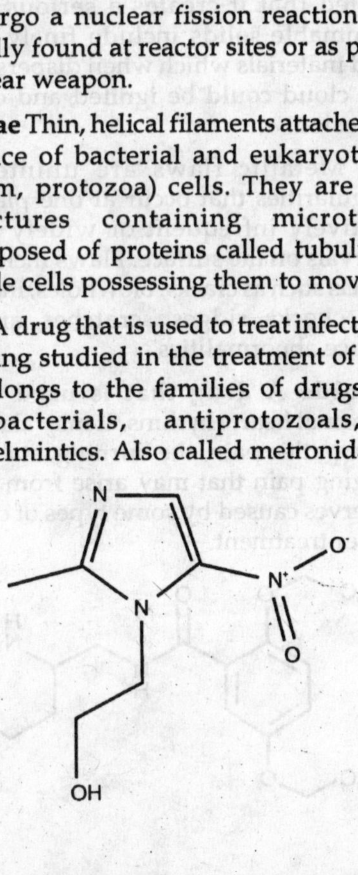

Flammable liquid A liquid having a closed cup flash point below 100°F (37.8°C). Flammable liquids do not include compressed gases or cryogenic fluids. Flammable liquids are subdivided as follows: 1. Class I-A - Liquids having a closed cup flash point below 73°F (22.8°C) and having a boiling point below 100°F (37.8°C).

2. Class I-B - liquids having a closed cup flash point below 73°F (22.8°C) and having a boiling point at or above 100°F (37.8°C).

3. Class I-C - liquids having a closed cup flash point at or above 73°F (22.8°C) and below 100°F (37.8°C).

Flammable solid A solid substance, other than one which is defined as a blasting agent or explosive, that is liable to cause fire through friction or as a result of retained heat from manufacture, which has an ignition temperature below 212°F (100°C), or which burns so vigorously or persistently when ignited that it creates a serious hazard. Flammable solids include finely divided solid materials which when dispersed in air as a cloud could be ignited and cause an explosion.

Flaws Metallic flaws are unintentional irregularities that occur at one place or at relatively infrequent or widely varying intervals on the surface. Flaws include such defects such as cracks, blowholes, inclusions, pits, checks, ridges, scratches, and other surface abnormalities.

Flecainide A drug that is used to treat abnormal heart rhythms. It may also relieve neuropathic pain, the burning, stabbing, or stinging pain that may arise from damage to nerves caused by some types of cancer or cancer treatment.

F_3C, O, O, H, N, N, H, F_3C, O

FLIPR Fluorometric Laser Imaging Plate Reader system.

Floc Mass having a fluffy or wooly appearance.

Flocculation A technique for liquid/solids separation. Cationic or anionic polyelectrolytes (e.g. polyacrylamides) are added to highly colloidal water causing coagulation and subsequent settling. The phenomena could be charge neutralization or a bridging effect between separate particles.

Flow chart (ANSI/IEEE) A graphical representation of the definition,analysis or solution of a problem in which symbols are used torepresent operations, data, flow, and equipment.

Flow cytometry Analysis of biological material by detection of light-absorbing or fluorescing properties of cells or subcellular fractions (i.e., chromosomes) passing in a narrow stream through a laser beam. An absorbance or fluorescence profile of the sample is produced. Automated sorting devices, used to fractionate samples, sort successive droplets of the analyzed stream into different fractions depending on the fluorescence emitted by each droplet.

Flow decay Measuring the decline in flow rate through a filter to establish a Silt Index for the water being filtered. The Silt Index is a measure of suspended solids and their ability to clog the filter.

Flow restrictor A flow-limiting orifice used to control flow rate or pressure drop in a liquid stream.

Fluconazole (Diflucan) Indications: Treatment and secondary prophylaxis of mucosal candidiasis; secondary prophylaxis of cryptococcal infection.

Contraindications: Known hypersensitivity.

Dosage: Treatment of oral candidiasis: 50-100 mg po qd x 7-14 days; candida esophagitis: 200 mg po qd x 14-21 days;

vaginal candidiasis: 150 mg po x one. Secondary prophylaxis of mucosal candidiasis: 50-200 mg po qd. There are many potential drug interactions, some of which require dosage modification

Cryptococcal infection maintenance therapy (secondary prophylaxis): 200 mg po qd. Most experts recommend initial treatment of cryptococcal infection with amphotericin B; if using fluconazole, dose 400 mg po qd x 8 weeks.

Toxicity: Nausea, headache, hepatotoxicity.

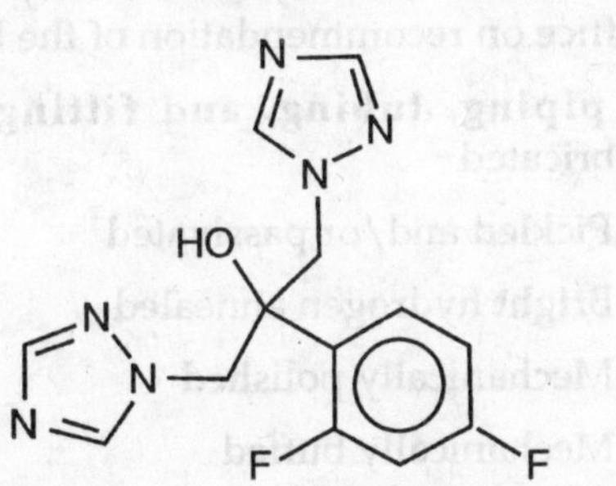

Fluid service (piping) As defined in ASME B31.3, fluid service is a general term concerning the application of a piping system, considering the combination of fluid properties, operating conditions, and other factors, which establish the basis for design of the piping system. 1. Category D Fluid Service: A fluid service in which all the following apply: (a) the fluid handled is nonflammable, nontoxic, and not damaging to human tissues . (b) The design gage pressure does not exceed 1035 kPA (150 psi). (c) The design temperature is from -29°C (-20°F) through 186°C (366°F).

2. Category M Fluid Service: A fluid service in which the potential for personnel exposure is judged to be significant and in which a single exposure to a very small quantity of a toxic fluid, caused by leakage can produce serious irreversible harm to persons upon breathing or bodily contact, even when prompt restorative measures are taken.

3. High Pressure Fluid Service: A fluid service for which the owner specifies the use of (High Pressure Piping) for piping design and construction.

4. Normal Fluid Service: A fluid service pertaining to most piping covered by ASME B31.3, i.e., not subject to the rules for Category D, Category M, or High Pressure Fluid Service, and not subject to severe cyclic conditions.

Damaging to human tissues for the purpose of the Code, describes a fluid service in which exposure to the fluid, caused by leakage under expected operating conditions, can harm skin, eyes, or exposed mucous membranes so that irreversible damage may result unless prompt restorative measures are taken. These measures may include, flushing with water, administration of antidotes, or medication.

Fluidized bed A container holding powder coating material which is aerated from below so as to form an air-supported expanded cloud of such material through which the preheated object to be coated is immersed and transported.

Fluorescein An orange-red compound, $C_{2}0H_{12}O_{5}$, which exhibits intense fluorescence in alkaline solution.

Fluorescence The relatively slow (but not nearly as slow as phosphorescence) emission of longer-wavelength light following the absorption of shorter-wavelength radiation. Fluorescence is common in aromatic compounds with several rings joined together or in any compound with alternating carbon-carbon double bonds. Fluorescence can be a highly sensitive mode of detection in certain assays and is suitable for automation, but can be susceptible to interference due to cells and chemicals other than the target.

Fluorinated plastics Fluorinated plastics are thermoplastic paraffinic polymers where the hydrogen has been replaced by fluorine, and in some cases, chlorine. These materials are some of the more popular in the CPI because of good chemical resistance to a wide variety of aggressive chemicals, and relatively high heat resistance of 400°F to 500°F. They include FEP, PTFE, PFA, PCTFE, ETFE, PVDF, and PVF.

Fluorine F 18 EF5 A substance that is being studied in positron emission tomography (PET) imaging to detect tumor hypoxia (a low level of oxygen in the tumor).This may help predict how the tumor will respond to treatment. It belongs to the family of drugs called radiopharmaceuticals. Also called 18F-EF5.

Fluoropyrimidine One of a group of substances used to treat cancer. Fluoropyrimidines belong to the family of drugs called antimetabolites. Examples are capecitabine, floxuridine, and fluorouracil (5-FU).

Fluorouracil A much-used anticancer drug that belongs to the family of drugs called antimetabolites .

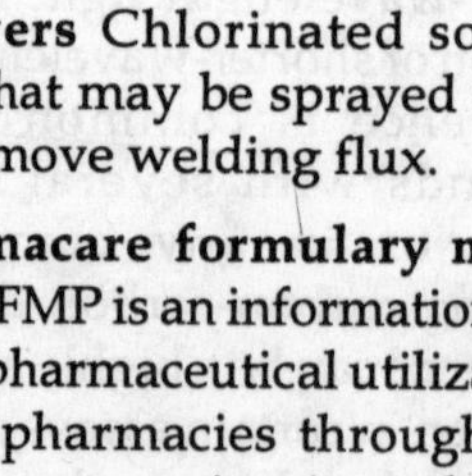

Flux removers Chlorinated solvents with alcohols that may be sprayed from aerosol cans to remove welding flux.

FMP (pharmacare formulary management program) FMP is an information system that manages pharmaceutical utilization at retail and mail pharmacies through facilitating clinical communications between the patient, physician, and pharmacist.

Food and drug administration(USA) An agency of the Department of Health, and Human Services which is responsible for ensuring compliance with the amended federal Food, Drug and Cosmetic Act. This agency must pass judgment on the safety of drugs, the labels affixed to drug packages, and all printed material accompanying a packaged drug before that drug may be introduced to interstate commerce. The law empowers the F.D.A. to pass on the efficacy of a new drug or pharmaceutical preparation and gives the agency ultimate jurisdiction over the clinical testing of a drug before it is approved for general sale and use. Prosecution of violation of the F.D. and C. Act is carried out by the Attorney General's Office on recommendation of the F.D.A.

For piping, tubing, and fittings: 1. As fabricated

2. Pickled and/or passivated

3. Bright hydrogen annealed

4. Mechanically polished

5. Mechanically buffed

6. Chemically polished

7. Electropolished.

For sheet, strip, and plate: 1. As fabricated. Without any specific surface treatments.

2. Rolled Finish. Manufactured by either hot or cold rolled process.

3. No. 1. A dull, hot rolled finish, annealed and pickled.

4. No. 2D. A dull, cold rolled finish, annealed and pickled.

5. No. 2B. A bright, cold rolled finish, annealed and pickled.

6. No. 4. A general purpose polished finish widely used for architectural panels, trim, and sanitary equipment. Following initial grinding with coarse abrasives, the surface is finally finished with lubricated 150 grit abrasive belts.

7. No. 4S. Processed as No. 4 except the final surface is polished to a smother finish. The purchaser must specify this alternative

finish; the specification must state a No. 4 finish, using a 240 or 320 grit mechanical polish, whose particular surface roughness must meet the specified Ra value.

8. No. 6. A dull finish having a lower reflectivity than No. 4. It is produced by a tampico brushing in a medium of abrasive and oil and is used primarily for architectural applications.

9. No. 7. A finish with a high degree of reflectivity, produced by buffing to a finely ground surface without removing the grit lines.

10. No. 8. The most reflective finish, obtained by polishing with successively finer abrasives and buffing extensively with very fine buffing rouges. This finish is most widely used for press plates, mirrors, etc.

For wrought and cast forgings: 1. As fabricated or machined

2. Mechanically ground, polished, or buffed

3. Abrasive blast cleaned, using one of the following methods: a. Sand blast b. Shot blast c. Glass blast d. Wet blast

4. Slurry polished

5. Roll deburred

6. Chemically cleaned a. Acid washed (pickled and passivated) b. Solvent washed

7. Electropolished.

Formaldehyde A colorless, highly irritating, pungent compound used in the pharmaceutical and cosmetic industries as an antimicrobial agent.

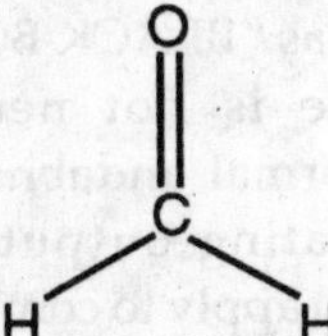

Formulary A formulary is a list of prescription drugs that may be preferred under a pharmacy benefits plan. Drugs included on the formulary may have a lower co-pay than drugs that are not included on the list. Formularies typically include both brand-name and generic drugs that have been approved by the U.S. Food and Drug Administration.

Formulary excluded drugs These are the medications not covered for members in closed formulary benefits plan unless a medical exception is obtained. Formulary-excluded drugs are covered for members in open formulary benefits plans. Depending on their plan, some members pay a higher copayment for these drugs.

Formulary exclusion list This is a list of prescription drugs that a pharmacy benefits plan does not cover if a member belongs to a closed-formulary prescription plan. If it is medically necessary for a member enrolled in a closed-formulary plan to use a drug on the Formulary Exclusion List, the member's physician must contact the Pharmacy Management Precertification Unit to request coverage as a medical exception. Also, there often are alternatives to drugs on the formulary exclusion list that are covered.

Formulation A combination of an active drug and pharmacologically inactive ingredients used to achieve adequate bioavailability.

Forward flow test An objective and quantitative method of determining filter integrity. A test in which the filter is wetted and a predetermined constant air pressure is applied. A measurement of pure diffusional airflow through the wetted membrane is made. If the diffusional airflow across the membrane is below the maximum allowable value given, then the filter is acceptable.

Foscarnet (Foscavir) Indications: Treatment of CMV infection, including ganciclovir-resistant strains.

Contraindications: Known hypersensitivity, significant renal dysfunction.

Dosage: Initial therapy: 60 mg/kg IV q8h or 90 mg/kg IV q12h x 14 days.

Maintenance therapy (secondary prophylaxis): 90-120 mg/kg IV qd.

Toxicity: Nephrotoxicity, hypocalcemia, hypophosphatemia, hypokalemia, headache, fatigue, nausea, anemia, seizures.

Fouling Occurs when gelatinous coatings, colloidal masses, or dense bacterial growth form a compacted crust on membrane or filter surfaces which blocks further flow.

Frank starling relationship One of the mechanisms by which the heart can increase cardiac output. The heart muscle intrinsically increases its strength of contraction when its fibers are stretched. A plot of tension generated as a function of fiber length (EDV) is known as a Frank-Starling curve. Myocardial fiber stretch is increased by an increase in venous return (preload).

Free radical A highly chemically reactive atom, molecule or molecular fragment with a free or unpaired electron. Free radicals are produced in many different ways such as, normal metabolic processes, ultraviolet radiation from the sun, nuclear radiation and the breakdown in the body of spoiled fats. Free radicals have been implicated in aging, cancer, cardiovascular disease and other kinds of damage to the body, .

Free radical scavenger The cascade of chemical reactions that occurs when a free radical reacts with another molecule in order to gain an electron. The molecule that loses an electron to the free radical then becomes a free radical, repeating the process until the energy of the free radical is spent, or the reaction is stopped by an antioxidant. In biological systems, this cascade can damage important molecules like DNA.

Frozen software This is software which is under configuration controland may not be altered without change control.

FTE Full Time Equivalent.

Fulvestrant A drug that blocks estrogen activity in the body and is used in the treatment of estrogen-dependent tumors such as breast cancer. It belongs to the family of drugs called antiestrogens.

Fume hoods Units that collect fumes from chemicals, solvents, acids, and other hazardous materials. Hoods may include HEPA filters if powders are present, or carbon filters to filter fumes from the work surface and return cleaned air to the room. Most fume hoods are 100% exhausted to outdoors. A glass, Plexiglas or acrylic front panel may be included for worker safety.

Functional Description A written description of what a system is to do with sequence of operation relating activities to Critical Parameters (Why the system does what it does for GMP reasons). A non-GMP system should also have a functional specification to aid designers and software development.

Functional gene tests Biochemical assays for a specific protein, which indicates that a specific gene is not merely present but active.

Functional genomics The analysis of genetic information and its biological function. An important step in the identification of targets.

Functional requirement (ANSI/IEEE) A requirement that specifies afunction that a system or system component must be capable ofperforming.

Functional testing (Bluhm, Myers, Hetzel) Also known as "BLACK BOX" testing, since source code is not needed. Involves inputting normal andabnormal test cases; then, evaluating outputs against those expected.Can apply to computer software or to a total system.

Functionality Suitability for the intended purpose.

Fungi Plural of fungus. Low forms of plant life unable to form protein and carbohydrates (heterotrophs) that are widespread in nature. Fungal cells are larger than bacterial cells, and their typical internal structures, such as nucleus and vacuoles, can be seen easily with a light microscope. On the basis of their mode of sexual reproduction, fungi are grouped in four classes: Phycomycetes, Ascomycetes, Deuteromycetes (Fungi Imperfectii), and Basidiomycetes. Two major groups of fungi are the yeasts and molds.

Fungicide An agent that destroys fungi.

Fusion The melting together of filler metal and base metal, or of base metal only, that results in coalescence.

Fusion welding Welding in which the base material is fused together without the addition of filler material to the weld.

G

G If followed by a number, a chromatographic phase; e. g., G4 is diethylene glycol succinate polyester. Defined in USP/NF.

G protein One of a group of proteins involved in signal transduction - the intercellular or intracellular transfer of activation or inhibition signals through a so- called signaling pathway. within cells.

GABA (gamma aminobutyric acid) An amino acid which acts as an inhibitory neurotransmitter.

Gabapentin A substance that is being studied as a treatment for relieving hot flashes in women with breast cancer. It belongs to the family of drugs called anticonvulsants.

Gadolinium texaphyrin A substance that is being studied in the treatment of cancer. It may make tumor cells more sensitive to radiation therapy, improve tumor images using magnetic resonance imaging (MRI), and kill cancer cells. It belongs to the family of drugs called metalloporphyrin complexes. Also called motexafin gadolinium.

Gamete Mature male or female reproductive cell (sperm or ovum) with a haploid set of chromosomes (23 for humans).

Gamma globulin A blood protein that plays a major role in the process of immunity. Sometimes the term "gamma globulin" refers to a whole group of blood proteins that are known as antibodies or immunoglobulins (Ig). Most often, however, it applies to a particular immunoglobulin, designated as IgG, believed to be the most abundant type of antibody in the body.

Ganciclovir (Cytovene) Indications: Treatment and prophylaxis of CMV infection.

Contraindications: Known hypersensitivity, neutropenia, thrombocytopenia.

Dosage: Initial therapy: 5 mg/kg IV q12h x 14-21 days.

Maintenance therapy (secondary prophylaxis): 5 mg/kg IV qd or oral ganciclovir

1 gm po tid.

Also available as vitreal implant requiring ophthalmologic surgery.

Toxicity: Neutropenia, thrombocytopenia, anemia, nausea, abdominal pain, headache, confusion.

teratogenic in animals.

Ganciclovir An antiviral agent used to prevent or treat cytomegalovirus infections that may occur when the body's immune system is suppressed. In gene therapy, ganciclovir is used with an altered herpes simplex virus-1 gene to kill advanced melanoma cells and brain tumor cells.

Gas chromatography (GC) A process by which the components of a mix are separated from one another by volatilizing the sample into a carrier gas stream and passing the gas through a column containing a substance that selectively retains (adsorbs) and releases the volatile constituents.

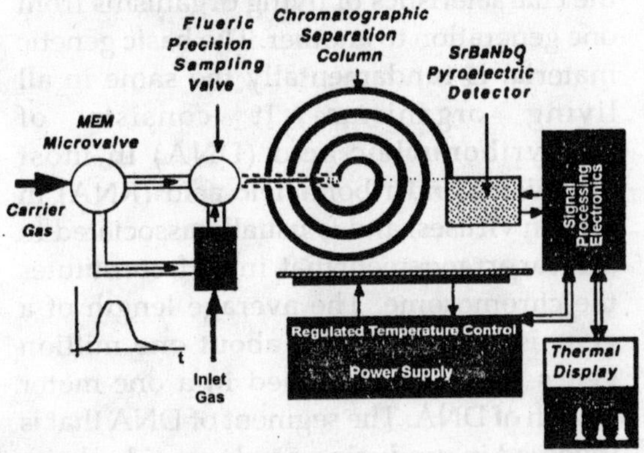

Fig.Gas chromatography

Gas metal arc welding (GMAW) An arc welding process that produces coalescence of metals by heating them with an arc between a continuous filler metal (consumable) electrode and the work. Shielding is obtained entirely from an externally supplied gas or gas mixture. Some variations of this process are called MIG (Metal Inert Gas) Or CO_2 welding, nonpreferred terms.

Gas room A separately ventilated, fully enclosed room in which only toxic and highly toxic compressed gases and associated equipment and supplies are stored or used.

Gas tungsten arc welding (GTAW) An arc welding process that produces coalescence of metals by heating them with an arc between a tungsten (nonconsumable) electrode and the work. Shielding is obtained from a gas or gas mixture. Pressure may or may not be used and filler material may or may not be used. (This process is sometimes called TIG (Tungsten Inert Gas) welding, a nonpreferred term).

Gastric neurostimulator Also called a "pacemaker," it is designed to assist people with gastroparesis. The pacemaker is a battery-operated, electronic device that is surgically implanted. It emits mild electrical pulses that stimulate stomach contractions so food is digested and moved from the stomach into the intestines. The electrical stimulation also helps control nausea and vomiting associated with gastroparesis.

Gastro intestinal Affecting the gastro (stomach) intestinal tract

Gastroesophageal reflux disease (GERD) The return of stomach contents back up into the esophagus, which frequently causes discomfort, indigestion, and/or heartburn because of irritation of the esophagus by stomach acids. GERD can lead to scarring and stricture of the esophagus, requiring stretching (dilating) of the esophagus.

Gastrointestinal (GI) tract Includes the oral cavity and proceeds to the esophagus, stomach, small intestine, large intestine, rectum and anus.

Gastroparesis A condition in which the stomach takes too long to empty its contents (due to abnormal gastric motility), often seen as a complication of diabetes. Symptoms include bloating, nausea, vomiting and constipation. Treatment includes dietary modification and the use of cholinergic medications and metoclopromide.

GCP Good Clinical Practices: Describes the practices, responsibilities and actions of the sponsor, investigator, and monitor, that must be followed in any clinical trial to ensure the safety of study participants and the quality of the data.

Gefitinib A drug that is used to treat non-small cell lung cancer and is being studied in the treatment of other types of cancer. It belongs to the family of drugs called epidermal growth factor receptor (EGFR)-tyrosine kinase inhibitors.

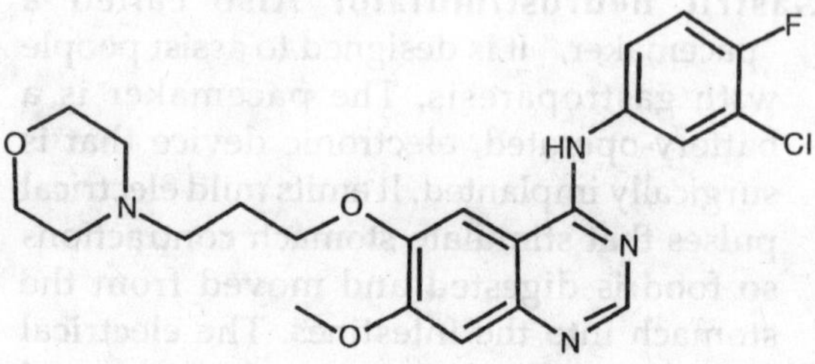

Gel A colloid, where the dispersed phase is liquid and the dispersion medium is solid.

Gel electrophoresis A DNA separation technique that is very important in DNA sequencing. Standard sequencing procedures involve cloning DNA fragments into special sequencing cloning vectors that carry tiny pieces of DNA. The next step is to determine the base sequence of the tiny fragments by a special procedure that generates a series of even tinier DNA fragments that differ in size by only one base. These nested fragments are separated by gel electrophoresis, in which the DNA pieces are added to a gelatinous solution, allowing the fragments to work their way down through the gel. Smaller pieces move faster and will reach the bottom first. Movement through the gel is hastened by applying an electrical field to the gel.

Gel polarization The phenomenon of formation of a layer of insoluble/semi-soluble material at a liquid/filter interface. It is a common occurrence with excessive linear velocity flow through filters of colloidal suspensions and macromolecular solutions.

Gelatin A derived protein formed from the collagen of the tissues by boiling in water, sometimes called an albuminoid, though it lacks the characteristic albuminoid properties. Glue, size, and isinglass are forms of gelatin.

Genasense A substance that is being studied in the treatment of cancer. It may kill cancer cells by blocking the production of a protein that makes cancer cells live longer and by making them more sensitive to anticancer drugs. It belongs to the family of drugs called antisense oligodeoxyribonucleotides.

Gene A natural unit of hereditary material that is the physical basis for the transmission of the characteristics of living organisms from one generation to another. The basic genetic material is fundamentally the same in all living organisms. It consists of deoxyribonucleic acid (DNA) in most organisms and ribonucleic acid (RNA) in certain viruses, and is usually associated in a linear arrangement that, in part, constitutes the chromosome. The average length of a gene is 1μm and thus, about one million genes could be contained in a one-meter stretch of DNA. The segment of DNA that is involved in producing a polypeptide chain, it includes regions preceding (leader) and following (trailer) the coding region as well as intervening sequences (introns) between individual coding segments (exons).

Gene expression The process by which a gene's coded information is converted into the structures present and operating in the cell. Expressed genes include those that are transcribed into mRNA and then translated into protein and those that are transcribed into RNA but not translated into protein

Gene family Group of closely related genes that makes similar products.

Gene mapping Determination of the relative positions of genes on a DNA molecule (chromosome or plasmid) and of the distance, in linkage units or physical units, between them.

Gene markers Landmarks for a target gene, either detectable traits that are inherited along with the gene, or distinctive segments of DNA.

Gene product The biochemical material, either RNA or protein, resulting from expression of a gene. The amount of gene product is used to measure how active a gene is; abnormal amounts can be correlated with disease causing alleles.

Gene sequencing The determination of the sequence of bases in a DNA strand. The two most widely used methods are the chain-termination method, developed by Sanger in the mid-seventies, and the chemical method developed by Maxam & Gilbert around the same time.

Gene splicing The enzymatic attachment of one gene or part of a gene to another.

Gene target A gene or its product (protein) which plays a critical role in pathologyA

Gene therapy The insertion of normal DNA directly into cells to correct a generic defect.

GeneBloc molecules Specific antisense molecule consisting of DNA and RNA building blocks and blocking groups at the 5' and 3' ends to enhance stability against molecular degradation.

Generic drugs Drug formulations of identical composition with respect to the active ingredient, i.e., drugs that meet current official standards of identity, purity, and quality of active ingredient. Drug dosage forms considered as "generically equivalent" are more properly considered as "chemically equivalent" in that they contain a designated quantity of drug chemical in specified stable condition and meet pharmacopoeial requirements for chemical and physical properties.

Each of a number of preparations of a given drug entity may carry a different "proprietaryname" or "trademark"; such a name is registered with the U.S. Patent Office and identifies the special brand of the drug with the firm owning the name. All such preparations - identical with respect to content and specification of active ingredient - may be looked upon as comprising a "genus"; they are generically equivalent and are generic drugs. department of health regulations require manufacturers of generic drugs to establish biological equivalence of their product to the original patented drug product.

It is well recognized that a number of factors other than quantity of drug present in a dose can determine the ultimate therapeutic usefulness of the drug preparation, and even the availability of drug to the site of action once the preparation has been given. Drugs may be generically equivalent but not therapeutically equivalent. Factors which affect therapeutic usefulness or efficacy of drug preparations include appearance, taste, disintegration and dissolution properties of the preparation, interaction of active materials with other ingredients including binders and solvents, pH, particle size, age of preparation, conditions of manufacture such as degree of tablet compression, and the nature and amount of coating of enteric-coated tablets.

When the patent of a proprietary drug expires, a manufacturer must establish the biological equivalence of its generic formulation in order to market the product. To do so, the bioavailability if the generic formulation is compared to the proprietary product in a cross-over experiment.

Generics Drugs containing the same active ingredient after expiration of the patent for the active ingredient

Genetic code The sequence of nucleotides, coded in triplets (codons) along the mRNA that determines the sequence of amino acids in protein synthesis. The DNA sequence of a gene can be used to predict the mRNA sequence, and the genetic code can in turn be used to predict the amino acid sequence.

Genetic diseases Diseases that occur because a mutation in the genetic material.

Genetic engineering The selective, deliberate alteration of genes by technological means.

Genetic map Genome/B>

The full complement of chromosomes and extra-chromosomal DNA coding for cellular proteins, contained within each cell of a given species. Its size is generally given as total number of base pairs.

Genetics The scientific study of heredity: how particular qualities or traits are transmitted from parents to offspring.

Genome DNA sequence of an organism; its size is generally given as its total number of base pairs.

Genome project Research and technology development effort aimed at mapping and sequencing some or all of the genome human beings and other organisms.

Genomic library A collection of clones made from a set of randomly generated overlapping DNA fragments representing the entire genome of an organism.

Genomic sequence The order of the subunits, called bases, that makes up a particular fragment of DNA in a genome. DNA is a long molecule made up of four different kinds of bases, which are abbreviated A, C, T, and G. A DNA fragment that is 10 bases long might have a base sequence of, for example, ATCGTTCCTG. The particular sequence of bases encodes important information in an individual's genetic blueprint, and is unique for each individual (except identical twins).

Genotype The "internally coded, inheritable information" carried by all living organisms. This stored information is used as a "blueprint" or set of instructions for building and maintaining a living creature. These instructions are found within almost all cells (the "internal" part), they are written in a coded language (the genetic code), they are copied at the time of cell division or reproduction and are passed from one generation to the next ("inheritable"). These instructions are intimately involved with all aspects of the life of a cell or an organism. They control everything from the formation of protein macromolecules, to the regulation of metabolism and synthesis.

Genotype to phenotype Investigators start with a set of genes that are known (or strongly suspected) to be important in modulating the response to drugs, and search for variation in their sequences (that is, their genotype.)

Germicidal lamps Light sources that emit ultraviolet radiation at a wavelength of 254 nanometers. These lights are commonly found in biological safety cabinets and used to inactivate bacteria, viruses and fungi which are either airborne or on exposed surfaces.

Germicide An agent that destroys microorganisms, especially pathogenic microorganisms ("germs"). Sterilants, disinfectants, and antiseptics are germicides.

Germplasm The total genetic variability, represented by germ cells or seeds, available to a particular population of organisms.

GGTP The earliest liver function to become abnormal.

Globulin Globulin helps to combat infection on a normal level. It is the total protein value minus albumin value.

GLP Good Laboratory Practice: in the pharmaceutical context, requirements for 'nonclinical' tests on animals. It does not cover chemical or microbiological testing of raw materials or products.

Glucagonoma A rare pancreatic tumor that produces a hormone called glucagon. Glucagonomas can produce symptoms similar to diabetes.

Glucocorticoid A compound that belongs to the family of compounds called corticosteroids (steroids). Glucocorticoids affect metabolism and have anti-inflammatory and immunosuppressive effects. They may be naturally produced (hormones) or synthetic (drugs).

Glucose The main sugar that the body makes from the three energy-providing nutrients — proteins, fats, and carbohydrates — but mostly from carbohydrates. Glucose is the major source of energy for living cells and is carried to each cell through the bloodstream. However, the cells cannot use glucose without the help of insulin.

Glutamine An amino acid used in nutrition therapy. It is also being studied for the treatment of diarrhea caused by radiation therapy to the pelvis.

H
O H
C — C — N
HO H
CH_2
CH_2
C
H_2N O

Glutathione A substance found in plant and animal tissues that has many functions in a cell. These include activating certain enzymes and destroying toxic compounds and chemicals that contain oxygen.

Glutathione S transferase A family of enzymes involved in metabolism and in making toxic compounds less harmful to the body.

Glycinamide ribonucleotide formyltransferase inhibitor A drug that blocks DNA synthesis and may prevent tumor growth. It is being studied as a treatment for cancer.

Gmp critical parameter A parameter that has a direct effect on product quality.

GMP Good Manufacturing Practice: in the pharmaceutical context,these are the requirements covering all aspects of pharmaceutical manufacture, including chemical and microbiological testing of raw materials and products.

GMP facility A production facility or clinical trial materials pilot plant for the manufacture of pharmaceutical products. It includes the manufacturing space, the storage warehouse for raw and finished product, and support lab areas.

Golgi bodies Very small particles composed of membrane aggregates and responsible for the secretion of certain enzymes and macromolecules. Golgi bodies are the deposition and packaging site for many excreted products.

Good clinical practice (GCP) A standard for the design, conduct, performance, monitoring, auditing, recording, analyses, and reporting of clinical trials that provides assurance that the data and reported results are credible and accurate, and that the rights, integrity, and confidentiality of trial subjects are protected.

Good clinical research practice (GCRP) Term sometimes used to describe GCP.

Good engineering practice (GEP) A combination of standards, specifications, codes, regulatory and industrial guidelines as well as accepted engineering and design methods intended to design, construct, operate, and maintain pharmaceutical and/or biotechnology facilities taking into account not only regulatory compliance but also safety, economics, environmental protection and operability. Standards and specifications are provided by recognized sources such as established engineering and architectural contractors as well as pharmaceutical companies. Codes are provided by local, state, jurisdictions and/or insurance companies. Guidelines are issued by professional societies, industrial organizations, or regulatory agencies. Engineering design methods have been established throughout the engineering educational system.

Good large scale practice organism (GLSP) The National Institutes of Health (NIH) specifies physical containment levels and defines Biosafety Levels for Large Scale in their "Guidelines for Research Involving Recombinant DNA Molecules" - Appendix K - May 1999. Level of physical containment recommended for large-scale (more than 10 liters of culture) research or production involving viable, non-pathogenic, and non-toxigenic recombinant strains derived from host organisms that have an extended history of safe large scale use. Likewise, the GLSP level of physical containment is recommended for organisms that have a built-in environmental limitation that permits optimum growth in large-scale bioreactors, but limited survival if released to the environment.

Goserelin Drug for long-term palliation and symptom control of prostate cancer. Also used in some breast cancer patients.

Grade (in cancer) The grade of a cancer reflects how abnormal it looks under the microscope. There are several grading systems for different types of cancer.

Granisetron Anti-nausea drug widely used for chemotherapy side effects.

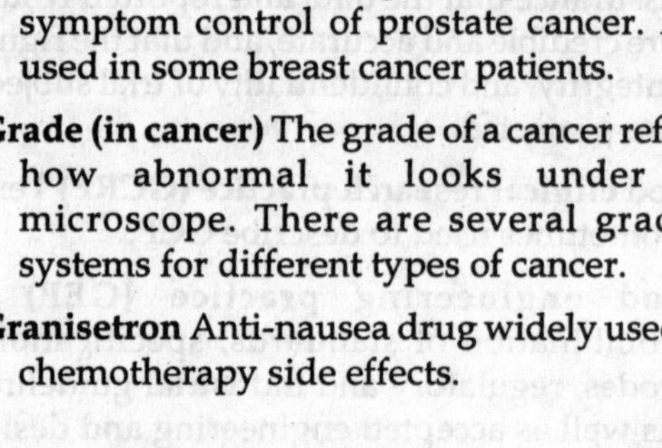

Granulocyte colony stimulating factor (G-CSF, Filgrastim) Indications: Treatment of neutropenia, defined as ANC < 500-750/ mm3, as a result of HIV disease, chemotherapy, or other drugs (hydroxyurea, ganciclovir, ZDV, TMP-SMX).

Contraindications: Known hypersensitivity to drug or Escherichia coli-derived products.

Dosage: 5-10 mcg/kg/day SC. Complete blood count should be checked twice a week, and ANC should be maintained at > 1,000-2,000/ml. G-CSF should be stopped if there is no response after 7 days at a dose of 10 mcg/kg/day.

Toxicity: Bone pain.

Growth hormone (GH) A hormone secreted by the pituitary gland. GH stimulates growth and repair of the body as well as the activities of the immune system. With age, GH release diminishes (also known as hGH or human growth hormone).

GTP binding proteins Regulatory proteins that act as molecular switches. They control a wide range of biological processes including: receptor signaling, intracellular signal transduction pathways, and protein synthesis. Their activity is regulated by factors that control their ability to bind to and hydrolyze GTP to GDP.

GxP A collective term used to refer to the regulations and guidances governing the research, development, testing, and manufacturing of drugs, medical devices, and biologics.

Gynecologic Oncology The study and treatment of cancers of the female reproductive organs.

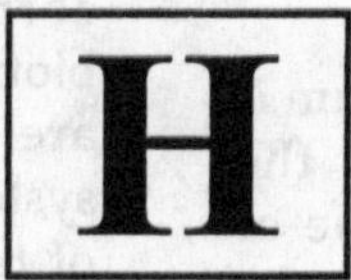

HA20 A monoclonal antibody that is being studied in the treatment of refractory B-cell non-Hodgkin's lymphoma. Monoclonal antibodies are made in the laboratory and can locate and bind to cancer cells. hA20 binds to the protein CD20, which is found on B cells (a type of immune system cell), and some types of lymphoma cells. Also called IMMU-106 and HCD20.

HAART Highly active antiretroviral therapy. Treatment for human immunodeficiency virus (HIV) infection that uses a combination of several antiretroviral drugs. The drugs inhibit the ability of the virus to multiply in the body, and they slow down the development of AIDS.

Habituation A condition characterized by a psychological craving for the effects produced by the administration of a drug.

The Expert Committee on Addiction-Producing Drugs of the World Health Organization defines habituation (1957) as: "...a condition resulting from the repeated consumption of a drug. Its characteristics include: 1. A desire (but not compulsion) to continue taking the drug for the sense of improved well-being which it engenders;

2. little or no tendency to increase the dose;

3. some degree of psychic dependence on the effect of drug; but absence of physical dependence and hence of the abstinency syndrome;

4. detrimental effects, if any, primarily on the individual."

Hairpin A double helical region formed by base pairing between adjacent (inverted) complementary sequences in a single strand of RNA or DNA.

Half life The period of time required for the concentration or amount of drug in the body to be reduced to exactly one-half of a given concentration or amount. The given concentration or amount need not be the maximum observed during the course of the experiment, or the concentration or amount present at the beginning of an experiment, since the half-life is completely independent of the concentration or amount chosen as the "starting point". Half-lives can be computed and interpreted legitimately only when concentration or amount varies with time according to the law appropriate to the kinetics of a first order reaction: the common logarithm of the concentration or amount is related linearly to time, e.g.:

$\log C = a + bt$

where C is concentration at time t, a (in logarithmic units) is the intercept of the line with the ordinate, and b (which has a negative sign) is the slope of the line. The parameters of the equation can be estimated from the plot of experimental values of log C and t. The half-life can be computed simply by dividing the slope of the curve into 0.301, the difference between the logarithm of a number (C) and the logarithm of number half as large (C/2); the symbol for half-life is t1/2.

The half-life of a drug in plasma or serum is frequently taken as indicating the persistence of the drug in its volume of distribution; this interpretation may be incorrect unless the material can move freely and rapidly from one fluid compartment of the body to another, and is not bound or stored in one or another tissue. The term "biological half-life" should not be used instead of the specific terms "plasma half-life" or "serum half-life". The tissue for which the half-life of a drug is determined should always be specified, e.g., "serum half-life"; the half-life of a drug in muscle, kidney, etc., or in the whole organism can be determined. Drug half-lives are frequently based on the results of chemical analyses, i.e., the results of the reaction of a reagent with a specific chemical group of a drug molecule; it should be remembered that detection of the group per se does not necessarily imply its continuous existence as part of a biologically active drug molecule.

A drug molecule that leaves the plasma may have any of several fates: it can be destroyed in the blood; it can be eliminated from the body; or it can be translocated to a body fluid compartment other than the intravascular to be stored, biotransformed, or to exert its pharmacodynamic effects.

When the plot of log plasma or serum concentration (during the period of its decline) against time is composed of two straight line segments, the inference may be made that two first order processes are involved in the distribution and biotransformation and elimination of the drug. The earlier phase - represented by the line segment of greater slope - is termed the distributive phase, and corresponds to the period during which translocation of the drug to its ultimate volume of distribution occurs and is the dominant process; the later phase - represented by the line of lesser slope - is termed the eliminative phase, and corresponds to the period when biotransformation and elimination of drug are dominant processes. For two-phase systems, three phase systems, etc., half-lives of the drugs in the various phases can be determined only after more sophisticated analysis of the data than that described above.

Haloenzyme An enzyme that contains a non-protein component.

Halogen One of the chlorine group (bromine, chlorine, fluorine, iodine) of elements, all univalent; they form monobasic acids with hydrogen, and their hydroxides (fluorine forms none) are monobasic acids. The radioactive element, astatine, also belongs to the halogen group.

Halophile An organism that displays accelerated growth or is dependent on high salt concentrations.

Handedness Chirality and handedness are concepts that apply to the structure of molecules. Chirality is defined by the lack of certain features of symmetry, which lead to an object not being superimposable on its mirror image. Handedness is a different phenomenon relating to the ability to classify chiral objects into right-handed and left-handed objects. All handed objects are chiral, but not all chiral objects are handed. In 1968 through 1970, Ruch and coworkers developed a theory of chirality that provided a mathematical basis for the handedness of chiral objects. Handed chiral objects are considered to be analogous to shoes, which are readily classified into right and left shoes regardless of the size, material, style, or other attributes of the shoes in question. Nonhanded chiral objects are considered to be analogous to potatoes, which have no symmetry because of their irregular patterns of "bumps" and "eyes," thereby meeting the lack of symmetry requirements for chirality. There is, however, no unambiguous way to classify a set of potatoes into "left" and "right" potatoes.

Handshake Requires the recipient of an electronic data record to acknowledge to the sender that the record has been received.

Handwritten signature The scripted name or legal mark of an individual handwritten by that individual and executed or adopted with the present intention to authenticate a writing in a permanent form. The act of signing with a writing or marking instrument such as a pen or stylus is preserved. The scripted name or legal mark, while conventionally applied to paper, may also be applied to other devices that capture the name or mark.

Haploid A single set of chromosomes (half the full set of genetic material), present in the egg and sperm cells of animals and in the egg and pollen cells of plants. Human beings have 23 chromosomes in their reproductive cells.

Hapten A molecule (usually a small organic molecule) which can be bound to an antigenic determinant/ epitope. Usually they are too small to give a response of their own. They become antigenic if they are coupled to a suitable macromolecule, such as a protein.

Small antigenic determinants capable of eliciting an immune response only when coupled to a carrier. Haptens bind to antibodies but by themselves cannot elicit an antibody response.

Hardness Concentration of calcium and magnesium salts in water. Hardness originally referred to the soap-consuming power of water; as such it is sometimes also taken to include iron and manganese. "Permanent hardness" also known as "noncarbonated hardness " is the excess of hardness over alkalinity. "Temporary hardness" also known as "carbonated hardness" is equal or less than the alkalinity. Permanent hardness can cause boiler or pipe scale and failure of reverse osmosis membranes.

Hardware acceptance test specification . Documented verification that all key aspects of hardwareinstallation adhere to appropriate codes and approved design intentionsand that the recommendations of the manufacturer have been suitablyconsidered.

Hardware design specification (APV) Description of thehardware on which the software resides and how it is to be connected toany system or equipment.

Harrison act A federal law passed in 1916 that regulated the manufacture, importation, transportation, and distribution (wholesale, retail, dispensing) of all "narcotics " defined by the act. Coca leaves and derivatives, opium and derivatives, and various synthetic agents were subject to the act and are officially designated as "narcotics". The effect of the law was to regulate possession and use of the materials designated as narcotics. Since regulation was achieved through taxation, the law was enforced by the Treasury Department, Bureau of Internal Revenue. Traffic in marihuana was first controlled by the Marijuana Tax Act of 1937.

More recently, additional materials, e.g., barbiturates, amphetamines, etc., were recognized by Congress as requiring legal control, and were included with narcotics and marihuana in the Controlled Substances Act of 1970. The law is implemented by placing a nominal tax on certain materials under the law, and by requiring that physicians, dentists, etc., be specially licensed, annually, to legally prescribe materials covered by the law. The Act of 1970 is enforced by the Drug Enforcement Administration of the U.S. Department of Justice.

Harvesting The separation of cells from growth media. It can be accomplished by filtration, precipitation, or centrifugation.

Hazard The potential for causing harm; that which is a potential cause of harm. With respect to chemicals which are capable of causing harm, "hazard" is about equivalent in meaning to "toxicity"; measuring the hazard or toxicity of a chemical is to measure its potency in producing harm: the lower the dose required to produce harm, the greater the hazard or toxicity, the more hazardous or toxic is the substance.

Since the time of Paracelsus, in the early 16th century, it has been recognized that all chemicals, given in sufficient doses, are capable of producing harm. Therefore, it is not very meaningful simply to call a chemical a hazard, or to speak of a chemical as hazardous, without qualification or definition. Three categories of information are needed to define a hazard: specific descriptions of the harms it can produce, specific identification of the species or kinds of subjects that can be harmed, and specification of the kinds of exposure to the chemical (including dose) which can result in the respective harms.

Observe that hazard is the potential for causing harm. However hazardous a chemical might be, it may present no risk if potential victims are not exposed to it! Risk management is the effort to limit the likelihood that the hazard of a chemical will be realized or manifested.

For chemicals, such as drugs, it is frequently more informative to consider their hazards relative to their potential for producing benefit, rather than relative to the hazards of other chemicals. An extremely potent therapeutic agent may also be potent in producing harm, but it may be a useful drug because of its large therapeutic index or standardized safety margin.

Hazardous chemical reaction A reaction which generates pressure or byproducts which could cause injury, illness or harm to humans, domestic animals, livestock or wildlife.

Hazardous occupancy - group H - (California building code) Group H occupancies include buildings or structures, or portions thereof, that involve the manufacturing, processing, generation or storage of materials that constitute a high fire, explosion, or health hazard. There are eight divisions in this Group: 1. Division 1 - Occupancies with a quantity of material in the building exceeding regulation set limits and that present a high explosion hazard, such as blasting agents, fireworks, black powder, certain oxidizers and detonatable unstable (reactive) materials, and other materials (refer to Code for more details).

2. Division 2 - Occupancies where combustible dust is manufactured, used, or generated in such a manner that concentrations and conditions creates fire or explosion potential, or occupancies where materials exceeding regulation set limits present a moderate explosion hazard or a hazard from accelerated burning, such as some organic peroxides, pyrophoric gases, flammable or oxidizing gases, some nondetonatable unstable (reactive) materials, and other materials (refer to Code for more details).

3. Division 3 - Occupancies where flammable solids, other than combustible dust, are manufactured, used or generated, or occupancies where materials exceeding regulation set limits present a high physical hazard, such as some organic peroxides and oxidizers, pyrophoric liquids or solids, flammable solids in storage, flammable or

oxidizing cryogenic fluids, and other materials (refer to Code for more details).

4. Division 4 - Repair garages not classified as Group S, Division 3 Occupancies.

5. Division 5 - Aircraft repair hangars not classified as Group S, Division 5 Occupancies, and heliports.

6. Division 6 - Semiconductor fabrication facilities and comparable research and development areas in which hazardous production materials (HPM) are used and the aggregate quantity of materials exceeds those set by regulations. Such facilities and areas shall be designed and constructed following a different set of regulations.

7. Division 7 - Occupancies having quantities of materials in excess of those set by regulations, and that are health hazards, such as corrosives (except stationary lead-acid battery systems), toxic and highly toxic materials, irritants, sensitizers, and other health hazards (refer to Code).

8. Division 8 - Laboratories and similar areas used for scientific experimentation or research having quantities of materials not in excess of those set by regulations, and not otherwise classified as Group B, Division 2 Occupancies (refer to Code for more details).

Hazardous substance A substance which by reason of being explosive, flammable, toxic, poisonous, corrosive, oxidizing, irritant or otherwise harmful, is likely to cause injury.

Haze The abnormal appearance of a localized diminishing in brightness or luster of a surface when compared to the adjacent surfaces.

Health hazard Classification of a chemical for which there is statistically significant evidence based on at least one study conducted in accordance with established scientific principles that acute or chronic health effects may occur in exposed persons. The term "health hazard" includes chemicals that are carcinogens, toxic or highly toxic agents, reproductive toxins, irritants, corrosives, sensitizers, hepatotoxins, nephrotoxins, neurotoxins, agents that act on the hematopoietic system, and agents that damage the lungs, skin, eyes or mucous membranes.

Health level 7 (HL7) A clinical data interchange messaging system in which messages are structured according to a predefined format and sent from one system to another. The sending system needs to know only how to convert its data into an HL7 message; the receiving system needs to know only how to extract the data.

Healthy volunteer A healthy person who agrees to participate in a clinical trial for reasons other than medical and receives no direct health benefit from participating.

Heart palpitation A subjective sensation of a rapid, irregular or forceful beating of the heart.

Heat A form of energy associated with the motion of atoms or molecules in solids and capable of being transmitted through solid and fluid media by conduction, through fluid media by convection, and through empty space by radiation. Two important characteristics of heat are: 1. Heat cannot be destroyed, only transferred from on body to another, or converted to another form of energy.

2. Heat always flows from the warmer to the colder substance.

Heat affected zone (HAZ) That portion of the base metal that has not been melted but whose microstructure or mechanical properties have been altered by the heat of welding, brazing, soldering, forming, or cutting.

Heat labile Able to be destroyed or altered by high temperature. Heat labile pharmaceuticals are sterilized by filtration.

Heat number An alphanumeric identification of a stated tonnage of metal obtained from a continuous melting in a foundry furnace.

Heat of Vaporization The amount of heat needed to change a unit volume from a liquid to a vapor at a given pressure without a temperature change.

Heavy metals High molecular weight metal ions, such as lead. Known for their interference with many processes, and "poisoning" of catalysts, membranes, and resins.

Hela cells An established line of human cervical carcinoma cells used to study the biochemistry and genetics of human cell growth.

Helix A spiral, staircase-like, structure with a repeating pattern described by two simultaneous operations, rotation, and translation. It is the natural conformation of many biological polymers.

Hematin An iron protoporphyrin differing from heme in that the central iron atom is in the ferric (Fe+++) rather than the ferrous (Fe++) state; the prosthetic group of methemoglobin.

Hemoglobin The red, respiratory conjugated protein of erythrocytes, consisting of approximately 6 percent heme and 94 percent globin (a protein).

Hemophilia A hereditary, plasma-coagulation disorder, principally affecting males but transmitted by females, and characterized by excessive, sometimes spontaneous, bleeding.

Hemopoietic Pertaining to or related to the formation of blood cells.

Hemostasis Blood (hemo) stopping of flow (stasis). The termination of bleeding due to clotting and vasoconstriction.

HEPA (High efficiency particulate air) filters Filters with a minimum efficiency of 99.97% for 0.3μm particle size as determined by test. The test can be by the monodispersed dioctyl phthalate (DOP) method or other equally sensitive method. When operated at design velocity, larger and smaller particles are captured at higher efficiencies. HEPA filters are made of compressed and bonded micro-fiberglass or Teflon® corrugated to produce a high surface area in a small area panel of filter medium. Employed in unidirectional airflow benches, air handlers, and as terminal air supply filters in cleanrooms.

Heparin A sulphur containing polysaccharide that stops blood from clotting by preventing the conversion of prothrombin to thrombin and by neutralizing thrombin. It is contained in the mast cells and is extractable from various tissues, notably the lung.

$CH_2OSO_3^-$
CO
OH^2
O
O
—O—
—O—
OSH_3^-
$NHSO_3^-$

Hepatics General identification of drugs used in liver treatment.

Hepatoprotective drugs Substantives used in the treatment of hepatic diseases; they improve the function of hepatic cells while protecting them from further impairment.

Hepatotoxin A toxin that is destructive to parenchymal (specific tissue) cells of the liver.

HER-2/neu A cancer gene found in some breast and ovarian cancer patients that is associated with a poor prognosis. In about 30% of breast cancers, a specific protein found on the surface of a cancer cells - called Her-2/neu (pronounced 'her two new') - is overexpressed, meaning it is 'overactive'. This condition causes cancer cells to multiply.

Herceptin This is the brand name for the drug trastuzumab, a genetically engineered substance, which attacks breast cancer by interfering with the production of cancerous cells. Herceptin binds to the Her-2/neu protein and prevents cancer cells from multiplying. Recent studies have indicated that a combination of Herceptin plus chemotherapy may prove to be a significant advance in the treatment of breast cancer.

Heredity Transfer of genetic information from parent cells to progeny.

Heterologous Consisting of different elements, or of elements in differing proportions.

Heteromeric Made of at least two different subunits.

Heterotrophs One of two categories in which microorganisms are classified on the basis of their carbon source. Heterotrophs use organic compounds such as carbohydrates, lipids, and hydrocarbons as a carbon and energy source.

Heterozygosity The presence of different alleles at one or more loci on homologous chromosomes.

Hexyl 5-aminolevulinate A substance that is used to find and kill tumor cells. It enters tumor cells and becomes activated when exposed to a special type of light. A chemical reaction causes the cells to produce fluorescent light and die.

HGB A1C (Glycohemoglobin) Indicates blood sugar activity for the past two to three months.

High level review of software Purposes: determine if programs meetdesign specs as described by such documents as modular flow diagrams, HIPO charts, pseudo code and operating manuals. Characteristics:involves comparing design specs and acceptance criteria with cognitivemechanisms which depict the program in terms more easily understood byautomation practitioners and non-computer scientists. Uses: qualityacceptance review by QA software auditing, for example to complement"walk-through", for inspections, and for troubleshooting problems.

High purity process systems The equipment that includes the stainless steel vessels, tube, pipe, fittings, and valves used to manufacture and transport drug products.

High throughput screening Rapid evaluation of large numbers of chemical compounds to determine which one(s) interact with a given biologic target.

Hippocampus An area of the brain believed responsible for memory and personality.

Histamine Histamine is a chemical present in cells throughout the body that is released during an allergic reaction. Histamine is one of the substances responsible for the symptoms on inflammation and is the major reason for running of the nose, sneezing, and itching in allergic rhinitis. It also stimulates production of acid by the stomach and narrows the bronchi or airways in the lungs.

HIV antibody Presence of antibody is associated with having been infected by the virus known to cause AIDS (Acquired Immune Deficiency Syndrome).

HMG CoA reductase inhibitor Hydroxymethylglutaryl-coenzyme A reductase inhibitor. A substance that blocks an enzyme needed by the body to make cholesterol and lowers the amount of cholesterol in the blood. HMG-CoA reductase inhibitor drugs are called statins.

HMO A Health Maintenance Organization is a health plan that receives a discount from hospitals, physicians, and other providers based upon the volume of patients each provides. The HMO's members receive comprehensive preventative, hospital, and medical care from specific medical providers who have agreed upon pre-set rates. Members select a Primary Care Physician or medical group from the HMO's list of affiliated doctors and generally have no deductibles or claim forms. Members make a small co-payment, usually between $3 and $20. Some HMO's have capitated contracts with providers and some pay providers on a single discounted fee-for-service basis.

Hold up volume The volume of liquid remaining in a vessel or piping system after it has been allowed to drain.

Hollow fiber Refers to reverse osmosis and ultrafiltration membranes formed into small diameter (about 0.05" I.D.) tubes. The inner surface is a very thin (RO or UF) membrane skin supported by a thicker porous outer layer that gives the tube its strength. Hollow fibers are used in bundles of 1,000 or more in a single cartridge shell. Water is forced through the center (upstream surface) of each tube and purified permeate is collected from the outer wall (downstream surface).

Home brew Reagents or the combination of reagents made in a laboratory, or purchased reagents used by that laboratory for clinical tests and not for sale to other laboratories.

Homeobox A short stretch of nucleotides whose base sequence is virtually identical in all the genes that contains it. It has been found in many organisms from fruit flies to human beings. In the fruit fly, a homeobox appears to determine when particular groups of genes are expressed during development.

Homeopathics Drugs obtained in a specific way by diluting a single or multiple substances which, if they were not diluted, would induce in a healthy individual such symptoms, against which they are being administered; the homeopathic method of treatment is based on the principle that "similar is treated by similar" the word homeopathy was created by its founder, a physician Samuel Hahnemann, from the Greek words "homos" - the same and "pathos" - disease.

Homologous chromosome Chromosome containing the same linear gene sequences as another, each derived from one parent.

Homologue Used to describe a compound belonging to a series of compounds differing from each other by a repeating unit, such as a methylene group, a peptide residue, etc.

Homology Similarity in DNA or protein sequences between individuals of the same species or among different species.

Hormone A substance produced by endocrine glands, released in very low concentration into the bloodstream, and which exerts regulatory effects on specific organs or tissues distant from the site of secretion.

Chemical substances having a specific regulatory effect on the activity of a certain organ or organs. The term was originally applied to substances secreted by various endocrine glands and transported in the bloodstream to the target organs. It is sometimes extended to include those substances that are not produced by the endocrine glands but that have similar effects.

Hormone therapy Treatment that adds, blocks, or removes hormones. For certain conditions (such as diabetes or menopause), hormones are given to adjust low hormone levels. To slow or stop the growth of certain cancers (such as prostate and breast cancer), synthetic hormones or other drugs may be given to block the body's natural hormones. Sometimes surgery is needed to remove the gland that makes a certain hormone. Also called hormonal therapy, hormone treatment, or endocrine therapy.

Hormone treatment Treatment that adds, blocks, or removes hormones. For certain conditions (such as diabetes or menopause), hormones are given to adjust low hormone levels. To slow or stop the growth of certain cancers (such as prostate and breast cancer), synthetic hormones or other drugs may be given to block the body's natural hormones. Sometimes surgery is needed to remove the gland that makes a certain hormone. Also called hormonal therapy, hormone therapy, or endocrine therapy.

Hospital Is an institution that: a. is primarily engaged in providing, by or under the supervision of physicians, inpatient diagnostic, surgical and therapeutic services for the diagnosis, treatment and rehabilitation of injured, disabled or sick persons; b. Maintains clinical records on all patients; c. has bylaws in effect with respect to its staff of physicians; d. has a requirement that every patient be under the care of a physician;provides 24 hour nursing service rendered or supervised by a registered nurse; e. has in effect a hospital utilization review plan; f. is licensed pursuant to any state or agency of the state responsible for licensing hospitals; and g. has accreditation under one of the programs of the Joint Commission on Accreditation of Hospitals and Healthcare Organizations.

The term hospital does not include any institution, or part thereof, that is used principally as a rest facility, nursing facility, convalescent facility or facility for care of the aged. Nor does it include any facility when used for the treatment of alcohol or chemical dependency, except as may be authorized by the program administrator, ValueOptions.

Host vector (HV) system The host is the organism into which a gene from another organism is transplanted. The guest gene is carried by a vector, which is a larger DNA molecule, such as a plasmid, or a virus into which that gene is genetically engineered and which then propagates in the host. NIH Guidelines under Appendix E. - Certified Host-Vector Systems contains a list of derivatives host-vector systems previously classified as Host-Vector 1 Systems or Host-Vector 2 Systems, they are: Bacillus subtilis, Saccharomyces Cerevisiae, Escherichia coli, Neurospora crassa, Streptomyces, and Pseudonomas putida.

HPLC (High pressure liquid chromatography) Sometimes called high-performance liquid chromatography, is a separation technique based on a solid stationary phase and a liquid mobile phase. Separations (into distinct bands) are achieved by partition, adsorption, or ion-exchange processes, depending upon the type of stationary phase used. Each band is then profiled as the solvent flows through a UV detector, or by fluorescence, or refractive index detectors.

HSA (Human serum albumin) The main protein constituent of human serum. It has no prosthetic group and is soluble in water and dilute salt solution. It is sometimes used in the treatment of shock, hypoproteinemia, and erythroblastosis fetalis.

hsCRP A screening test for heart disease.

Human factors The study of how people use technology. It involves the interaction of human abilities, expectations, and limitations, with work environments and system design. The term "human factors engineering" (HFE) refers to the application of human factors principles to the design of devices and systems. It is often interchanged with the terms "human engineering," "usability engineering," or "ergonomics." The goal of HFE is to design devices that users accept willingly and operate safely in realistic conditions. In medical applications, HFE helps improve human performance and reduce the risks associated with use error.

IND Investigational New Drug Application: A request for Food and Drug Administration (FDA) authorization to administer an investigational drug to humans. Such authorization must be secured prior to interstate shipment and administration of any new drug that is not the subject of an approved new drug application.

Human gene therapy Insertion of normal DNA directly into cells to correct a genetic defect.

Human Genome Initiative Collective name for several projects begun in 1986 by DOE to: 1. Create an ordered set of DNA segments from known chromosomal locations.

2. Develop new computational methods for analyzing genetic map and DNA sequence.

3. Develop new techniques and instruments for detecting and analyzing DNA.

This DOE initiative is now known as the Human Genome Program. The national effort, led by DOE and NIH, is known as the Human Genome Project.

Human genome The full collection of genes needed to produce a human being.

Human growth hormone (somatropin, serostim) Indications: Hormonal treatment of AIDS wasting syndrome.

Contraindications: Known hypersensitivity, presence of an actively growing intracranial tumor.

Dosage: For patients > 55 kg, dose is 6 mg SC qd; for patients 45-55 kg, dose is 5 mg SC qd; for patients 35-45 kg, dose is 4 mg SC qd.

Toxicity: Arthralgia, edema, hypertension, hyperglycemia.

Human subject A human subject, is an "individual who is or becomes a participant in research, either as a recipient of the test article or as a control. A subject may be either a healthy human or a patient." Synonym: subject/ trial subject.

Huntington disease Is an hereditary disorder characterized by mental and physical deterioration that ultimately leads to death. It is sometimes referred to as Hungtinton's chorea due to the involuntary rapid movement of limbs (chorea), which are a symptom of the disease. The characteristic symptoms of the disease are caused by loss of neurons (nerve cells) in the brain. Huntington's is caused by a faulty gene known as HD, which is located on chromosome 4. Diagnosis is by genetic testing. Currently, there is no cure, although medication may be used to control symptoms of the illness.

HVLP Acronym used for medicinal preparations produced in bulk, it means via industrial production.

Hybrid systems Combination of electronic and paper records, common in today's analytical labs, in which raw data is recorded electronically to reconstruct the analysis, but the final results are printed and signed on paper. department of health does not prohibit hybrid systems but has expressed some concerns about their usefulness.

Hybridization The process of joining two complementary strands of DNA or one each of DNA and RNA to form a double-stranded molecule.

Hybridoma A hybrid cell resulting from the fusion of a specific antibody producing spleen cell with a myeloma cell. The hybrid cell has the growth characteristics of the myeloma component and the antibody secreting characteristics of the spleen cell and will multiply to become a source of large quantities of pure, monoclonal antibody.

Hydration therapy The replacement of fluids and electrolytes to the body.

Hydrogen peroxide (H2O2) A colorless, heavy, strongly oxidizing, unstable liquid used principally in aqueous solutions as an antiseptic, bleaching agent, oxidizing agent, and laboratory reagent. In the vapor phase, as an airborne sterilant.

Hydrolysis A chemical reaction between water and organic compounds, particularly esters, ketones, and alcohols. This reaction can lead to breakdown of some proteins.

Hydrophilic Tending to dissolve in water. Describes the polar interactions between two molecules, e.g. a small molecule and a protein or any molecule and a solvent. Hydrophilic portions of molecules are those that are charged or contain oxygen or nitrogen atoms. The opposite of hydrophobic.

'Water loving'. The capacity of a molecular entity or of a substituent to interact with polar solvents, in particular with water, or with other polar groups.

Hydrophobic Definition: Literally - water fearing, from the Greek hydro - "water" and phobo - "fear" i.e. -tending to avoid water. Describes the non-polar interactions between two molecules, e.g., a small molecule and a protein or any molecule and a solvent. Non-polar portions of molecules are uncharged and tend to contain hydrocarbon moieties. The "hydrophobic effect" is the entropy driven force that causes oil to separate from water. It is notoriously strong, though not as strong as covalent forces. This force is one of the main determinants of the structure of globular protein molecules, since the hydrophilic (water loving) parts of the molecule tend to surround the hydrophobic parts that cluster in the center, away from the aqueous (polar) solvent .The opposite of hydrophilic.

Hydrotest A pressure test of piping, pressure vessels, or pressure-containing parts, usually performed by pressurizing the internal volume with water at a pressure determined by the applicable code or to test the integrity of a process system.

Hydroxychloroquine A substance that decreases immune responses in the body. It is used to treat some autoimmune diseases, and is being studied as a treatment for graft-versus-host disease. Hydroxychloroquine belongs to the family of drugs called antiprotozoals.

Hydroxymethylglutaryl coenzyme a reductase inhibitor HMG-CoA reductase inhibitor. A substance that blocks an enzyme needed by the body to make cholesterol and lowers the amount of cholesterol in the blood. HMG-CoA reductase inhibitor drugs are called statins.

Hydroxyurea (Hydrea) Indications: Has been shown to act synergistically with ddI and possibly d4T; not department of health-approved for management of HIV infection.

Contraindications: Known hypersensitivity, significant bone marrow suppression, pregnancy.

Dosage: 500 mg po bid.

Toxicity: Bone marrow suppression, stomatitis, nausea, vomiting, rash; severe pancreatitis has been described infrequently.

Hydroxyurea Drug used for some types of leukaemia.

Hygienic clamp joint A tube outside diameter union consisting of two neutered ferrules having flat faces with a concentric groove and mating gasket that is secured with a clamp, providing a nonprotruding, recessless product contact surface. Tri-clamp is a Tri-Clover proprietary name; consequently, it should not be used to describe the above-mentioned fitting unless that particular brand is used.

Hygienic Of, or pertaining to, equipment and piping systems that by design, materials of construction, and operation provide for the maintenance of cleanliness (pyrogen free but not sterile) so that products produced by these systems will not adversely affect human or animal health.

Hygroscopicity The property of a substance that enables it to absorb water vapor from the surrounding atmosphere. Hygroscopic materials will change weight as the relative humidity of their environment changes. In the case of hygroscopic chemicals, this will change the formula weight.

Hyperalgesia The excessive sensibility to low intensity noxious stimuli.

Hypersensitivity reaction A state of altered reactivity, possibly life threatening, in which the body reacts with an exaggerated immune response to a foreign substance.

Hypersensitivity The physiological state necessary for a subject's manifesting an allergic response or reaction; the state is dependent on the administration of a hapten or allergen to a susceptible individual, and the development of antibodies and immune mechanisms capable of being activated by a subsequent administration of the haptene.

Hypersensitivity may exist but not be manifested until a second administration of hapten occurs. The dose of hapten (or drug) required to produce the allergic response may be smaller, larger, or the same size as the dose required for the drug to produce its characteristic pharmacologic effects; hence hypersensitivity is not the same as sensitivity and the two words should not be used as synonyms. The nature of the response to haptene in a hypersensitive subject is determined by the immune mechanisms and effector organs and is not, in general, related to the nature of the hapten; the allergic response in the hypersensitive subject is generally qualitatively different from the expected pharmacodynamic response to the hapten or drug, being determined by the immune system, rather than by the receptor(s) that mediate that drug's pharmacodynamic effect.

Hypersomnia A condition that means "someone who sleeps too much."

Hypertension Persistently high blood pressure, known as a risk factor for the development of heart disease, peripheral vascular disease, stroke and kidney disease.

Hypertext Links in a document that permit you to jump immediately to another document. In most Web browsers links are displayed as colored, underlined text.

Hypertext Markup Language (HTML) A set of codes that describe the way type, graphics, and other elements are displayed on a Web page.

Hypertrophic cardiomyopathy One of three forms of cardiomyopathy, the main feature of which is an excessive thickening of the heart muscle without an obvious cause. The thickening may obstruct blood flow and symptoms include shortness of breath on exertion, dizziness, fainting and chest pain.

Hypnotic A drug that produces a state clinically identical to sleep by means of action in the central nervous system.

Hypochlorite A weak, unstable salt of hypochlorous acid used in aqueous solutions as a bleach, oxidizer, deodorant, and disinfectant.

Hypokalemia Low potassium levels in the blood: This can be caused by excessive secretion of aldosterone which promotes the excretion of potassium in the urine, sweat and saliva. When potassium levels drop to about half the normal levels muscle, weakness results.

Hypotensives Drugs reducing blood pressure.

Hypothalamus An area of the brain that is believed to be the command center for instructions to the endocrine system.

Hypoxia A condition of lowered oxygen levels in the blood. Hypoxia promotes free radical activity in the body.

I

Ibandronate A drug that is used to prevent and treat osteoporosis, and is being studied in the treatment of cancer that has spread to the bones. It belongs to the family of drugs called bisphosphonates.

IBC (intermediate bulk container) A container for storing, transporting, and handling dry materials. Normally bigger than ½ cubic meter but smaller than 3 cubic meters, dust free, able to receive and discharge a variety of materials, and capable of automation.

Ibuprofen A non-steroidal anti-inflammatory drug (NSAID) commonly used to treat pain, swelling, and fever

ICH International Committee on Harmonization.

ICI 182780 A drug that blocks estrogen activity in the body and is used in the treatment of estrogen-dependent tumors such as breast cancer. It belongs to the family of drugs called antiestrogens. Also called fulvestrant and Faslodex.

ICI D1694 An anticancer drug that stops tumor cells from growing by blocking the ability of cells to make DNA. Also called raltitrexed. It belongs to the family of drugs called thymidylate synthase inhibitors.

Idarubicin An anticancer drug that belongs to the family of drugs called antitumor antibiotics. Also called 4-demethoxydaunorubicin.

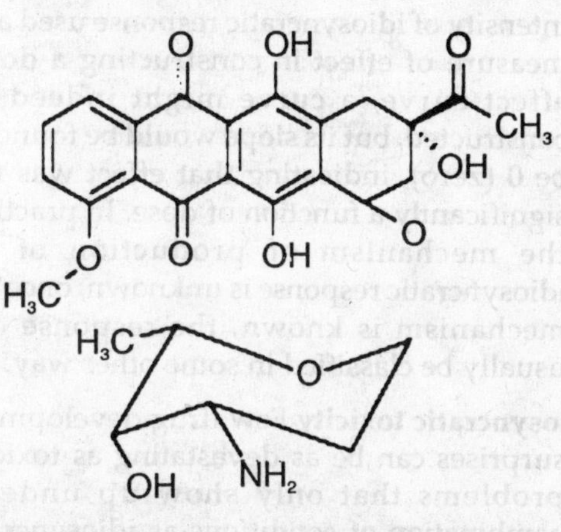

IDEC Y2B8 An anticancer drug that is a combination of a monoclonal antibody and a radioisotope (yttrium-90). Monoclonal antibodies are laboratory-produced substances that can locate and bind to cancer cells. Also called yttrium Y90 ibritumomab tiuxetan.

IDEC Y2B8 monoclonal antibody An anticancer drug that is a combination of a monoclonal antibody and a radioisotope (yttrium-90). Monoclonal antibodies are laboratory-produced substances that can locate and bind to cancer cells. Also called yttrium Y90 ibritumomab tiuxetan.

Identification In USP, a relatively quick presumptive test to verify that a material is what the label says it is. These are not final proof of identity, and related substances may have the same tests.

Idiosyncratic response A qualitatively abnormal or unusual response to a drug which is unique, or virtually so, to the individual who manifests the response. "Idiosyncratic Response" usually applies to a response that is not allergic in nature and cannot be produced with regularity in a substantial number of subjects in the population, and which is ordinarily not produced in a greater intensity in an individual, or in a greater fraction of the population, by the expedient of increase in the dose. In other words, were frequency or intensity of idiosyncratic response used as a measure of effect in constructing a dose-effect curve, a curve might indeed be constructed, but its slope would be found to be 0 (zero), indicating that effect was not significantly a function of dose. In practice, the mechanism of production of an idiosyncratic response is unknown; once the mechanism is known, the response can usually be classified in some other way.

Idiosyncratic toxicity Few drug development surprises can be as devastating as toxicity problems that only show up under a combination of conditions as idiosyncratic toxicity. Because of the role of variations in human drug metabolizing enzymes there may only be subtle (or no) evidence of such problems during pre-clinical safety studies. Such problems are also unlikely to show up in all but the largest clinical trials, but if the side effects are serious, it can result in product withdrawal.

IDLH (immediately dangerous to life and health) A concentration of airborne contaminants, normally expressed in parts per million (ppm) or milligrams per cubic meter, which represents the maximum level from which one could escape within 30 minutes without any escape-impairing symptoms or irreversible health effects. This level is established by the National Institute of Occupational Safety and Health (NIOSH).

IH636 grape seed extract A substance that is being studied for its ability to prevent damage to normal tissue caused by radiation therapy. It belongs to a family of compounds called antioxidants.

IL 1 alfa Interleukin-1-alfa. A type of biological response modifier (a substance that can improve the body's response to infection and disease). IL-1-alfa stimulates the growth and action of immune system cells that fight disease. IL-1-alfa is normally produced by the body, but it can also be made in the laboratory. Also called IL-1-alpha.

IL 1 Interleukin-1. A type of biological response modifier that stimulates immune system cells that fight disease, and is involved in inflammatory responses. There are two forms of IL-1, IL-1 alfa and IL-1 beta. Both forms of IL-1 are produced by the body, and can also be made in the laboratory.

IL 2 Interleukin-2. A type of biological response modifier (a substance that can improve the body's natural response to disease) that enhances the ability of the immune system to kill tumor cells and may interfere with blood flow to the tumor. These substances are normally produced by the body. Aldesleukin is IL-2 that is made in the laboratory for use in treating cancer and other diseases.

IL 3 Interleukin-3. A type of biological response modifier (a substance that can improve the body's natural response to disease) that enhances the immune system's ability to fight tumor cells. These substances are normally produced by the body. They are also made in the laboratory for use in treating cancer and other diseases.

IL 4 Interleukin-4. A type of biological response modifier (a substance that can improve the body's natural response to disease) that enhances the immune system's ability to fight tumor cells. These substances are normally produced by the body. They are also made in the laboratory for use in treating cancer and other diseases.

IL 6 Interleukin-6. A type of biological response modifier (a substance that can improve the body's natural response to infection and disease). These substances are normally produced by the body, but they can also be made in the laboratory.

IL 11 Interleukin-11. A type of biological response modifier (a substance that can improve the body's natural response to disease) that stimulates immune response and may reduce toxicity to the gastrointestinal system resulting from cancer therapy. These substances are normally produced by the body. They are also made in the laboratory for use in treating cancer and other diseases. Also called oprelvekin.

IL 12 Interleukin-12. A type of biological response modifier (a substance that can improve the body's natural response to disease) that enhances the ability of the immune system to kill tumor cells and may interfere with blood flow to the tumor. These substances are normally produced by the body. They are also made in the laboratory for use in treating cancer and other diseases.

Illness Means a sickness, disorder or disease and includes pregnancy.

Imatinib mesylate A drug that is being studied for its ability to inhibit the growth of certain cancers. It interferes with a portion of the protein produced by the bcr/abl oncogene. Also called Gleevec and STI571.

Imipenem An antibiotic drug used to treat severe or very resistant infection. It belongs to the family of drugs called carbapenems.

Imiquimod A substance that improves the body's natural response to infection and disease. It is used to treat early basal cell skin cancer and other conditions. It is being studied as a topical agent (something used on the surface of the body) for the prevention of some types of cancer. It belongs to the family of drugs called biological response modifiers.

Immobilized enzymes Enzymes which are immobilized on or in a variety of water-soluble or water- insoluble matrices with little or no loss of their catalytic activity. Since they can be reused continuously, immobilized enzymes have found wide application in the industrial, medical and research fields.

Immune response The production of antibodies (humoral response) or particular types of cytotoxic lymphoid cells (cell-mediated response) on challenge with an antigen.

Immune system The immune system is a collection of cells and proteins that works to protect the body from potentially harmful, infectious microorganisms (microscopic life-forms), such as bacteria, viruses and fungi. The immune system plays a role in the control of cancer and other diseases, but also is the culprit in the phenomena of allergies, hypersensitivity and the rejection of transplanted organs, tissues and medical implants.

Immune therapy Enhancement of the body's immune system via intravenous (IV) infusion or intramuscular vaccination. This therapy helps the body fight disease and infection.

Immunity The state of an organism in which protection from many infectious diseases is afforded by prior exposure to the infectious agents.

Immuno electrophoresis The separation of different antigen-antibody systems by diffusion in an agar gel; a separate precipitation band in the gel detects each system.

Immunogen A substance that elicits a cellular immune response and/ or antibody production .

Immunoglobulin (IG) A member of a class of proteins that functions as an antibody. The wide range of different specifities of antibodies depends on subtle differences in their structure.

Immunoglobulin (IgA, IgD, IgE, IgG, and IgM) A class of serum proteins rich in antibodies. Often used, along with the more specific monoclonal antibodies, in diagnostic reagents in the health field.

Immunoglobulin A (IgA) The body's first line of defense against infectious diseases and is present in seromucous secretions such as saliva, tears, nasal fluids, sweat and secretions of the lung and genito-urinary and gastro-intestinal tracts.

Immunoglobulin Ig A protein of the globulin-type found in serum or other body fluids that possesses antibody activity. An individual Ig molecule is built up from two light (L) and two heavy (H) polypeptide chains linked together by disulfide bonds. Igs are divided into five classes based on antigenic and structural differences in the H chains.

Immunoglobulins Immunoglobulins, also known as antibodies, are proteins found in blood and in tissue fluids. Immunoglobulins are produced by cells of the immune system called B-lymphocytes. Their function is to bind to substances in the body that are recognized as foreign antigens (often proteins on the surface of bacteria and viruses). This binding is a crucial event in the destruction of the microorganisms that bear the antigens. Immunoglobulins also play a central role in allergies when they bind to antigens that are not necessarily a threat to health and provoke an inflammatory reaction.

Immunology The study of how the body defends itself against disease.

Immunophenotyping The recording of observable immunological characteristics of an individual, which result from interaction between the genes of that individual and the environment.

Immunoproteins All the proteins concerned with the immune system (antibodies, interferon, and cytokines).

Immunostimulancia Drugs inducing increased activity of the immune system thus increasing the body's immunity.

Immunosuppressives Drugs reducing the natural immunity of the body used, for example, after transplantation.

Immunotherapy Immunotherapy ("allergy shots") is a form of preventive and anti-inflammatory treatment of allergy to substances such as pollens, house dust mites, fungi, and stinging insect venom. Immunotherapy involves giving gradually increasing doses of the substance, or allergen, to which the person is allergic. The incremental increases of the allergen cause the immune system to become less sensitive to the substance, perhaps by causing production of a particular "blocking" antibody, which reduces the symptoms of allergy when the substances is encountered in the future.

Immunotoxins Semi-synthetic conjugates of various toxic molecules, including radioactive isotopes and bacterial or plant toxins, with specific immune substances such as immunoglobulins, monoclonal antibodies, and antigens. The antitumor or antiviral immune substance carries the toxin to the tumor or infected cell where the toxin exerts its poisonous effect.

Impartial witness A person, who is independent of the trial, who cannot be unfairly influenced by people involved with the trial, who attends the informed consent process if the subject or the subject's legally acceptable representative cannot read, and who reads the informed consent form and any other written information supplied to the subject.

Imprinting A biochemical phenomenon that determines, for certain genes, which one of the pair of alleles, the mother's or the father's, will be active in that individual.

Impurity Any component present in the intermediate or API (Active Pharmaceutical Ingredient) that is not the desired entity. It may be either process or product related.

Impurity profile A description of the identified and unidentified impurities present in a typical batch of API (Active Pharmaceutical Ingredient) produced by a specific controlled production process. It includes the identity or some qualitative analytical designation (e.g. retention time), the range of each impurity observed, and type of each identified impurity. For each API there should be an impurity profile describing the identified and unidentified impurities present in a typical batch. The impurity profile is normally dependent upon the process or origin of the API.

In hospital drug Drug administered during hospital confinement, not usually considered in studies of prescription drugs.

In line An integral part of the flow path. In a fluid stream, something is said to be in-line if the entire fluid stream flows directly through or past it.

In process control Checks performed during production in order to monitor and if necessary to adjust the process and/or to ensure that the intermediate or API (Active Pharmaceutical Ingredient) conforms to its specification. (also called Process Control)

In silico pharmacology Bioinformatics is used in drug target identification and validation and in the development of biomarkers and toxicogenomic and pharmacogenomic tools to maximize the therapeutic benefit of drugs. Now that the 'parts list' of cellular signalling pathways is available, integrated computational and experimental programmes are being developed, with the goal of enabling in silico pharmacology by linking the genome, transcriptome and proteome to cellular pathophysiology.

In situ Literally "in place" - in the natural or original position. For example, experimental treatments performed on organs or tissues in the body rather than after removal from the body (ex vivo) or on extracts from them (in vitro). An in situ model, e.g. rat brain perfusion, retains many of the natural physiological features of the whole animal, while minimizing or eliminating some of the variables inherent in performing an experiment in vivo.

In vivo Literally, "in the living being" (Latin). The term refers to a reaction or process that occurs in the body of a living organism. The advantage of in vivo studies is that they are performed in the most physiologically relevant setting, compared with in vitro, ex vivo, or in situ studies. On the other hand, in vivo studies suffer from the inherent complexity of a living organism, a multitude of variables and inter-individual variation. In vivo studies are necessary because many complex processes cannot be modeled in a simpler setting. In addition, the department of health requires that, prior to human clinical trials of a new chemical entity, some in vivo testing, e.g. toxicology, must be performed in animals. All researchers operate under an ethical and legal mandate to minimize the number of animals sacrificed in the name of research.

Inactivation Any process that destroys the ability of a specific microbiological agent or eukaryotic cell to self-replicate.

Inactive ingredient Any component other than an active ingredient.

Incidental release The discharge of a microbilogical agent or eukaryotic cell from a containment system that is expected when the system is appropriately designed and properly operated and maintained. Incidental releases are de minimis in nature.

Inclusion body Condensed particles of protein formed inside E. coli and other bacteria formed when the cells are forced to make large amounts of a product protein. The cells must be broken to harvest inclusion bodies.

Inclusion criteria The criteria that prospective subjects must meet to be eligible for participation in a study.

Inclusions Particles of foreign material in a metallic matrix. The particles are usually compounds such as oxides, sulfides, or silicates, but may be any substance foreign to and essentially insoluble in the matrix.

Incontinence Inability to retain urine

IND (investigational new drug) application A document filed with the department of health prior to clinical trial of a new drug. It gives a full description of the new drug, where and how is manufactured, all QC information, etc. The IND is followed by NDA (New Drug Application).

IND application Investigational new drug application authority given by the department of health following application to test drug products in patients

Independent data monitoring committee (IDMC)/Data and safety monitoring board (DSMB)/monitoring committee/Data monitoring committee An independent data monitoring committee that may be established by the sponsor to assess at intervals the progress of a clinical trial, the safety data, and the critical efficacy endpoints, and to recommend to the sponsor whether to continue, modify, or stop a trial.

Independent ethics committee (IEC)/ Institutional review board (IRB) An independent body (a review board or a committee, institutional, regional, national, or supranational), constituted of medical/ scientific professionals and nonmedical/ nonscientific members, whose responsibility it is to ensure the protection of the rights, safety, and well-being of human subjects involved in a trial and to provide public assurance of that protection, by, among other things, reviewing and approving/providing favorable opinion on the trial protocol, the suitability of the investigator(s), facilities, and the methods and material to be used in obtaining and documenting informed consent of the trial subjects. The legal status, composition, function, operations, and regulatory requirements pertaining to IECs / IRBs may differ among countries, but should allow the IECs / IRBs to act in agreement with good clinical practice (GCP).

Indication Indication is a circumstance, or a set of circumstances signalling the initiation of a certain treatment or diagnostic procedure, for example, drug administration; it is the opposite to contraindication.

Indinavir (Crixivan) Indications: Treatment of HIV infection in combination with other agents.

Contraindications: Known hypersensitivity.

Dosage: 800 mg po q8h on an empty stomach or with a non-fat meal. Patients should drink at least 48 ounces of fluid a day. Of note, bid dosing has decreased efficacy and should be avoided. When coadministered with ritonavir (100-200 mg po bid) as pharmacologic booster, dose is 800 mg po bid without food restrictions. There are many potential drug interactions, some of which require dosage modification

Toxicity: Nephrolithiasis, gastrointestinal intolerance, hyperbilirubinemia.

Indirect amine (agent) Compounds that can cause displacement of NA from storage vesicles (ie. amphetamine, tyramine). Note agents that inhibit neuronal uptake (uptake 1) can diminish the actions of indirect amines by preventing their uptake into the nerve terminal.

Indirect impact system An engineering system considered having no direct impact on product quality.

Indirect parasympathomimetic Agent that causes inhibition of acetylcholinesterase (AchE) to elevate Ach levels (ie. organophosphates).

Individualized medicine Another term for pharmacogenomics. One key issue for pharmacogenomics is just how individualized drug therapies are going to become. There is fundamental tension between the economics of faster and cheaper medical care and customized prescriptions and therapies. Haplotypes offer hope, as does the tradeoffs between liability for patients likely to encounter adverse events who can be screened out before they take a drug and the prospect of overly fragmented pharmaceutical segments.

Indomethacin A drug that belongs to the family of drugs called nonsteroidal anti-inflammatory drugs (NSAIDs). Indomethacin reduces pain, fever, swelling, and redness. It is also being used to reduce tumor-induced suppression of the immune system and to increase the effectiveness of anticancer drugs.

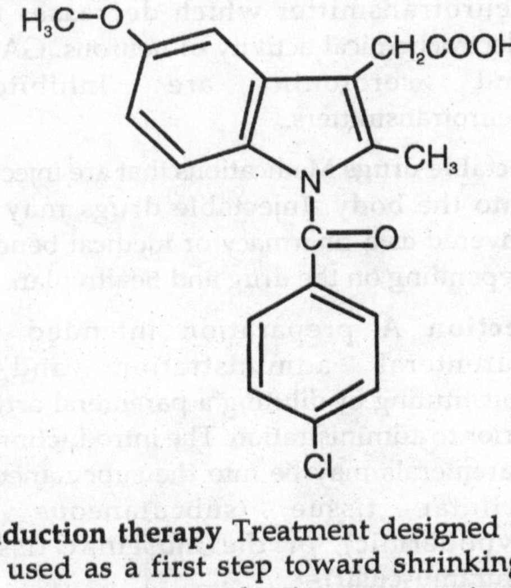

Induction therapy Treatment designed to be used as a first step toward shrinking the cancer and in evaluating response to drugs and other agents. Induction therapy is followed by additional therapy to eliminate whatever cancer remains.

Inert Does not dissolve in water or react chemically with other substances.

Infarct Tissue which has died due to a lack of oxygen resulting from a blood clot or blocking of an artery.

Infected Contaminated with extraneous biological agents and therefore capable of spreading infection.

Infectious Able to cause disease in a susceptible host.

Infectious agent A biological organism that can establish a process of infection.

Infiltration The entry of air from an adjoining room or from outdoors through wall and ceiling openings due to a difference in air pressure between the two areas.

Inflammation A localized protective response elicited by injury or destruction of tissues, which serves to destroy, dilute or isolate both the injurious agent and the injured tissue. It is characterized in the acute form by the classical signs of pain (dolor), heat (calor), redness (rubor), swelling (tumor) and loss of function. Histologically, it involves a complex series of events, including dilatation of arterioles, capillaries and venules, with increased permeability and blood flow, exudation of fluids, including plasma proteins and leucocytic migration into the inflammatory focus.

Infliximab A monoclonal antibody that blocks the action of a cytokine called tumor necrosis factor alfa. It is being studied in the treatment and prevention of weight loss and loss of appetite in patients with advanced cancer. It belongs to the family of drugs called monoclonal antibodies.

Informatics The study of the application of computer and statistical techniques to the management of information. In genome projects, informatics includes the development of methods to search databases quickly, to analyze DNA sequence information, and to predict protein sequence and structure from DNA sequence data.

Informed consent A process by which a subject voluntarily confirms his or her willingness to participate in a particular trial, after having been informed of all aspects of the trial that are relevant to the subject's decision to participate. Informed consent is documented by means of a written, signed, and dated informed consent form.No informed consent may include any "language through which the subject or the representative is made to waive or appear to waive any of the subject's legal rights, or releases or appears to release the investigator, the sponsor, the institution, or its agents from liability for negligence."

Infusion The introduction of parenterals into a vein (intravenous).

Infusion kinetics Infusion, as a means of drug administration, involves an effectively continuous flow of a drug solution into the blood stream over a relatively long period of time. (Intravascular injections are separate administrations of drug solutions, each over a short period of time.) A major purpose of an infusion is to maintain a steady blood or plasma concentration of drug over a long period of time, i.e. to achieve and maintain Css.

The Css achieved during infusion of a drug is directly proportional to the rate of drug administration (D/T, or k0), and inversely proportional to both the rate of elimination (kel), and to the volume of body throughout which the drug is distributed: Css = (D/T)/ kelVd. Since, kelVd equals total clearance: Css = (D/T)/ClT, or Css = k0/ClT. The concentration finally achieved varies directly with the infusion rate and indirectly with the total clearance of the drug (always assuming first-order elimination and a single compartment system).

For a drug given by infusion, and eliminated by first-order kinetics from a one-compartment system, the rate at which Css is achieved depends only on the half-life of the drug. In the absence of other doses (such as a loading dose [q.v.]) the plasma concentration at any time after beginning the infusion (CT), expressed as a fraction of the Css to be achieved, is given by (1 - f):

$$CT/Css = 1 - 0.5^{T/t½}$$

After duration of infusion of one half-life, 50% of the final concentration will have been achieved; after a duration of infusion of 4 half-lives, about 95% of the final concentration will have been achieved.

Infusion pumps When receiving an intravenous (IV) solution, infusion pumps can time, infuse and flush IVs automatically.

Inhibitors A substance that diminishes the rate of a chemical reaction. The process is called inhibition. Inhibitors are sometimes called negative catalysts but since the action of an inhibitor is fundamentally different from that of a catalyst this terminology is discouraged. In contrast to a catalyst, an inhibitor may be consumed in the course of a reaction.

Inhibitory neurotransmitter A neurotransmitter which decreases the electrochemical activity of neurons. GABA and serotonin are inhibitory neurotransmitters.

Injectable drugs Medications that are injected into the body. Injectable drugs may be covered as a pharmacy or medical benefit, depending on the drug and health plan.

Injection A preparation intended for parenteral administration and/or constituting or diluting a parenteral article prior to administration. The introduction of parenterals may be into the subcutaneous cellular tissue (subcutaneous or hypodermic), or the muscular tissue (Intramuscular).

Injury Means accidental bodily injury which is sustained directly and which is independent of all other causes.

Inoculum 1. Fermentation: an aliquot of a pure culture of microorganism added to the primary .

Inotropic therapy This therapy works to increase the force of the heart muscle so it pumps harder. Used mainly for weak or injured hearts, the medication works to relax the blood vessels so blood can move more freely allowing patients to perform daily activities more easily.

Inspection The act by a regulatory authority(ies) of conducting an official review of documents, facilities, records, and any other resources that are deemed by the authority(ies) to be related to the clinical trial and that may be located at the site of the trial, at the sponsor's and/or contract research organization's (CROs) facilities, or at other establishments deemed appropriate by the regulatory authority(ies).

Installation qualification [IQ] (PMA CSVC) Documented verificationthat all key aspects of [software and] hardware installation adhere toappropriate codes and approved design intentions and that therecommendations of the manufacturer have been suitably considered.

Institution (medical) Any public or private entity or agency or medical or dental facility where clinical trials are conducted.

Institutional review board (IRB) An independent body constituted of medical, scientific, and non-scientific members, whose responsibility is to ensure the protection of the rights, safety and well-being of human subjects involved in a trial by, among other things, reviewing, approving, and providing continuing review of trial protocol and amendments and of the methods and material to be used in obtaining and documenting informed consent of the trial subjects.

Insulin A hormone secreted by a group of cells in the pancreas in response to high blood sugar levels. Defective secretion of or response to insulin is the cause of diabetes.

Integration testing (IEEE) An orderly progression of testing in whichsoftware elements, hardware elements, or both are combined and testeduntil the entire system has been integrated.

Integrative and organ systems pharmacology "Pharmacological research using in vivo animal models or substantially intact organ systems that are able to display the integrated responses characteristic of the living organism that result from complex interactions between molecules, cells, and tissues."

Interaction Interaction means the mutual effect of drugs and of other substances coming into the organism (food, alcohol, nicotine, etc.); certain drugs or substances mutually increase their effects, while others on the contrary reduce them; the attending physician should always be informed about all drugs (including OTC drugs) which are being or will be administered to the patient; drugs with frequent interactions include, for example, certain anti-coagulants, antacids, anti-epileptics, laxatives and others.

Interface (ANSI/IEEE) A shared boundary. To interact or communicatewith another system component.

Interim Clinical Trial/Study ReportA report of intermediate results and their evaluation based on analyses performed during the course of a trial.

Internal consistency A property of data that does not contradict itself.

Internal standard A reference compound, known as an internal standard, is often added to biological samples, such as blood, plasma, urine or tissue samples, in order to diagnose and/or account for several potential sources of variability that can occur during sample preparation and analysis. These include:

normalization for initial volume of each sample,

verification of liquid transfer during robotic sample preparation,

verification of autosampler injection and normalization for injection volume,

normalization for instrument tuning and response,

verification of chromatographic retention time,

normalization for instrument drift over the course of the analysis, and

normalization for percent recovery during sample preparation.

Whenever possible, the structure of the internal standard should be similar to that of the analyte. Deuterated versions of the analyte are typical of this type of internal standard. When this is not possible, structurally dissimilar standards which elute with retention times similar to the analyte can be used.

Internet A global system of computer networks that provides the infrastructure for e-mail, the World Wide Web, and other online activities.

Internet service provider (ISP) A company that provides access to the Internet for individuals and organizations. ISPs range in size from small local services to huge national providers, like Netcom and AT&T, and international full-service providers.

Intervention Type The type of treatment used in a trial as specified by the protocol, e.g. Drug, Vaccine, Medical Device.

Intrathecal Refers to drugs administered into the cerebrospinal fluid bathing the spinal cord and brain.

Intrinsic activity The maximal stimulatory response induced by a compound in relation to that of a given reference compound .This term has evolved with common usage. It was introduced by Ariëns as a proportionality factor between tissue response and receptor occupancy. The numerical value of intrinsic activity (alpha) could range from unity (for full agonists, i.e., agonist inducing the tissue maximal response) to zero (for antagonists), the fractional values within this range denoting partial agonists. Ariëns' original definition equates the molecular nature of alpha to maximal response only when response is a linear function of receptor occupancy. This function has been verified. Thus, intrinsic activity, which is a drug and tissue parameter, cannot be used as a characteristic drug parameter for classification of drugs or drug receptors. For this purpose, a proportionality factor derived by null methods, namely, relative efficacy, should be used. Finally, "intrinsic activity" should not be used instead of "intrinsic efficacy". A "partial agonist" should be termed "agonist with intermediate intrinsic efficacy" in a given tissue.

Intrinsic asthma Intrinsic asthma is asthma that has no apparent external cause.

Intrinsic efficacy (or intrinsic activity) The property of a drug that determines the amount of biological effect produced per unit of drug-receptor complex formed. Two agents combining with equivalent sets of receptors may not produce equal degrees of effect even if both agents are given in maximally effective doses; the agents differ in their intrinsic activities and the one producing the greater maximum effect has the greater intrinsic activity. Intrinsic activity is not the same as "potency" and may be completely independent of it. Meperidine and morphine presumably combine with the same receptors to produce analgesia, but regardless of dose, the maximum degree of analgesia produced by morphine is greater than that produced by meperidine; morphine has the greater intrinsic activity. Intrinsic activity - like affinity - depends on the chemical natures of both the drug and the receptor, but intrinsic activity and affinity apparently can vary independently with changes in the drug molecule.

The fraction of C0 remaining at some specified time after drug administration; more generally, the fraction of C, or AB, remaining after some specified time interval. For first-order, single compartment systems (i.e. those yielding a single straight line when log C is plotted against t), f can be determined from the relationship: log C = log C0 - b t. When t is the time after drug administration, or the interval between two administrations, and t½ is the elimination half-life of the drug, f is 0.5 raised to a power that is the ratio of the time interval to the elimination half-life, i.e., 0.5t/t½.

The fraction of a dose which is absorbed and enters the systemic circulation following administration of a drug by any route other than the intravenous route; the availability of drug to tissues of the body, generally. When the total clearance and the dose of drug administered are known, F can be determined from the relationship: (AUC x CIT)/D = F. When identical doses of a drug have been given by the intravenous and by some other route (x), and the AUCs have been determined, the bioavailability of the drug after administration by route X can be determined: F=AUCx/AUCiv. The amount of free drug recovered in the urine (AU) after administration of identical doses given intravenously and by route X can also be used to determine

Intrinsic sympathomimetic activity Beta-blocker that has partial agonist action. Has potential to prevent bradycardia or negative inotropy in resting heart (if 1 partial agonist) and to prevent bronchoconstraction (if 2 partial agonist). Pindolol is prototype agent.

Invasion Refers to the direct migration and penetration by cancer cells into neighboring tissues.

Investigational new drug The purpose of an IND application is to provide data showing that it is reasonable to begin tests of a new drug in humans.

There are three IND types:

An Investigator IND is submitted by a physician who both initiates and conducts an investigation, and under whose immediate direction the investigational drug is administered or dispensed. A physician might submit a research IND to propose studying an unapproved drug, or an approved product for a new indication or in a new patient population.

An Emergency Use IND allows the department of health to authorize use of an experimental drug in an emergency situation that does not allow time for submission of an IND in accordance with the normal process. It is also used for patients who do not meet the criteria of an existing study protocol, or if an approved study protocol does not exist.

A treatment IND is submitted for experimental drugs showing promise in clinical testing for serious or immediately life-threatening conditions while the final clinical work is conducted and department of health review takes place.

There are two IND categories:

Commercial

Research (non-commercial)

The IND application must contain information in three broad areas:

Animal pharmacology and toxicology studies

Manufacturing information

Clinical protocols and investigator information

Once the IND is submitted, the sponsor must wait 30 calendar days before initiating any clinical trials. During this time, the department of health has an opportunity to review the IND for safety to ensure that research subjects will not be subjected to unreasonable risk.

Investigational product A pharmaceutical form of an active ingredient or placebo being tested or used as a reference in a clinical trial, including a product with a marketing authorization when used or assembled (formulated or packaged) in a way different from the approved form, or when used for an unapproved indication, or when used to gain further information about an approved use.

Investigator A person responsible for the conduct of the clinical trial at a trial site. If a trial is conducted by a team of individuals at a trial site, the investigator is the responsible leader of the team and may be called the principal investigator.

Investigator/institution An expression meaning "the investigator and/or institution, where required by the applicable regulatory requirements." (ICH)

Investigator's brochure A compilation of the clinical and nonclinical data on the investigational product(s) that is relevant to the study of the investigational product(s) in human subjects.

Ion channels Enable ions to flow rapidly through membranes in a thermodynamically downhill direction after an electrical or chemical impulse.

Gated, ion-selective glycoproteins that traverse membranes. The stimulus for channel gating can be a membrane potential, drug, transmitter, cytoplasmic messenger, or a mechanical deformation. Ion channels which are integral parts of ionotropic neurotransmitter receptors are not included.

IP Intellectual Property.

IPL Acronym used for individually produced drugs; it means the drugs prepared in the pharmacy usually according to a breakdown specified by the physician on the prescription.

IPO Initial Public Offering.

IRB Institutional review board.

Irinotecan Newer drug used for large bowel cancers.

Isoniazid (INH) Indications: Treatment of TB in combination with other agents; prophylaxis of TB in context of positive PPD.

Contraindications: Known hypersensitivity, significant hepatic disease.

Dosage: Treatment: 300 mg po qd (or 900 mg twice a week [DOT]); prophylaxis: 300 mg po qd for nine months. Pyridoxine should be given concurrently for prevention of peripheral neuropathy.

Toxicity: Hepatotoxicity, especially in alcoholics and persons older than 50; peripheral neuropathy; fever; rash.

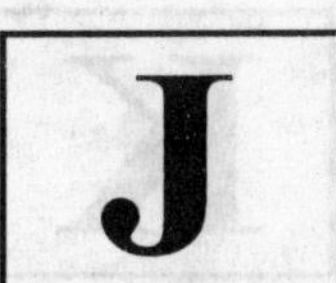

Joint venture Specific kind of cooperation between different companies.

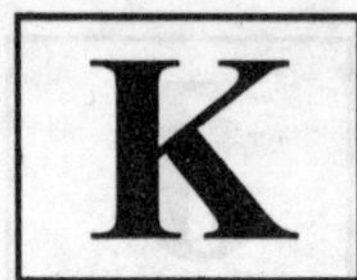

K0 The "absorption rate constant" when rate of absorption (D/T) does not vary. k0 describes the rate at which drug enters the body during constant-rate intravenous infusions, or during use of "sustained" release preparations for oral or transdermal drug administration.

Ka The "absorption rate constant" for a drug administered by a route other than the intravenous. The rate of absorption of a drug absorbed from its site of application according to first-order kinetics. ka is determined directly, or indirectly, as the slope of the linear relationship between the logarithm of the amount un absorbed and t, when natural logarithms, i.e. logarithms to the base e, are used. The half-time for absorption is computed as 0.693/ka, i.e. ln 2/ka.

Karenitecin A drug being studied in the treatment of cancer. It belongs to a family of drugs called topoisomerase inhibitors. It is related to the anticancer drug camptothecin.

Karyotype A photomicrograph of an individual's chromosomes arranged in a standard format showing the number, size, and shape of each chromosome type. It is used in low-resolution physical mapping to correlate gross chromosomal abnormalities with the characteristics of specific diseases.

Kel The "elimination rate constant" for a drug eliminated according to the laws of first-order reaction kinetics; the slope of the plot of the logarithm of concentration against time, when natural logarithms, i.e. logarithms to the base e, are used.

$t_{1/2} = 0.693/kel$. $kel = 2.303b$. $ClT = kel\ Vd$. AUC from Tn to infinity = Cn/Kel.

Keratins Insoluble protective or structural proteins consisting of parallel polypeptide chains in a-helical or b-conformation.

Ketoconazole A drug that treats infection caused by a fungus. It is also used as a treatment for prostate cancer because it can block the production of male sex hormones.

Ketorolac A drug that belongs to a family of drugs called nonsteroidal anti-inflammatory agents. It is being studied in cancer prevention.

Ketose A simple monosaccharide having its carbonyl groups at other than a terminal position. Kilobase (kb) Unit of length for

DNA fragments equal to 1000 nucleotides (kilo base pairs of DNA).

Kinase A class of enzymes that catalyze the transfer of a terminal phosphate group from ATP to another molecule. Kinases are involved in a wide variety of intracellular signalling pathways, and as such are targets for many therapeutic approaches.

LC/MS/MS

liquid chromatography - tandem mass spectrometry

Mass spectrometry (MS) is an analytical technique to measure the mass-to-charge ratio (m/z) of ions. It is most generally used to find the composition of a physical sample by generating a mass spectrum representing the masses of the components of a sample. It has several broad applications: 1. Identifying unknown compounds by the mass of the compound and/or fragments thereof.

2. Determining the isotopic composition of one or more elements in a compound.

3. Determining the structure of compounds by observing the fragmentation of the compound.

4. Quantitating the amount of a compound in a sample using carefully designed methods (mass spectrometry is not inherently quantitative).

5. Studying the fundamentals of gas phase ion chemistry (the chemistry of ions and neutrals in vacuum).

6. Determining other physical, chemical or even biological properties of compounds with a variety of other approaches.

A mass spectrometer is a device used for mass spectrometry, and produces a mass spectrum of a sample to find its composition. This is normally achieved by ionizing the sample and separating ions of differing masses and recording their relative abundance by measuring intensities of ion flux. A typical mass spectrometer comprises three parts: an ion source, a mass analyzer, and a detector.

Liquid chromatography (LC) is the science of separating molecules, applied in a liquid mobile phase, based on differences in affinity for a solid stationary phase relative to the mobile phase, often while varying the composition of the mobile phase.

In LC/MS/MS, molecules are partially resolved by rapid LC, followed by detection via tandem mass spectrometry (MS/MS). This mode of detection is exquisitely sensitive due to the operator's ability to tune the instrument to a particular m/z value to the exclusion of other molecular species that may be present.

Kinetic outliers Intersubject variability - in particular, the presence of kinetic outliers - is encountered during the course of a drug development program. Often, these outliers can be explained by genetic variability or polymorphism in cytochrome CYP450 genes responsible for drug metabolism. Genetic analysis of outliers could help explain the variability in metabolism and possibly influence the development and labeling of the drug in question.

Knock down A modulated reduction of gene expression.

Knockout models Models, such as laboratory mice, which have had a normal gene replaced by a marker, providing clues as to the missing or "knocked-out" gene's relation to organ development, viability and reproduction.

Knockout or gene knockout Informal term for the generation of a mutant organism in which the function of a particular gene has been eliminated.

KRN5500 An anticancer drug that belongs to a family of drugs called antitumor antibiotics. It is an anthracycline.

KRN7000 A drug being studied in the treatment of cancer. It is a biological response modifier that belongs to the family of drugs called glycosphingolipids or agelasphins.

KUDCO Kremers Urban Development Company is the wholly owned U.S. generic drug business of SCHWARZ PHARMA Inc., U.S.A.

L

L If followed by a number, a chromatographic column packing. E. g.: L1 is octadecyl silane chemically bonded to porous silica or ceramic particles 3 to 10 µm in diameter. Defined in USP/NF.

Label The information on the 'immediate' container of an item.

Labeling Information on the label and all other material accompanying the product.

Labile Unstable or unsteady; not fixed; characterized by adaptability to alteration or modification, i.e., relatively easily changed, as in cleavage of a molecule or molecular rearrangement in a compound or complex chemical material.

Laboratory study Research done in a laboratory. These studies may use test tubes or animals to find out if a drug, procedure, or treatment is likely to be useful. Laboratory studies take place before any testing is done in humans.

Laboratory test A medical procedure that involves testing a sample of blood, urine, or other substance from the body. Tests can help determine a diagnosis, plan treatment, check to see if treatment is working, or monitor the disease over time.

LAL (limulus amoebocyte lysate) A material obtained by rupturing the cellular components of the blood of a horseshoe crab (Limulus Poliphemus). This material coagulates in the presence of LPS (lypopolysaccharides) and is a test used to quantitate bacterial endotoxins (pyrogens).

Laminar airflow - clean work station A workstation in which the unidirectional airflow characteristics predominate throughout the entire airspace with a minimum of eddies (turbulence) to jeopardize critical surfaces.

Laminar flow Non-turbulent fluid flow is usually considered laminar if the Reynolds number is less than 2000 in a pipe. Depending upon many possible varying conditions, the flow may be laminar at a Reynolds number as low as 1,200 or as high as 40,000; however, such conditions are not experienced in normal practice. In the pharmaceutical industry, this term incorrectly refers to the air discharge of a clean air bench or wall.

Lamivudine (3TC, Epivir) Indications: Treatment of HIV infection in combination with other agents. Also has activity against hepatitis B virus.

Contraindications: Known hypersensitivity.

Dosage: 150 mg po bid. Also available as Combivir, a fixed dose combination of ZDV

300 mg with 3TC 150 mg; and Trizivir, a fixed dose combination of ZDV 300 mg, 3TC 150 mg, and abacavir 300 mg.

Toxicity: Uncommon. Headache, gastrointestinal intolerance, and insomnia have been reported.

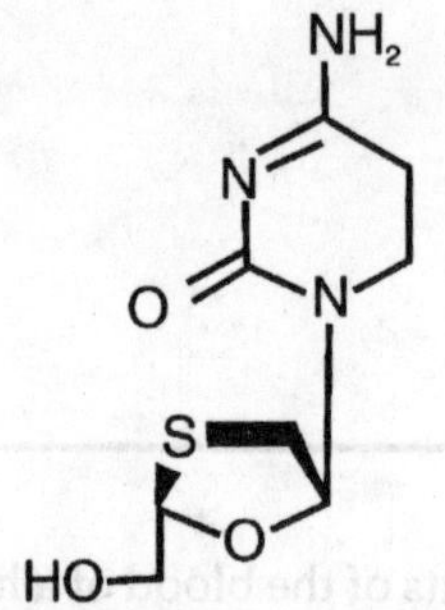

LAN (local area network) Networks with computers geographically close together (that is, in the same building).

Langelier index A measure of the degree of saturation of calcium carbonate in water that is based on pH, alkalinity and hardness. If the Langelier Index is negative, the water is corrosive (pH value below 7 or acidic). If the Langelier Index is positive, calcium carbonate can precipitate out of solution to form scale (pH value above 7 or basic). The Langelier Index will vary for cold water and for warm water.

Latency period The period of time which must elapse between the time at which a dose of drug is applied to a biologic system and the time at which a specified pharmacologic effect is produced. In general, the latent period varies inversely with dose; the relationship between dose and latent period for a given agent is described by a time-dose or time-concentration curve.

Latent heat The amount of heat needed to change a unit of substance, such as water, from a solid to a liquid without change in temperature or pressure.

Latent period or latency The period of time that must elapse between the time at which a dose of drug is applied to a biologic system and the time at which a specified pharmacologic effect is produced. In general, the latent period varies inversely with dose; the relationship between dose and latent period for a given agent is described by a time-dose or time-concentration curve.

Laxatives Laxatives are natural or synthetic substances stimulating the emptying of the intestines; some people can develop dependence, therefore their administration should be limited.

Lay In metallurgy, the direction of the predominant surface pattern ordinarily determined by the production method used.

LD 50 The dose of a substance that will kill half (50%) of the treated test animals when given as a single dose. A measure of acute toxicity.

LDH LDH is a material found in blood cells and liver cells. Breakdown of the blood cells as in heart disease or liver damage may increase values.

Leach To dissolve by the action of a moving liquid. For example, high purity water leaches trace impurities from glass vessels.

Lead optimization A portion of the drug discovery continuum, lead optimization is the complex process of refining the chemical structure of a "hit" to improve its drug characteristics, with the goal of producing a pre-clinical drug candidate. Typically, by the lead optimization stage many compounds have been screened and many "hits" discarded for various reasons. At this stage, analogues of a biologically active compound or a series of structurally related compounds are synthesized, the goal being to find a molecule with the most favorable combination of physicochemical, e.g. solubility, pharmacologic, e.g. therapeutic efficacy, pharmacokinetic, e.g. metabolic stability, and toxicologic, i.e. safety, properties.

Learning A change in neural function as a consequence of experience.

Leg A leg, in the context of an in vivo study, refers to the dosing of an animal or group of animals that is an independently executed part of a multi-part study. Thus, a five-legged dog study does not mean that the experiment is done using dogs having five legs; rather, it might be a study with a control (untreated) group and four dose levels of a test compound.

Legacy systems Hardware and software applications in which a company has already invested considerable time and money. Legacy systems typically perform critical operations in companies for many years even though they may no longer use state-of-the-art technology. Replacing legacy systems can be disruptive and therefore requires careful planning and appropriate migration support from the manufacturer.

Legally acceptable representative An individual or juridical or other body authorized under applicable law to consent, on behalf of a prospective subject, to the subject's participation in the clinical trial.

Leptospira A genus of the family Treponemataceae, thin coiled organisms, flagellated at the extremities, one or both of which are bent back like a hook. Both pathogenic and innocent forms have been isolated.

Letrozole An anticancer drug that belongs to the family of drugs called nonsteroidal aromatase inhibitors. Letrozole is used to decrease estrogen production and suppress the growth of estrogen-dependent tumors.

Leucovorin A drug used to protect normal cells from high doses of the anticancer drug methotrexate. It is also used to increase the antitumor effects of fluorouracil and tegafur-uracil, an oral treatment alternative to intravenous fluorouracil.

H_2N N H N H N N N HO O H COOH N O COOH

Leukemia Cancers of the immature blood cells that grow in the bone marrow and tend to accumulate in large numbers in the bloodstream. Precision does not currently accept these specimens for testing with ChemoFx.

Leukocyte A general name for white, nucleated blood cells found in the blood and lymphatic tissue.

Leuprolide A drug that belongs to the family of drugs called gonadotropin-releasing hormone analogs. It is used to block hormone production in the ovaries or testicles.

Leuvectin An agent that delivers the gene for interleukin-2 (IL-2) into cells to increase production of IL-2 by the cells.

Levamisole An antiparasitic drug that is also being studied in cancer therapy with fluorouracil.

Level of evidence 1ia Randomized, controlled, double-blinded clinical trial with total mortality as an endpoint.

Level of product protection The level of protection required for an area based on an assessment by the manufacturer of contamination risk.

Levocarnitine A form of carnitine, which is a substance made in the muscles and liver. It can be given as a supplement to prevent and treat carnitine deficiency in patients who are receiving chemotherapy for cancer or undergoing dialysis for kidney disease. Also called L-carnitine.

Levofloxacin A substance used to treat bacterial infections. It belongs to the family of drugs called quinolone antibiotics.

LGD1069 An anticancer drug used to decrease the growth of some types of cancer cells. It belongs to the family of drugs called retinoids. Also called bexarotene.

LH RH Luteinizing hormone-releasing hormone. A hormone that stimulates the production of sex hormones in men and women.

Lidocaine A substance that is used to relieve pain by blocking signals at the nerve endings in skin. It can also be given intravenously to stop heart arrhythmias. It belongs to the families of drugs called local anesthetics and antiarrhythmics.

H
N
N
O

2-(diethylamino)–N-(2,6-dimethylphenyl) acetamide monohydrochloride

Life cycle concept (PMA CSVC) An approach to computer systemdevelopment that begins with identification of the user's requirements,continues through design, integration, qualification, user validation, control and maintenance, and ends only when commercial use of thesystem is discontinued.

Ligand Any molecule that binds to another, in normal usage a soluble molecule such as a hormone or neurotransmitter, that binds to a receptor.

Ligand gated ion channel A transmembrane ion channel whose permeability is increased by the binding of a specific ligand, typically a neurotransmitter at a chemical synapse. The permeability change is often drastic, such channels let through effectively no ions when shut, but allow passage at up to 107 ions/sec when a ligand is bound.

Ligase An enzyme used to catalyze the joining of single-stranded DNA segments.

Like Many other physiological "constants," renal plasma clearance varies regularly and exponentially with body weight, across mammalian species (Science 109: 757, 1949). Renal plasma clearances, in normal animals, can be predicted using the following relationships, where Cl R is in ml/hr, and body weight (B) is in grams:

ClR (inulin) = 1.74B0.77

ClR (PAH) = 5.40B0.80

Nonrenal Clearance:

Clearance by the fecal route (ClF), respiratory route (ClL), salivary route (ClS), biliary route (ClB), can be computed in a fashion analogous to computation of ClR: measuring the amount of substance excreted in the feces, expired air, saliva, etc., over an interval and dividing by the plasma concentration at mid-interval and the length of the interval. Following oral administration of a substance, measurement of fecal clearance may be confounded by the presence, in feces, of unabsorbed substance or of substance absorbed but excreted into the lumen of the gastrointestinal tract in, e.g., bile. Specialized techniques exist for estimating clearance of substances by the liver (ClH), by biotransformation and/or biliary excretion.

Unlike half-lives, clearances are directly additive and for any substance:

ClT = ClR + ClL + ClH + ClS + ClF + . . . etc.

Limit of detection The lowest concentration of an analyte that can be detected reliably (present or absent) in a particular sample. Exact definitions vary.

Limit of quantitation The lowest concentration of an analyte that can be determined quantitatively (at acceptable precision) in a particular sample. Exact definitions vary.

Limit tests Typically qualitative tests which show whether the concentration of a particular substance is above or below the USP/NF limit (usually for arsenic, calcium, sodium, potassium, chloride, sulfate, heavy metals, iron, or selenium). Some limit tests are much more extensive, notably those for lead and mercury. Microbial limit tests are usually for total aerobic count, or for presence of Staphylococcus aureus, Pseudomonas aeruginosa, Salmonella, or Escherichia coli in substances which are not required to be sterile.

Limits of quantitation The lowest and highest concentrations of analyte in a sample that can be quantitatively determined with suitable precision and accuracy. The lower limit of quantification (LLOQ) is often defined by an arbitrary cut-off, e.g., the concentration at which the signal-to-noise ratio is equal to 10:1 or the signal is equal to the mean of the negative control plus 5 times the standard deviation of the negative control values. The upper limit of quantification (ULOQ) is the highest concentration value for which the precision meets a pre-determined standard, or the highest concentration on the standard curve, whichever is lower.

LIMS Laboratory Information Management System.

Linearity For an analytical method, linearity is the ability of the assay to return values that are directly proportional to the concentration of the analyte in the sample. Mathematical data transformations, to obtain linearity, may be allowed if there is scientific evidence that the transformation is appropriate for the method. For a biological assay, linearity often refers to a time course in which the measured response is proportional to incubation time. The time course of all biological assays reaches a plateau (i.e., becomes non-linear) at some point, due to depletion of substrate or cofactors, denaturation of enzyme, etc. Many biological assays are conducted such that a single measurement is obtained in the linear portion of the time course, thereby allowing the determination of a reaction rate from a single time point.

Linkage map A map of the relative positions of genetic loci on a chromosome, determined on the basis of how often the loci are inherited together. Distance is measured in centimorgans (cM).

Linkage The proximity of two or more markers (e.g., genes, RFLP markers) on a chromosome; the closer together the markers are, the lower the probability that they will be separated during DNA repair or replication processes (binary fission in prokaryotes, mitosis or meiosis in eukaryotes), and hence the greater the probability that they will be inherited together.

Lipids Hydrophobic biological compounds (fats and fatlike materials) that are insoluble in water, but soluble in nonpolar solvents such as benzene, chloroform, and ether. The major components in most lipids are fatty acids.

Lipofuscin The brown waste material deposited in skin and nerve cells that is commonly called "age spots." Lipofuscin is made of free radical damaged proteins and fats.

Lipoprotein A conjugated protein containing a lipid, prosthetic group.

Lipoproteins Proteins combined with lipids that serve as carriers of cholesterol. LDL ("Bad" Cholesterol); HDL ("Good" Cholesterol). The higher the value, the less likely that cholesterol deposits are in the blood stream and the less likely the chance of coronary heart disease. Cholesterol/HDL ratio measures the coronary risk factors.

Liposome An artificial phospholipid vesicle. Liposomes can be useful for the enclosure of macromolecules such as nucleic acids or, after loading with an appropriate drug. They may be used therapeutically to achieve slow release of the drug into circulation.

Liver spots Deposits of lipofuscin in the skin.

Loading dose A larger than normal dose (D*) administered as the first in a series of doses, the others of which are smaller than D* but equal to each other. The loading dose is administered in order to achieve a therapeutic amount in the body more rapidly than would occur only by accumulation of the repeated smaller doses. The smaller doses (D) which are given after D* are called "maintenance doses". The effect of D* on C becomes relatively less with each succeeding maintenance dose; finally Css,max and Css,min are determined by D, and are uninfluenced by D*.

The relative sizes of D and D* can be adjusted so that peak plasma concentrations (Cmax) are the same following every dose, including the first with D*, and all are equal to Css,max. These conditions are met when D/D* = 1-f.

Local anesthesia Drugs that cause a temporary loss of feeling in one part of the body. The patient remains awake but has no feeling in the part of the body treated with the anesthetic.

Localize Determination of the original position (locus) of a gene or other marker on a chromosome.

Locus (pl. loci) The position on a chromosome of a gene or other chromosome marker; also, the DNA at that position. The use of locus is sometimes restricted to mean regions of DNA that are expressed.

Log D Log D is the base 10 logarithm of the partition coefficient of a compound between a buffer of fixed pH and an organic solvent, typically octanol or hexane. Both the solvent and the pH of the buffer must be specified in order to correctly interpret the value. Log D is considered one of the most useful basic physicochemical measurements of a compound.

Long range restriction mapping Restriction enzymes are proteins that cut DNA at precise locations. Restriction maps depict the positions on chromosomes of restriction enzyme cutting sites. These are used as biochemical "signposts", or markers of specific areas along the chromosomes. The map will detail the positions on the DNA molecule that are cut by particular restriction enzymes.

Longitudinal study Investigation in which data are collected from a number of subjects over a long period of time (a well-known example is the Framingham Study).

Loop testing Checking the installed combination of elementscharacterising each type of input/output loop.

Lopinavir/Ritonavir (Kaletra) Indications: Treatment of HIV infection in combination with other agents.

Lopinavir is a new protease inhibitor combined with ritonavir, which significantly augments its blood level.

Contraindications: Known hypersensitivity, concurrent use of ritonavir.

Dosage: Three (133 mg lopinavir/33 mg ritonavir) po bid. . There are many potential drug interactions, some of which require dosage modification

Toxicity: Diarrhea, nausea, weakness, headache.

Low level review of software Purposes: .

Detect possible coding errors.

Dtermine adherence to design specs.

Dtermine adherence to standards.

Implement path analyses Characteristics: .

Requires highly trainedexperts who are familiar with software/hardware systems on whichprogram is based. .

To conduct low-level line-by-line source code inspection requires ateam of experts working no more that two 2 hour sessions/ day; thismeans about 100-150 lines of code per man-day (1.5 million lines = 40man years)Use: chiefly during software development.

Lower flammability level (LFL) The minimum concentration of vapor in air at which propagation of flame will occur in the presence of an ignition source. LFL is sometimes referred to as LEL or Lower Explosive Limit.

LPS (Lipopolysaccharide) Molecule found in the outer cell walls of some bacteria that trigger the immune response resulting in fever. Also referred to as pyrogens or as endotoxins, though, strictly speaking, they are not endotoxins but predominant components of endotoxins produced by gram-negative bacteria. Common cause of pyrogenic reactions in parenteral products.

LY231514 A drug that is used to treat malignant pleural mesothelioma and advanced non-small cell lung cancer and is being studied in the treatment of other types of cancer. It belongs to the family of drugs called enzyme inhibitors. Also called Alimta and pemetrexed disodium.

LY293111 A substance that is being studied as a treatment for cancer. It belongs to the family of drugs called leukotriene B4 receptor antagonists.

LY317615 A substance that is being studied in the treatment of cancer. It belongs to the families of drugs called protein kinase C inhibitors and angiogenesis inhibitors. Also called enzastaurin.

Lymphocyte A lymphocyte is any of a group of white blood cells of crucial importance to the adaptive part of the body's immune system. The adaptive portion of the immune system mounts a tailor-made defense when dangerous invading organisms penetrate the body's general defenses.

Lymphoma Cancers that arise in the lymph nodes and tissues of the body's immune system. Lymphomas are divided into two categories: Hodgkin's and non-Hodgkin's lymphomas. Precision does not currently accept these specimens for testing with ChemoFx.

Lyophilization Also known as freeze drying, it is a means of stabilizing wet substances by freezing them, then evaporating the resulting ice, to leave a substantially dry, porous residue which has the same size and shape of the original frozen mass.

Lyophilizer A freeze dryer.

Lysate A product of lysis, which is the disintegration or dissolution of the cell walls.

Lysergic acid diethylamide (LSD) A semi-synthetic drug, was first synthesised by Albert Hofmann in 1938. Basic material for the semi-synthetically production of LSD are the lysergic acid compounds of the ergot (sclerotia/spore capsule of a parasite mushroom). .

On the illicit drug market LSD has been sold in the form of impregnated paper (blotters/ trips), microdots, thin squares of gelatine (window panes), or impregnated on sugar cubes. Stamps or blotters are the common dose form. They are made by impregnating paper with a solution of LSD in alcohol. These papers are "trade marked" with various designs.

Lysine As essential, basic amino acid obtained from many proteins by hydrolysis.

Lysis The dissolution or destruction of red blood cells, bacteria, or other antigens by a specific lysin (antibody), or by the action of detergents, thus allowing the cell contents to escape.

Lysosome A membrane-surrounded organelle in the cytoplasm of eukaryotic cells; it contains many hydrolytic enzymes.

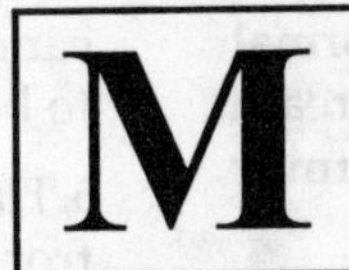

MAb Monoclonal Antibody)

Machine code (ANSI/IEEE) A representation of instructions and datathat is directly executable by a computer (machine language).

Machine lines/process lines Surface topography created from machining or honing/polishing lines will normally run parallel but bisecting (perpendicular) lines may occur when the honing stone mandrel is removed from the work piece.

Machine welding Welding with equipment that performs the welding operation under the constant observation and control of a welding operator. The equipment may or may not perform the loading and unloading of the works.

Macromolecules Molecules whose molecular weights are greater than about 5,000 Daltons.

Macroparticle Particle with an equivalent diameter greater than 5 µm. ISO/FDIS 14644-1.

Macrophage A phagocytic cell of the immune system found in blood and connective tissue and involved in removing debris after injury.

Macrorestriction map Map depicting the order of and distance between sites at which restriction enzymes cleave chromosomes.

Macroreticular resin An ion exchange resin with a reticular porous matrix that makes it effective for removing colloids and bacteria from process streams, as well as dissolved anions. It is especially useful for preventing colloidal and organic fouling of mixed-bed resins and premature clogging of final filters.

Magnesium An element absorbed in the intestine. Abnormal levels are found in pancreatitis, alcoholism and Addison's disease.

Maintainability Ease with which maintenance can be performed.

Maintenance drug Any prescription drug that requires more than a 34-day supply. Most are used on a steady, year-round basis for a long-term illness.

Major change (PMA CSVC) A change to a validated system that, in theopinion of change-control reviewers, necessitates a revalidation of thesystem.

Makeup air External air introduced to the air handling system for ventilation and pressurization.

Malignant effusion An abnormal fluid collection containing cancerous cells.

Malignant Malignant characterizes cells that can be distinguished from normal cells based on their microscopic appearance, expression of abnormal proteins and capacity to invade and spread to other portions of the body via invasion or metastasis. By definition, the term "cancer" applies only to malignant tumors.

Malignant tumor A cancerous tumor, which may spread from its original location to invade normal tissues and interfere with organ functions. If it is not treated, abnormal cells may spread through the blood stream or lymphatic system and form a tumor elsewhere in the body.

Manual welding Welding in which the entire operation is performed and controlled completely by hand.

Manufacture All operations of receipt of materials, production, packaging, repackaging, labelling, relabelling, quality control, release, storage and distribution of APIs and the related controls.

Manufacturing process (biotechnology) The basic processes for rDNA fermentation and purification normally include the following steps: 1. Inoculum Preparation: The aim is to develop for the production stage fermentation a pure inoculum in sufficient volume and in the fast-growing (logarithmic) phases so that a high population density is obtained. This is accomplished through a seed fermentation train.

2. The Medium: This is designed to provide the microorganism with all the nutrients it requires. Provision is usually made to add nutrients during fermentation.

3. Oxygen Supply: An adequate supply of oxygen is required. As oxygen is only slightly soluble in water, a number of methods are used to make oxygen more readily available to the microorganisms in the broth, including sparging, mechanical agitators, and dispersion baffles in the fermenter tank.

4. Temperature Control: Heat is generated both by the metabolism of nutrients and by the power dissipated in stirring and has to be removed by controlled cooling. Tank jackets or internal coils are used to control temperature.

5. Antifoam Agents: Microbiological systems that are vigorously stirred and aerated usually produce foam. Excessive foam cannot be tolerated and so provisions have to be made for adding antifoam agents.

6. Harvesting: This is the removal of the cells from the broth. This can be accomplished by cross-flow filtration or centrifugation.

7. Cell Lysis: With E. coli fermentations, the product protein is contained within the cell in the form of an inclusion body. High-pressure homogenizers are often used to chop up the E. coli bacteria into fine fragments, liberating the inclusion bodies for further processing.

8. Purification: This is the separation of the desired product from the other constituents in the harvested broth. Various processes including refolding, ultrafiltration/diafiltration, centrifugation, and chromatographic columns are employed to purify the product.

Marker An identifiable physical location on a chromosome (e.g., restriction enzyme cutting site, gene) whose inheritance can be monitored. Markers can be expressed regions of DNA (genes) or some segment of DNA with no known coding function but whose pattern of inheritance can be determined.

Market capitalization Indicator for a company's current value.

Mast cell Mast cells play an important role in the body's allergic response. Mast cells are present in most body tissues, but are particularly numerous in connective tissue, such as the dermis (innermost layer) of skin. In an allergic response, an allergen stimulates the release of antibodies, which attach themselves to mast cells. Following subsequent allergen exposure, the mast cells release substances such as histamine (a chemical responsible for allergic symptoms) into the tissue.

Master seed lot A culture of a microorganism distributed from a single bulk into containers in a single operation in such a manner as to ensure uniformity, to prevent contamination and to ensure stability. A master seed lot in liquid form is usually stored at or below -70ºC. A freeze-dried master seed lot is stored at a temperature known to ensure stability.

Matched pair design A type of parallel trial design in which investigators identify pairs of subjects who are "identical" with respect to relevant factors, then randomize them so that one receives Treatment A and the other Treatment B.

Material A general term used to denote raw materials (starting materials, reagents, process aids, solvents) intermediates, APIs (Active Pharmaceutical Ingredients) and packaging and labelling materials.

Material containment The method to incorporate suitable measures into design procedures and operational practices for the containment of materials that can harm personnel and the workplace environment, and minimize potential for cross contamination and housekeeping concerns in the fine chemical, bulk pharmaceutical and pharmaceutical industries. Solids and/or liquids are normally most hazardous in the form of powders and have been divided into the following three categories: 1. Biologically Hazardous additives are compounds that when contacting a living cell, will alter, endanger, or damage the cell in some shape or form. These should be treated as requiring total containment.

2. Chemically Hazardous additives are compounds that when coming into contact with an oxidant, will cause harm to its surroundings due to reaction and/or oxidation. These products usually require containment and/or blanketing with an inert gas.

3. General Intermediates are compounds that are neither biologically nor chemically hazardous additives but they will cause a housekeeping problem. They usually require dusting prevention.

Maximum Cr/Fe ratio The maximum ratio of chromium to iron and the depth at which it occurs are the most direct measures of the chromium enrichment in a material oxide layer. Typical ratios are about 1.5 or greater for well-electropolished 316L stainless steel. The depth at which the maximum Cr/Fe ratio is found varies but is usually about one-half the oxide thickness.

Maximum depth of enrichment In stainless steel the chromium enrichment layer comprises all depths at which the chromium concentration is greater than the iron concentration. For well electropolished 316L stainless steel, the maximum depth of this layer is typically 20 to 25 angstroms (⊕). Chromium Enrichment Layer Thickness).

Maximum drug benefit The maximum amount a particular benefits plan will pay to cover the costs of prescription drugs for a member or member's family during a specific period of time (a quarter year, a calendar year or a contract year).

Maximum working pressure The pressure at which the system is capable of operating for a sustained period.

Maximum Working Temperature The maximum temperature at which the system may operate for a sustained period. The maximum working temperature should relate to the maximum working pressure and the fluids involved.

Maze procedure Also known as the Cox-Maze procedure, a surgical approach to treatment of atrial fibrillation with a success rate of over 90%. The procedure uses strategically-placed incisions in both atria to interrupt the circular electrical patterns that are responsible for this arrhythmia. (Alternative procedures used surgically to treat atrial fibrillation include radiofrequency, microwave, and cryothermy. The goal of all three is to scar heart tissue to block the abnormal electrical impulses from being conducted through the heart and promote the normal conduction of impulses through the proper pathway.)

MDR protein Multi-drug resistance protein 1 is the protein product of the human MDR1 gene and is a member of the ABC (ATP-binding cassette) superfamily of plasma membrane transporter proteins that pump drugs (such as some anti-cancer drugs) and other xenobiotics out of the cytoplasm of cells. This particular family of transporters is expressed by mammalian cells, but analagous proteins are expressed by bacteria, where they contribute to antibiotic resistance. As the name suggests, the gene encoding the MDR1 protein was discovered in drug-resistant tumors. MDR1 is synonymous with human P-glycoprotein (Pgp), a name that was actually first applied to the bacterial version of the protein. In the context of drug discovery in general,the MDR1 protein can have a major impact on the pharmacokinetic properties of drugs by reducing absorption from the gastrointestinal tract, limiting distribution from the blood into the brain, and/or contributing to biliary excretion from hepatocytes. MDR1 protein can also be a locus of drug-drug interactions in patients taking an inhibitor and a substrate of the transporter at the same time. Because MDR1 protein is expressed in so many locations in the human body that play key roles in pharmacokinetics, the effects of modulation of its activity (induction or inhibition) are complex and difficult to predict. Absorption Systems offers a highly sensitive in vitro functional assay in MDR1-transfected MDCK cells, which is used to determine whether a test compound is a substrate for MDR1 protein. We can also assess the involvement of rodent mdr1 at the blood-brain barrier with an in situ rat brain perfusion assay or human MDR1 in the small intestine with an in vitro Caco-2 cell assay or an ex vivo intestinal tissue assay.

MDR1 MDCK MDR1-MDCK are Madin Darby Canine Kidney cells transfected with the human multi-drug resistance gene. Confluent monolayers made from these cells can be used to access a test compound's potential role as a P-gp substrate.

Mean The sum of the values of all observations or data points divided by the number of observations, an arithmetical average.

Mean effective dose (ED50) The dose of a drug predicted (by statistical techniques) to produce a characteristic effect in 50 percent of the subjects to whom the dose is given. The median effective dose (usually abbreviated ED50) is found by interpolation from a dose-effect curve. The ED50 is the most frequently used standardized dose by means of which the potencies of drugs are compared. Although one can determine the dose of drug predicted to be effective in one percent (ED1) or 99 percent (ED99) of a population, the ED50 can be determined more precisely than other similar values. An ED50 can be determined only from data involving all or none (quantal) response; for quantal response data, values for ED0 and ED100 cannot be determined. In analogy to the median effective dose, the pharmacologist speaks of a median lethal dose (LD50), a median anesthetic dose(AD50), a median convulsive dose (CD50), etc.

Mean kinetic temperature (MKT) The single calculated temperature at which the degradation of an article would be equivalent to the actual degradation that results from actual temperature fluctuations during the storage period. It is not a simple arithmetical mean. The MKT is calculated from average storage temperatures recorded over a one-year period, with a minimum of 12 equally spaced storage temperatures being recorded.

Mechanical code Uniform Mechanical Code

Mechanical completion The point in a project at which all equipment and materials have been installed, but not commissioned (started-up).

Mechanism of action A more detailed, molecular description of events.

The knowledge of mechanisms of action is important for two reasons: 1. you need secondary assays that are really associated with a mechanism of action in order to optimize leads in the best possible way, and

2. the department of health will increasingly require that you know the mechanism of action, before you go into clinical trials, to prevent possible toxic side effects. ... The good news is that an increasingly large percentage of drugs that are going through the pipeline now have known mechanisms of action (MOAs) at a molecular level, which is a contrast to 10 to 20 years ago. We now are understanding how therapies interact with the human body and with disease on a much more detailed level. Most drugs now have known targets, and most targets participate in known pathways. The caveat to that, as I mentioned earlier, is that biology is very complicated, and we're learning that the target isn't enough. It's not enough to simply know that a certain molecule binds to a certain protein and turns it off. What you really need to know about are the pathways, and the side pathways, and the domains, and the homologous targets

Media (plural of medium) Substances used to provide sterile nutrients to the fermentation or cell growth process supporting the growth of the live microorganisms. Media may be liquid (broth) or solid, and generally include sucrose or glucose as a carbon source, various minerals, a nitrogen source, and selected growth factors.

Media prep The act of preparing nutrient media for cell culture or fermentation.

Median effective dose The dose of a drug predicted (by statistical techniques) to produce a characteristic effect in 50 percent of the subjects to whom the dose is given. The median effective dose (usually abbreviated ED50) is found by interpolation from a dose-effect curve. The ED50 is the most frequently used standardized dose by means of which the potencies of drugs are compared. Although one can determine the dose of drug predicted to be effective in one percent (ED1) or 99 percent (ED99) of a population, the ED50 can be determined more precisely than other similar values. An ED50 can be determined only from data involving all or none (quantal) response; for quantal response data, values for ED0 and ED100 cannot be determined. In analogy to the median effective dose, the pharmacologist speaks of a median lethal dose (LD50), a median anesthetic dose(AD50), a median convulsive dose (CD50), etc.

Median The middle value in a data set; that is, just as many values are greater than the median and lower than the median value (with an even number of values, the conventional median is halfway between the two middle values).

Medical Devices Any health care product that does not achieve its principal intended purposes by chemical action in or on the body or by being metabolized. The term "devices" also includes components, parts, or accessories of medical devices, diagnostic aids such as reagents, antibiotic sensitivity disks, and test kits for in vitro diagnosis of diseases and other conditions. There are three classes of medical devices: 1. Class I, General Controls (registration of manufacturers, recordkeeping and labeling requirements, compliance with GMPs).

2. Class II, Special Controls (including performance standards, posmarket surveillance, and patient registries).

3. Class III, Premarket Approval (implanted and life supporting or life sustaining devices).

Medical Oncologist A physician who is specially trained to diagnose and treat cancer.

Medical practice computer system A PC- or network-based computer system used to manage electronic patient files. Defined by the European Forum for GCP, such a system is neither sponsor-supplied nor trial-specific.

Medical provider Is a licensed or board certified practitioner of the healing arts, including but not limited to, a physician, nurse, physiotherapist, speech therapist, chiropractor, acupuncturist, mid-wife, podiatrist or optometrist, acting within the scope of such license or certification and performing services that are medically necessary.

Medically necessary Describes any service, supply, treatment or hospital confinement, or part of a hospital confinement which is: a. effective and essential to the treatment of the injury or illness for which it is prescribed or performed; b. based on valid medical need according to accepted standards of medical practice and meets generally accepted standards of medical practice; c. an appropriate level of care provided in the most appropriate setting, based on the diagnosis and condition, and that could not have been omitted without an adverse effect on the person's condition or quality of medical care; d. not primarily for the comfort, convenience or administrative ease of the licensed doctor or other health care provider, or for you and/or your covered dependents; and e. ordered by a physician (except where the treatment is rendered by a medical provider and is generally recognized as not requiring a physician's order).

Medicinal product Any substance or combination of substances presented for treating or preventing disease in human beings or animals. Any substance or combination of substances that may be administered to human beings or animals with a view to making a medical diagnosis or to restoring, correcting or modifying physiological functions in human beings or in animals is likewise considered a medicinal product.

Medicines control agency (MCA) The United Kingdom regulatory authority that approves or rejects CTX/CTC and PL applications.

Medium (filter) The material from which a filter is constructed.

Megabase (MB) Unit of length for DNA fragments equal to 1 million nucleotides and roughly equal to 1Centimorgan (cM)

Megatrials Massive randomized clinical trials that test the advantages of marginally effective experimental drugs by enrolling 10,000 or more subjects. Synonym: large-sample trials.

Megestrol acetate (Megace) Indications: Appetite stimulant for treatment of AIDS wasting syndrome.

Contraindications: Known hypersensitivity, pregnancy.

Dosage: Oral suspension: 400-800 mg po qd; tablets: 80 mg po qid up to 800 mg/day.

Toxicity: Hypogonadism, adrenal insufficiency, diarrhea, impotence, hyperglycemia, rash.

Megohm-cm/B+A1888 A measure of ionic purity in water.

Meiosis The process of two consecutive cell divisions in the diploid progenitors of sex cells. Meiosis results in four rather than two daughter cells, each with a haploid set of chromosomes.

Melanoma A cancer that begins in skin cells called melanocytes and spreads to internal organs.

Melphalan Chemotherapy drug; can be given by mouth.

Member A person receiving the benefit coverage to whom the ID card is issued. A member can also be referred to as "insured", "covered member", or "plan member".

Member ID This number is assigned to serve as the identification number for the member. This number is usually indicated on your prescription ID card.

Membrane A barrier, usually thin, that only permits the passage of particles of a certain size or special nature. Filtration membranes are thin polymer films that are permeable to water and other fluids: 1. Microporous membrane filters have measurable pore structures that physically remove particles or microorganisms larger than pore size.

2. Ultrafiltration membranes (sometimes called molecular sieves) also remove molecules larger than a specified molecular weight.

3. Reverse osmosis membranes are permeable to water molecules and very little else, rejecting even dissolved ions and endotoxins in water.

Membrane stabilizing activity (Local anesthetic action) Beta-blocker that has the ability to decrease electrical conductance, particularly in heart (Quinidine-like effects).

Malignant hyperthermia (MH) is a pharmacogenetic disease of skeletal muscle. When exposed to inhalation anesthetics (those which are gases), muscle metabolism increases with a rapid rise in body temperature which if left untreated can lead to death. Triggering agents include succinylcholine (NMJ depolarizing blocker) and volatile anesthetic. Treatment: Drug of choice is Dantrolene (inhibits Ca++ release).

Membrane transport proteins Membrane proteins primary function is to facilitate the transport of molecules across a biological membrane. Included in this broad category are proteins involved in active transport, facilitated transport and ion channels. They play key roles in drug absorption, distribution and excretion, and are sometimes involved in drug toxicity and drug-drug interactions. They may be indirectly involved in drug metabolism as well, due to their involvement in drug uptake into hepatocytes.

Memorandum of understanding (MOU) An MOU between department of health and a regulatory agency in another country allows mutual recognition of inspections.

Mental health disorders Are those conditions categorized as mental disorders in the most recent edition of the International Classification of Diseases, whether or not involving a biological, chemical or other type of disorder which might not otherwise be considered mental or nervous. Conditions for which the primary diagnosis and treatment is for alcohol or chemical dependency are not included in mental health disorders but are covered separately.

Meristem The growing point or area of rapidly dividing cells at the tip of a stem, root, or branch.

Mesophile An organism that grows best in the temperature range of 20°C to 50°C (68°F to 122°F).

Messenger RNA (mRNA) RNA that serves as a template for protein synthesis.

Meta-analysis A statistical process for pooling data from many clinical trials and summarizing it through formal statistical means. Also called overview. (statistics).

Metabolism Metabolism, one mechanism of clearance of drugs and other xenobiotics, is the irreversible biochemical transformation of a compound to another chemical (metabolite). The metabolite is usually more polar (water-soluble) and, therefore, more readily excreted, than the parent compound; thus, metabolism facilitates drug excretion. Conceptually, metabolism is often divided into Phase I (oxidation or reduction) and Phase II (conjugation with negatively charged functional groups), which are closely coupled in intact cells such that Phase II metabolites are often present at much higher concentrations than Phase I metabolites. In the context of toxicology, metabolism is often referred to as activation; the same enzymes that facilitate excretion of compounds via metabolism can also produce highly reactive metabolites or metabolic intermediates, which bind to cellular proteins or DNA, leading to cell death or cancer. Many drug-drug interactions take place at the level of drug metabolism, via inhibition or induction of drug-metabolizing enzymes, leading to toxicity or therapeutic failure, respectively.

Metadata Electronic records that include processing parameters and audit trail logs. Metadata allows reviewers to replay the original result, or reconstruct a final report from raw data. In chromatography, metadata include integration parameters and calibration tables. An example of metadata can be in long division "1,000 ÷ 5" would be the raw data, the work you had to show on your paper in fourth grade math class would be the metadata, and "200" would be your result.

Metameter A term used to designate "the measurement or transformation of the measurement used in evaluating biological tests." Examples of metameters of dose include "milligrams," "moles," "log milligrams," "log milligrams per kilogram of body weight," etc. Metameters of response include "increase in blood pressure, in mmHg," "Maximum blood pressure achieved, in mmHg," and "percent increase in blood pressure." Metameters are frequently and erroneously chosen only to facilitate statistical summary and analysis of data; the metameter used may also obscure or influence the biological interpretation of the data in a manner not intended or expected by the investigator. For example, implicit in the calculation of "percent change in blood pressure " is the statement that the final state of the system is a function of the initial state that may or may not be true.

Metaphase A stage in mitosis or meiosis during which the chromosomes are aligned along the equatorial plane of the cell.

Metastasis The spread of disease from one part of the body to another. In cancer, metastasis is the migration of cancer cells from the original tumor site through the blood and lymph vessels to produce cancers in other tissues. Metastasis is also the term used for a secondary cancer growing at a distant site.

Metastasize In cancer, to spread, by transferring a malignancy (out-of-control growth) from the site of disease to another part of the body.

Metastatic cancer Cancer that has spread from its original site to one or more additional body sites.

Methaqualone and analogues Methaqualone was first synthesised in 1951 and introduced as a new drug that produced sedation and sleep in 1956. .

Methaqualone has been initially designed to counter the nervous damages caused by long-term consumption and to reduce the risk of the dependency potential of barbiturates. This did not succeed. .

Interest in methaqualone rose dramatically in recent years. Its popularity was due to its undeserved reputation as an 'aphrodisiac' often in combination with diphenhydramine. Because of its strong habit-forming properties the drug was placed in the list of controlled substances and the legal manufacturer stopped its production and removed it from the market in 1984.

Methods validation Establishing, through documented evidence, a high degree of assurance that an analytical method will consistently yield results that accurately reflect the quality characteristics of the product tested.

Methotrexate A drug that acts as an antimetabolite and specifically as a folic acid antagonist that inhibits the synthesis of DNA , RNA , and protein.

Methyl cellulose A common viscosity-increasing agent used in ophthalmics preparations. It is inversely soluble with temperature.

Metoclopramide A drug used to stimulate stomach muscle contractions to help empty food. It also helps reduce nausea and vomiting. Side effects include fatigue, sleepiness, and sometimes depression, anxiety, and problems with physical movement.

MHO Unit of measurement for conductance; the reciprocal of ohm (resistance).

Microbe A microscopic one-celled organism, animal or vegetable, a microorganism.

Microbiology The study of microscopic life such as bacteria and viruses.

Microencapsulated Surrounded by a thin, protective layer of biodegradable substance referred to as microsphere.

Microhmo A measure of conductance equal to one millionth of a mho.

Microinch A unit of length equal to one millionth of an inch (0.000001 inches).

Micron or micrometer A unit of length equal to one millionth of a meter (μm) or thousandth of a millimeter (25μm are approximately 0.001 inch.). Bacteria range in size from 0.5μm to 20μm.

Microorganism A microbe - A microscopic plant or animal, such as a bacterium, protozoan, yeast, virus, or algae.

Microwave A type of radiation used in treatment for atrial fibrillation. The use of microwave energy cures atrial fibrillation in approximately 80 percent of patients.

Milliequivalent To simplify the calculation of ion exchange resin capacity, total dissolved ion concentrations are usually converted into equivalent concentrations of calcium carbonate, the most common source of dissolved ions in water. Resin capacity is normally given in ppm as $CaCO_3$, or in grains per gallon as $CaCO_3$ (7,000 grains = 1 pound). However, it may also be given as milliequivalents per liter (meq/L). Since calcium carbonate has a molecular weight of 100 and an equivalent weight of 50 (because calcium has a valence of two) ppm as $CaCO_3$ can be converted to meq/L by dividing by 50. Thus, 1 ppm of $CaCO_3$ = 0.02 meg/L.

Minienvironment The actual localized control space limited by a defined enclosure that separates or isolates the inside from the outside environment, such that the transfer of potential contamination from one side to the other is minimized or completely eliminated, depending on the design. Minienvironments are not always isolators. ISO 14644-4.

Minocycline A tetracycline antibiotic used to treat many different bacteria in urinary tract infections, acne , gonorrhea , and chlamydia , and other injections.

Minor Change (PMA CSVC) A change to a validated system that, in theopinion of change-control reviewers, does not necessitate arevalidation of the system.

Mitochondria Structures in cells that act as power plants.

Mitomycin C Useful chemotherapy drug, often used as a radiosensitiser.

Mitosis The process of nuclear division in cells that produces daughter cells that are genetically identical to each other and to the parent cell.

Mitral valve prolapse (MVP) Also known as Barlow's syndrome or systolic click-murmur syndrome. When the valve between the left atrium and the left ventricle does not close smoothly or evenly during a normal heart contraction and a small amount of blood leaks backward through the valve.

Mixed airflow room Room which is supplied of air by conventional "turbulent" means, such as a diffuser or terminal HEPA filter but also includes an unidirectional flow zone (such as a hood over a critical area). Total air changes of the room are greatly enhanced by the operation of the hood.

Mixed bed ion exchange Mixing both anion and cation resins in the same deionizer results in higher efficiency, but lower capacity, than separate-bed deionizers.

Mode The most frequently occurring value in a data set. (statistics)

Modem From modulator/demodulator. A device that converts the digital data that your computer uses into analog data that can travel on telephone lines.

Modularity (Software) (ANSI/IEEE) The extent to which software iscomposed of discrete components such that a change to one component hasminimal impact on other components.

Moiety A part or portion of a molecule, generally complex, having a characteristic chemical or pharmacological property.

Moist air A binary mixture of dry air and water vapor. Each component behaves as if the other is not present and each occupies the complete volume of the mixture.

Molality The molal unit is not used nearly as frequently as the molar unit. A molality is the number of moles of solute dissolved in one kilogram of solvent. Be careful not to confuse molality and molarity. Molality is represented by a small "m," whereas molarity is represented by an upper case "M."

Molds Filamentous fungi that have a mycelial structure.

Mole One gram molecular weight of a compound.

Molecular genetics Deals with the study of the nature and biochemistry of genetic material. Includes the technologies of genetic engineering.

Molecular pharmaceutics A new journal from the American Chemical Society focusing on molecular mechanistic approaches to the development of bio- available drugs and delivery systems. ... research advancing the understanding of pharmaceutics at the molecular level while providing a forum for research among the fields of physical and pharmaceutical chemistry, biochemistry, molecular and cell biology, and materials science focused on drug delivery. With an emphasis on fundamental molecular concepts in chemistry and biology as applied to drug and drug delivery system activity, the journal will showcase emerging technologies used to advance the drug development process. Scientific areas include: physical and pharmaceutical chemistry, biochemistry, molecular and cellular biology, and polymer and materials science as they relate to drugs and drug development.

Molecular phenotyping The process of determining specific nucleic acids sequences inside a cell. .. Molecular phenotyping by in situ PCR combined with immuno-phenotyping is not yet completely reduced to practice, therefore, some development work is also necessary

Molecular weight Most drugs are composed of combinations of C, H, N, O, P, S, and the halogens. The molecular weight of a drug is obtained by adding the mass of each atom present in the drug. The units of MW are atomic mass units (u) or Daltons (D). 1 atomic mass unit = 1.660538 × 10 -27 kilograms

P-gp Inhibitor

A compound that binds to the multi-drug resistance (MDR) protein, P-glycoprotein (P-gp) and inhibits its transport activity. P-gp inhibitors are useful research tools; their clinical applications include reversal of resistance to cancer chemotherapy.

Molecule A group of atoms arranged to interact in a particular way; one molecule of any substance is the smallest physical unit of that particular substance.

Monitor Person employed by the sponsor or CRO who is responsible for determining that a trial is being conducted in accordance with the protocol. A monitor's duties may include, but are not limited to, helping to plan and initiate a trial, assessing the conduct of trials, and assisting in data analysis, interpretation, and extrapolation. Monitors work with the clinical research coordinator to check all data and documentation from the trial.

Monitoring report A written report from the monitor to the sponsor after each site visit and/or other trial-related communication according to the sponsor's standard operating procedures (SOPs).

Monitoring The act of overseeing the progress of a clinical trial, and of ensuring that it is conducted, recorded, and reported in accordance with the protocol, standard operating procedures (SOPs), GCP, and the applicable regulatory requirement(s).

Monoamine oxidase (MAO) An enzyme which, in the brain, breaks down certain neurotransmitters such as serotonin, dopamine and norepinephrine.

Monoclonal antibody (Mab or MoAb) Antibodies derived from a single source or clone of cells that recognize only one type of antigen. They are produced from hybridomas formed by the hybridization of two cells: a single antibody-producing cell and a cell that can be grown indefinitely in culture. Monoclonal antibodies have found markets in diagnostic kits and show potential for use in drugs and industrial purification processes.

Monoclonal antibody, humanized monoclonal antibody A highly specific protein that can bind to any single substance to register a presence or to deactivate it. Monoclonal antibodies can be used to detect disease or tag disease cells for attack with drugs, radiation, or toxins

Monograph The entry in USP or NF for a specific raw material or product.

Monomer The basic subunit from which, by repetition of a single reaction, polymers are made. For example, amino acids (monomers) condense to yield polypeptides or proteins (polymers).

Monosaccharides The building blocks of carbohydrates, hence known as "simple sugar". They are classified by the number of carbon atoms in the molecule, pentoses have five and hexoses six.

Morphine Strong opiate drug.

Mother liquor The residual liquid that remains after the crystallization or isolation processes. A mother liquor may contain unrecovered products (i.e., unreacted starting materials, intermediates, levels of the API and/or impurities). It may be used for further processing.

Motility Contractions of the muscles in the digestive tract that promote mixing and movement of digestive contents.

MRP II Manufacturing Resource Planning.

MRP Material Requirements Planning.

MSDS (material safety data sheet) Document describing the chemical and physical properties of a substance as related to its safe handling and storage. The substance manufacturer originates it.

Multi genic A biochemical pathway which requires more than one gene.

Multi use equipment Equipment used to process more than one product.

Multicellular Referring to organisms composed of more than one cell - often billions of them, arranged in various organs, tissues, and systems.

Multicenter trial A clinical trial conducted according to a single protocol but at more than one site, and, therefore, carried out by more than one investigator.

Multiple dose regimens The pharmacokinetic aspects of treatment schedules that involve more than one dose of a drug are discussed below. The relationships described involve assumptions of instantaneous intravenous administration and distribution of a drug that is eliminated by first-order kinetics from a single-compartment system, and is given in equal doses at equal time intervals. The relationships become less accurate in describing real situations to the extent that the real systems depart from the ideal model, i.e. to the extent that ka is not much greater than kel, and to the extent that Vda is not much smaller than Vdb.

When equal doses are administered at equal intervals, the peak plasma concentration after the nth dose, Cmax,n is given by the relationship:

Cmax,n = C0 (1 - f n)/(1- f)

The "trough" concentrations (Cmin) for the two conditions are:

Cmin,n = Cmax,n - C0, and

Css,min = Css,max - C0, respectively.

Knowing the half-life of a drug and the Css,max and Css,min desired to produce optimum therapy, the dose interval, τ (tau), necessary to achieve and maintain these maximum and minimum concentrations can be determined from the relationship:

τ= 1.443 (t1/2) ln(Css,max/Css, min).

(Remember that ln X = 2.303 log X, that t1/2 = 0.693/kel, and that 1/0.693 = 1.443.)

The doses to be administered at intervals, τ, to produce the desired Css,max and Css,min are inferred from experimental data relating the size of single doses to the peak plasma concentrations (Cmax) each produces, or are estimated from the relationship F · D/Vd = C, when the Vdand F of the drug are known. (The relationship among Css,max, Css,min and expected therapeutic outcome, including occurrence of side effects, are inferred from dose-effect relationships established in clinical pharmacologic experiments.)

With repeated doses, at equal intervals, peak plasma concentrations (Cmax) approach but, in theory, never reach Css,max. In practice, it is useful to know how long it takes for Cmaxto reach some specified level with respect to Css,max, i.e., how long it takes for Cmax/Css,max to reach, say, 0.95. Knowing the expected value of Css,max and the fractional achievement desired, e.g. 0.95, it is easy to compute the desired Cmax. Then, knowing the dose interval, τ, and the half-life of the drug, the time required to reach the desired Cmax is given by the relationship:

nτ = 1.443 (t1/2) ln [(Css,max - Cmax)/ Css,max]

where the time required (nτ) is expressed as the product of the number of doses and the duration of the dose interval (τ). The number of doses required to achieve the desired ratio of Cmax to Css,max may be determined by dividing the right hand member of the equation by the length of the dose interval.

When τ is long, relative to t1/2, many doses may have to be given, and much time may have to pass if a reasonable fraction of Css,max is to be achieved by administering identical doses at equal interval. Under such circumstances, prompt achievement of therapeutically effective blood levels may require beginning the treatment regimen with a "loading dose".

Multiplexing A sequencing approach that uses several pooled samples simultaneously, greatly increasing sequencing speed.

Murine Relating to a member of the rodent family Muridae, including rats and mice; such as murine monoclonal antibodies derived from mice.

Mutagen An agent that induces cellular DNA to undergo mutation (e.g. X-rays, mustard gas radiation).

Mutagenesis The induction of mutation in the genetic material of an organism; researchers may use physical or chemical means to cause mutations that improve the production of capabilities of organisms.

Mutant The altered cell resulting from mutation of the original wild type or any subsequent alteration.

Mutation An abrupt change of genotype involving either the structure or number of complete chromosomes or, more commonly, a change in the structure of a single gene so that its function is altered or lost. Certain chemicals called mutagens can induce it.

Mycelium The mat or complex group of protoplasmic units, or the entangled mass of tubelike or filamentous structures, i.e., hyphae, that represents the "body" of plant forms classified as Eumycetes (including Phycomycetes, Ascomycetes, Deuteromycetes (Fungi Imperfectii), and Basidiomycetes).

Mycobacterium A genus of the family Mycobacteriaceae containing slender, aerobic, usually acid fast, Gram positive, rod-shaped organisms of various forms, club shaped, swollen, but seldom branched or with filaments; it includes many species which were formerly and are still called bacilli, such as the pathogens of tuberculosis and leprosy.

Mycoplasma The smallest, free-living organism with a size range from 1.25μm to 0.5μm. Pleomorphic (many shapes) because of a lack of a cell wall. Cannot be quantitatively removed by 0.2μm filtration

Myeloma A malignant human plasma cell that can synthesize excessive amounts of whole antibody or single immunoglobulin chains.

Myorelaxans Drugs decreasing muscular tonus.

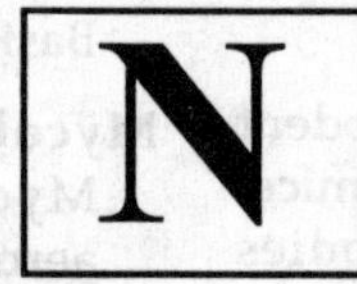

N The number of doses in a series; as a subscript, the last dose in a series or the number of the last dose.

N acetylcysteine An antioxidant drug that may keep cancer cells from developing or reduce the risk of growth of existing cancer.

N acetyldinaline A substance that is being studied as an anticancer drug in the treatment of non-small cell lung cancer. Also called CI-994.

N butyl-N-(4-hydroxybutyl) nitrosamine A substance that is used in cancer research to cause bladder tumors in laboratory animals. This is done to test new diets, drugs, and procedures for use in cancer prevention and treatment.

N of 1 study A trial in an individual subject is administered a treatment repeatedly over a number of episodes to establish the treatment's effect in that person, often with experimental and control treatments randomized.

Naproxen A non-steroidal anti-inflammatory drug (NSAID) used for the management of mild to moderate pain, fever, and inflammation . Naproxen blocks the enzyme cyclooxygenase that makes prostaglandins, resulting in lower concentrations of prostaglandins. As a consequence, inflammation, pain and fever are reduced.

Narcolepsy Is a condition when someone is often sleeping in the daytime.

Narcotic Formerly, an agent capable of producing coma or stupor (from Greek narke: torpor, numbness). Now, usually, any drug which produces analgesia and is capable of producing stupor: pain is relieved by a dose or narcotic before the occurrence of sleep or unconsciousness. Legally, the tern "narcotic" is applied only to those drugs the sale and use of which is regulated by the Harrison Narcotic Act.

National formulary (N.F.) A reference volume published formerly by the American Pharmaceutical Association containing standards of purity and methods of assay for some drugs, and formulae and methods of manufacture for a variety of pharmaceutical preparations. Drugs were included on the basis of demand as well as therapeutic value. The N.F. and the U.S.P. are recognized by the F.D.A. as official standards, and the two are now published as a single volume.

Natural drugs Are active ingredients, secondary metabolic products, of plants and other living systems, that may be isolated by extraction (morphine).

NCE New Chemical Entity.

NCI (National cancer institute) A Government organization that conducts and supports research, training, health information dissemination and other programs relating to the cause, diagnosis, prevention, and treatment of cancer. NDA New Drug Application.

Necrosis The pathological death of one or more cells, or of a portion of tissue or organ, resulting from irreversible damage to the nucleus.

Negative control drug or negative control procedure A treatment incorporated into an experiment with the intention that it have no effects on the experimental system like those expected of the independent variable. In a pharmacologic experiment, the negative control drug mimics in every way the drug preparation under investigation (including identity of dosage form, vehicle, mode of application, etc.) except that the negative control drug lacks the ingredient that is expected to be responsible for the biological effect of the test preparation. The negative control drug has two functions in an experiment: 1. To permit ascribing a causal relationship between treatment with the independent variable and changes in the experimental system which follow treatment. If the experimental system responds to both the negative control drug and the drug preparation under test, one cannot - in the absence of other information - legitimately infer that the effects of the test preparation are caused by the supposedly pharmacodynamically active test preparation.

2. To serve as a basis for quantitative estimation of the effects of the independent variable in excess of those effects produced by non-specific changes in the environment or the experimental system. A test drug preparation may have non-specific effects like those of the negative control drug, but may also have specific effects that can be attributed to the ingredient that is unique to the test preparation.

Careful use of a negative control drug in an experiment prevents erroneous conclusions about the apparent activity of a test preparation; use of a positive control drug prevents making erroneous conclusions about apparent inactivity of a test preparation.

Negligible Not more than 0.50 mg (US).

Nelfinavir (Viracept) Indications: Treatment of HIV infection in combination with other agents.

Contraindications: Known hypersensitivity.

Dosage: 1250 mg po bid or 750 mg po tid with food. There are many potential drug interactions, some of which require dosage modification

Toxicity: Diarrhea.

S HO O N H OH H N H N H

NEMA (national electrical manufacturers association) Enclosures As a way of standardizing enclosure performance, NEMA uses a rating system to identify the enclosure's ability to resist external environmental influences. Resistance to everything from dripping liquid to hose-down to total submersion is defined by this rating system. 1. Type 1 - Enclosures constructed for indoor use to provide a degree of protection to personnel against incidental contact with the enclosed equipment and to provide a degree of protection against falling dirt.

2. Type 2 - Enclosures constructed for indoor use to provide a degree of protection to personnel against incidental contact with the enclosed equipment, to provide a degree of protection against falling dirt, and to provide a degree of protection against dripping and light splashing of liquids.

3. Type 3 - Enclosures constructed for either indoor or outdoor use to provide a degree of protection to personnel against incidental contact with the enclosed equipment; to provide a degree of protection against falling dirt, rain, sleet, snow, and windblown dust; and that will be undamaged by the external formation of ice on the enclosure.

4. Type 3R - Enclosures constructed for either indoor or outdoor use to provide a degree of protection to personnel against incidental contact with the enclosed equipment; to provide a degree of protection against falling dirt, rain, sleet, and snow; and that will be undamaged by the external formation of ice on the enclosure.

5. Type 3S - Enclosures constructed for either indoor or outdoor use to provide a degree of protection to personnel against incidental contact with the enclosed equipment; to provide a degree of protection against falling dirt, rain, sleet, snow, and windblown dust; and in which the external mechanism(s) remain operable when ice laden.

6. Type 4 - Enclosures constructed for either indoor or outdoor use to provide a degree of protection to personnel against incidental contact with the enclosed equipment; to provide a degree of protection against falling dirt, rain, sleet, snow, and windblown dust, splashing water, and hose-directed water; and that will be undamaged by the external formation of ice on the enclosure.

7. Type 4X - Enclosures constructed for either indoor or outdoor use to provide a degree of protection to personnel against incidental contact with the enclosed equipment; to provide a degree of protection against falling dirt, rain, sleet, snow, and windblown dust, splashing water, hose-directed water, and corrosion; and that will be undamaged by the external formation of ice on the enclosure.

8. Type 5 - Enclosures constructed for indoor use to provide a degree of protection to personnel against incidental contact with the enclosed equipment; to provide a degree of protection against falling dirt; against settling airborne dust, lint, fibers, and flyings; and to provide a degree of protection against dripping and light splashing of liquids.

9. Type 6 - Enclosures constructed for either indoor or outdoor use to provide a degree of protection to personnel against incidental contact with the enclosed equipment; to provide a degree of protection against falling dirt; against hose-directed water and the entry of water during occasional temporary submersion at a limited depth; and that will be undamaged by the external formation of ice on the enclosure.

10. Type 6P - Enclosures constructed for either indoor or outdoor use to provide a degree of protection to personnel against incidental contact with the enclosed equipment; to provide a degree of protection against falling dirt; against hose-directed water and the entry of water during prolonged submersion at a limited depth; and that will be undamaged by the external formation of ice on the enclosure

11. Type 12 - Enclosures constructed (without knockouts) for indoor use to provide a degree of protection to personnel against incidental contact with the enclosed equipment; to provide a degree of protection against falling dirt; against circulating dust, lint, fibers, and flyings; and against dripping and light splashing of liquids.

12. Type 12K - Enclosures constructed (with knockouts) for indoor use to provide a degree of protection to personnel against incidental contact with the enclosed equipment; to provide a degree of protection against falling dirt; against circulating dust, lint, fibers, and flyings; and against dripping and light splashing of liquids.

13. Type 13 - Enclosures constructed for indoor use to provide a degree of protection to personnel against incidental contact with the enclosed equipment; to provide a degree of protection against falling dirt; against circulating dust, lint, fibers, and flyings; and against the spraying, splashing, and seepage of water, oil, and noncorrosive coolants.

Neoadjuvant chemotherapy Chemotherapy given prior to an operation to shrink the tumor with the aim of reducing the extent of surgery needed.

Neoplasm Any new growth of cells or tissues but the term is customarily used with rather specific reference to a focus (or a relatively large mass or region) of intermittently or constantly progressive, comparatively unlimited, or uncontrolled new growth that manifests varying degrees of autonomy.

Nephelometer Any apparatus used to measure the size and concentration of particles in a liquid by analysis of light transmitted through or reflected by the liquid.

Nephelometry The semiquantitative estimation of the concentration of particles in a suspension (e.g. bacterial cells in an antigenic preparation), by means of comparing it with the standard suspensions in a nephelometer.

Nephrotoxin A cytotoxin that is specific for cells of the kidney.

Nerve A cell which carries information to and from the central nervous system.

Nerve growth factor (NGF) A naturally occurring hormone that stimulates the growth of neurones.

Networks Organizations that are linked through contractual or ownership relationships. Many health plans consider themselves "network developers" because they contract with physicians and hospitals on behalf of their customers, employers, and carriers.

Network hospital Is a Hospital participating in a preferred provider network, in which the Covered Individual is enrolled by reason of his or her status under the Plan.

Network provider Is a medical provider, laboratory or radiology facility participating in a preferred provider network, in which the Covered Individual is enrolled by reason of his or her status under the Plan.

Neurites The tiny projections growing from each nerve cell which carries information between the cells. A nerve cell may have over 100,000 neurites growing out of it; each connected to another nerve cell.

Neurochemical A chemical that naturally occurs in the nervous system and plays a part in its functioning.

Neurodegenerative disease A type of neurological disorder marked by the loss of nerve cells. For example Alzheimer's Disease, Huntington's Disease, and Parkinson's Disease.

Neurofibrillary tangles Accumulation of twisted protein fragments inside neurons. Neurofibrillary tangles are one of the characteristic structural abnormalities found in the brains of patients with Alzheimer's disease patients. Upon autopsy, the presence of amyloid plaques and neurofibrillary tangles is used to positively diagnose Alzheimer's disease.

Neuroleptics A group of psychotropic drugs used mainly in the treatment of schizophrenia, having also a tranquilizing effect, suppressing anxiety, followed by anti-emetic effect, etc.

Neurology Medical specialty dealing with the disease or malfunction of the nerves.

Neuromuscular junction (NMJ) The junction between the terminal of a motor neuron and a skeletal muscle fiber is called the neuromuscular junction. It is simply one kind of synapse. Nerve impulses travel down the motor neurons and cause the skeletal muscle fibers at which they terminate to contract. This is part of the Somatic (Voluntary) Nervous System.

Neuron A nerve cell.

Neuropathy Disease or malfunction of the nerves.

Neurotransmitter One of the many chemicals that carry impulses between nerve cells.

Neurotrophic factor A molecule, typically a protein, such as nerve growth factor (NGF), that promotes nerve cell growth, repair, and survival.

Neurotrophin Neurotrophins are a family of structurally similar proteins that regulate the growth, differentiation, function, and plasticity of nerve cells.

Nevirapine (Viramune) Indications: Treatment of HIV infection in combination with other agents.

Contraindications: Known hypersensitivity.

Dosage: 200 mg po qd x two weeks; 200 mg po bid thereafter. Patients who develop rash during the first two weeks should not increase the dose until the rash resolves. There are many potential drug interactions, some of which require dosage modification

Toxicity: Rash is common (about 17% of patients, although fewer with dose escalation regimen) and does not require discontinuation of the drug unless accompanied by fever, mucous membrane involvement, or other systemic manifestations. Stevens-Johnson syndrome has been reported infrequently. Other side effects include nausea, headache, abnormal liver function tests.

O
N
N
N
N

New chemical entity (NCEs) A compound not previously described in medical literature.

New drug application (NDA) The New Drug Application contains most of the information included in the IND. Only after department of health approval of the NDA, can distribution and marketing of a new drug begin.

NF kappa B Ubiquitous, inducible, nuclear transcriptional activator that binds to enhancer elements in many different cell types and is activated by pathogenic stimuli. The NF-kappa B complex is a heterodimer composed of two DNA- binding subunits: NF-kappa B1 and relA.

NGF Nerve Growth Factor, a member of the neurotrophin family.

NHSA (normal human serum albumin) A blood plasma fraction usually prepared by Cohn cold ethanol precipitation. Dispensed as a 5% to 25% protein solution.

Niacin Is the active part of vitamin B3.

NIH (national institutes of health) Guidelines NIH Guidelines specify practices for constructing and handling recombinant deoxyribonucleic acid (DNA) molecules, and organisms and viruses containing recombinant DNA molecules.

Nitrates Salts of nitric acid used in the long-term treatment of coronary heart disease.

Nitrogen mustard (Mustine) Chemotherapy drug; a toxic agent but with impressive activity in lymphoma and certain types of solid cancer.

Nitrogenous base A nitrogencontaining molecule that has the chemical properties of a base.

Nominal A numerical identification of dimension, capacity, rating, or other characteristics used as a designation, not as an exact measurement.

Nociception A physiological protective mechanism that recognizes potentially harmful and injurious stimuli, which are perceived as pain.

Nociceptors, polymodal Small diameter sensory fibers involved in nociception and responding to stimuli of thermal, mechanical and chemical nature.

Nominal (rating of filter) An arbitrary micrometer value indicated by filter manufacturers. Based upon removal of some percentage of particles of a given size or larger, but rarely well defined and consequently not reproducible.

Nominal outside diameter A numerical identification of outside diameter to which tolerances apply.

Nominal pore size Based on retention efficiency, a filter should retain 99.9% of particles larger than its nominal rated pore size.

Nominal wall thickness A numerical identification of wall thickness to which tolerances apply.

Non desensitizing Refers to a receptor or ion channel, which remains activated as long as the agonist is present. In contrast, desensitizing receptors inactivate rapidly after activation even if the presence of the ligand.

Non GMP technology Facility design requirement resulting from decisions to address issues outside the realm of GMPs or manufacturer preferences. Often these do affect GMP related design features.

Non network hospital Is a Hospital that does not participate in a preferred provider network in which the Covered Individual is enrolled by reason of his or her status under the Plan.

Non network provider Is a medical provider, laboratory or radiology facility not participating in a preferred provider network, in which the Covered Individual is enrolled by reason of his or her status under the Plan.

Non participating dentist Is a dentist that is not within the DentalGuard Preferred provider network offered by The Guardian Life Insurance Company.

Non participating pharmacy Is a pharmacy that is not participating in a preferred provider network of pharmacies maintained by Medco Health Solutions.

Non specific esterase A class of enzyme that act on a particular chemical bond called an "ester." These enzymes are present in nearly all tissues and organs in the body.

Noncarbonate hardness Hardness in water caused by chlorides, sulfates, and nitrates of calcium and magnesium.

Nonclinical Study Biomedical studies not performed on human subjects.

Nonunidirectional airflow Air distribution where the first air entering the controlled space mixes with the internal air by means of induction. The airflow that does not meet the definition of unidirectional airflow; previously referred to as "turbulent" or "non-laminar" airflow.

Nootropics Drugs stimulating brain activity.

Norepinephrine (also known as Noradrenaline) An excitatory neurotransmitter involved in alertness, concentration, aggression and motivation, among other behaviors. Norepinephrine is made in the brain from the amino acid phenylalanine.

Normal saline A very common LVP that has a physiologic (0.9gm%) concentration of sodium chloride.

Northern blot A recombinant DNA technique used for the detection of specific RNA transcripts.

Not approvable letter An official communication from department of health to inform an NDA sponsor that the important deficiencies described therein preclude approval unless corrected.

Not exposed or closed Drug substance is protected from exposure to the environment during processing.

Notified body (NB) A private institution charged by the Competent Authority with verifying compliance with the applicable Essential Requirements stated in the Medical Device Directive. This process, called Conformity Assessment, has EU-wide validity once completed by the NB.

NPDWR water Potable water meeting EPA National Primary Drinking Water Regulations.

NSAID Non-Steroidal Anti-Inflammatory Drug.

Nuclease An enzyme that breaks down nucleic acids. Exonucleases cleave the nucleotides only at the ends of polynucleotide chains (e.g. phosphodiesterase). Endonucleases attack certain linkates wherever they occur in the polynucleotide chain.

Nucleic acid A large molecule composed of nucleotide subunits.

Nucleic acid hybridization Matching of either DNA or RNA (depending on the organism) from an unknown organism with DNA or RNA from a known organism. This method is used in tropical disease research for identifying species and strains of organisms.

Nucleolus A discrete region of the nucleus created by the transcription of rRNA genes. The nucleolus disappears during mitosis, or cell division.

Nucleotide sequence The chemical linkage of nucleic acids (adenine, guanine, cytosine or thymine) attached to a phosphate and a sugar group.

Nucleotide The structural unit of nucleic acids. A subunit of DNA or RNA consisting of purine bases (adenine, guanine), pyrimidine bases (thymine, or cytosine in DNA; uracil, or cytosine in RNA), a phosphate molecule, and a sugar molecule (deoxyribose in DNA and ribose in RNA). Thousands of nucleotides are linked to form a DNA or RNA molecule.

Nucleus The cellular organelle present in eukaryotes cells and separated from the cytoplasm by a nuclear membrane. It contains the genetic material and is essential for the continued life of the cell.

Null hypothesis A null hypothesis (for example, "subjects will experience no change in blood pressure as a result of administration of the test product") is used to rule out every possibility except the one the researcher is trying to prove, an assumption about a research population that may or may not be rejected as a result of testing. Used because most statistical methods are less able to prove something true than to provide strong evidence that it is false.

Nuremberg code Code of ethics for conducting human medical research set forth in 1947.

Nystatin Indications: Treatment of mucosal candidiasis.

Contraindications: Known hypersensitivity.

Dosage: Oral candidiasis: 5 ml suspension to be gargled and swallowed 5 times a day x 7-14 days; vaginal candidiasis: 100,000 unit tab intravaginally 1-2 times a day x 7-14 days.

Toxicity: Nausea, vomiting, diarrhea

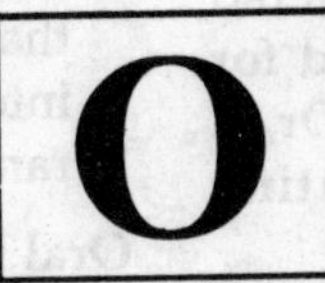

Object database management system (ODBMS) A database management system specifically designed to manage and store complex objects and their complex relationships; that is, such items are stored as objects rather than as tables or fields. They support modeling and creation of data as objects, allowing for greater flexibility in tracking parent method sets and subcomponents. Such systems may be better than relational database management systems at meeting the data integrity requirements.

Objective measurement A measurement that cannot be influenced by investigator bias; for example, blood glucose levels or ECG tracings.

Occupancy The purpose for which a building or part thereof is used or intended to be used.

Official Compendial; purported to comply with USP or NF

OHM Unit of electrical resistance in a circuit, such that a potential difference of one volt across a load of one ohm produces a current of one ampere.

Ointment A medication preparation that is applied topically (onto the skin). An ointment has an oil base whereas a cream is water-soluble.

Oligoucleotides A molecule made up of a small number of nucleotides, typically fewer than 25. These are frequently used as DNA synthesis primers.

Oncogene A gene that when expressed as a protein can lead cells to become cancerous, usually by removing the normal constraints on growth.

Oncologist A board certified medical specialist who specializes in treating cancer patients.

Oncology The branch of medicine concerned with the diagnosis and treatment of cancer.

Oncopharmacogenomics Identifying targets for anti- cancer drugs based on genomic vulnerability.

Ondansetron Anti-nausea drug widely used for chemotherapy side effects.

Open Exposed to the environment, not closed.

Open formulary A prescription benefits plan that has an open-formulary design generally will cover some drugs not included on the formulary.

Open formulary plan In this type of plan, pharmacy benefits cover medications on the Preferred Drug List as well as other drugs not listed.

Open study A trial in which subjects and investigators know which product each subject is receiving; opposite of double-blind study.

Open system A system that fails to meet one or more of the requirements that set the criteria for a closed system.

Operating environment All outside influences that interface with thecomputer system.

Operating parameter Any information entered into an automated system that is used for automated equipment operation. Or, a parameter indicative of the operating condition of a system.

Operating range The validated acceptance criteria within which a control parameter must remain, wherein acceptable product is being manufactured.

Operating system (OS) The most important program run on a computer because it manages all the other programs. Operating systems perform basic tasks, such as recognizing input from the keyboard, sending output to the display screen, keeping track of files and directories on the disk, and controlling peripheral devices such as disk drives and printers. For large systems, the OS has even greater responsibilities and powers. It regulates traffic, making sure that different programs and users running at the same time do not interfere with each other. The operating system also is responsible for security, ensuring that unauthorized users do not access a system. Microsoft Windows NT, LINUX, and UNIX are operating systems.

Operating variables All factors of operation, including control parameters that may potentially affect process state of control and/or fitness for use of the product.

Operation Room condition when normal process operations are undertaken.

Ophthalmics Pertaining to products for the eyes. GMP requirements for the preparation of ophthalmics are essentially identical to those for parenterals.

Ophthalmologics Drugs used in ophthalmology.

Opinion (in relation to Independent Ethic Committee) The judgement and/or the advice provided by an Independent Ethics Committee (IEC).

OQ (operational qualification) Documented verification that aspects of a facility system that can affect product quality perform as intended throughout anticipated operating ranges.

Oral Relating to the mouth.

Oral contraceptive A birth control pill taken by mouth. Most oral contraceptives include both estrogen and progesterone. When given in certain amounts and at certain times in the menstrual cycle, these hormones prevent the ovary from releasing an egg for fertilization.

Oral drug A drug that may be administered through ingestion (through the mouth).

Oral product A pharmaceutical product meant to be introduced through the mouth in the form of a tablet, capsule, or suspension.

Oral solid dosage drug Formulated in a solid or powder form for patient to ingest orally.

Orbital welding Automatic or machine welding of tubes or pipe in-place with the electrode rotating (or orbiting) around the work. Orbital welding can be done with the addition of filler material or as a fusion process without the addition of filler.

Organelles Membrane-surrounded structures found in eukaryotic cells; they contain enzymes and other components required for specialized cell function.

Organic Organic matter is a broad category that includes both natural and man-made molecules containing carbon and hydrogen. All living matter in water is made up of organic molecules. The most common are by-products of vegetative decay such as tannins, lignins, and humic acid.

Organic peroxide An organic compound that contains the bivalent -0-0- structure and which may be considered to be a structural derivative of hydrogen peroxide where on or both of the hydrogen atoms have been replaced by an organic radical. Organic peroxides can present an explosion hazard (detonation or deflagration) or they can be shock sensitive. They can also decompose into various unstable compounds over an extended period.

Organism A single, autonomous living thing. Bacteria and yeasts are organisms; mammalian and insect cells used in culture are not.

Origin Point or region where DNA replication is begun. Often abbreviated Ori.

Orphan drug Drugs developed for rare diseases and conditions which, in the U.S., affect fewer than 200,000 people or, in the European Union, affect 5 or fewer per 10,000 people. Because sales of orphan drugs are likely to be small compared to their development costs, pharmaceutical companies are awarded exclusive rights to market these medicines for a period of time as an incentive to develop them.

Orphan products The Orphan Drug Act (ODA) provides for granting special status to a product /indication combination upon request of a sponsor, and if the product/ indication combination meets certain criteria. This status is referred to as orphan designation. Orphan designation qualifies the sponsor of the product for the tax credit and marketing exclusivity incentives of the ODA.

Orthostatic (postural) hypotension The gravitational stress of sudden standing normally causes pooling of blood in the venous capacitance vessels of the legs and trunk. The subsequent transient decrease in venous return and cardiac output results in reduced BP and can cause the individual to faint. Baroreceptors in the aortic arch and carotid bodies sense the change in BP and activate autonomic reflexes that rapidly normalize BP by causing a transient tachycardia and vasoconstriction in the lower limbs. Agents that interfere with this reflex response can cause orthostatic (postural) hypotension ie. alpha-blockers, ganglionic blockers and guanethidine.

Pharmacokinetics the science and study of the factors which determine the amount of chemical agents at their sites of biological effect at various times after the application of an agent or drug to biological systems. Pharmacokinetics includes study of drug absorption and distribution ("biotranslocation"), study of the chemical alterations a drug may undergo in the body, ("biotransformation"), and study of the means by which drugs are stored in the body and eliminated from it. Simply put, pharmacokinetics considers how drugs move around the body and how quickly this movement occurs. This includes the processes which control the absorption, distribution, metabolism, and excretion of drugs (A.D.M.E.).

Pharmacodynamics the study of the relationship of drug concentration to drug effects

Pharmacogenetics the study of how people respond differently to medicines due to their genetic inheritance.The term has been pieced together from the words pharmacology (the study of how drugs work in the body) and genetics (the study of how traits are inherited). An ultimate goal of pharmacogenetics is to understand how someone's genetic make-up determines how well a medicine works in his or her body, as well as what side effects or toxicity are likely to occur.

Pheochromocytoma is a rare tumor that arises from tissue in the adrenal gland. The tumor increases production and release of epinephrine (adrenaline) and norepinephrine (noradrenaline), which raises blood pressure and heart rate. Most pheochromocytomas are removed surgically, individuals are initially stabilized with alpha-blockers (ie. phenoxybenzamine) or alpha/beta-blockers (labetalol or carvedilol). Beta-blockers alone should never be given alone prior to administration of an alpha-blocker.

Prototype drug is the 'lead agent' in a drug class (family). ie propranolol is the prototype of the beta-blockers and metoprolol is the prototype of the beta1-blockers. These are common agents used in exam questions.

Osmosis The diffusion of a solvent through a semipermeable membrane from a solution of higher concentration to one of lower concentration until there are equal concentrations of fluid on both sides of the membrane.

Osmotic pressure Pressure generated by the osmotic flow of water through a membrane into a (aqueous) phase containing a solute in a higher concentration.

OTC drug An OTC drug is available without a medical prescription, intended for self-healing; OTC stands for "Over the Counter". The OTC status of a drug is obtained by the producer for a certain drug form and for a certain indication, should his application for drug registration be positively assessed by the state authorities .

Out of pocket costs The portion of payments for health services that must be paid by the enrollee, including co-payments, co-insurance, or deductibles.

Out of Specification An examination, measurement, or test result that does not comply with preestablished criteria.

Overactive bladder syndrome (OAB) A symptom syndrome of urgency, which can lead to micturition and incontinence.

Overdosing Overdosing is a condition resulting from the administration of an excessive drug dose; the leaflet, which must be included with each drug, covers symptoms of overdosing and how to solve the potential consequences.

Oxaliplatin Newer platinum-derivative drug used in metastatic large-bowel cancer.

Oxandrolone (Oxandrin) Indications: Anabolic steroid for treatment of AIDS wasting syndrome.

Contraindications: Known hypersensitivity, history of breast or prostate cancer, significant hepatic dysfunction, nephrosis, pregnancy.

Dosage: 5-10 mg po bid.

Toxicity: Edema, hypertension, virilization, glucose intolerance, hyperlipidemia, abnormal liver function tests.

Oxidation (on metals) The formation of an oxide layer on a metal surface. When oxidation occurs because of welding, it is visible as discoloration. The discoloration or heat tint produced by oxidation has been associated with the onset of corrosion in stainless steel piping systems.

Oxide layer In welding, an area usually located in the heat-affected zone (HAZ) of the weldment where an oxidation reaction has taken place.

Oxide thickness The depth at which the oxide signal has fallen to half the maximum peak height. Typical values for well electropolished 316L stainless steel range from 20 to 50 angstroms (⊕).

Oxidizer A material other than a blasting agent or explosive, that readily yields oxygen or other oxidizing gas, or that readily reacts to promote or initiate combustion of combustible materials. Oxidizers are subdivided as follows: 1. Class 4 - An oxidizer that can undergo an explosive reaction due to contamination or exposure to thermal or physical shock. In addition, the oxidizer will enhance the burning rate and may cause spontaneous ignition of combustible materials.

2. Class 3 - An oxidizer that will cause a severe increase in the burning rate of combustible materials with which it comes in contact or that will undergo vigorous, self-sustained decomposition due to contamination or exposure to heat.

3. Class 2 - An oxidizer that will cause a moderate increase in the burning rate or that may cause spontaneous ignition of combustible materials with which it comes in contact.

4. Class 1 - An oxidizer whose primary hazard is that it slightly increases the burning rate but does not cause spontaneous ignition when it comes in contact with combustible materials.

Ozone Formed by an electric discharge or by the slow combustion of phosphorus, ozone is a modified and condensed form of oxygen, in which three atoms of oxygen are combined to form the molecule, O3. Because it is a powerful oxidizing agent it is used in deionized water systems to kill bacteria and to reduce by oxidation the amount of Total Organic Carbon (TOC) in the water. Air containing a perceptible amount of ozone has an odor suggesting chlorine or sulfurous acid gas.

P

P value The lowest level of significance at which a given null hypothesis can be rejected; that is, the probability of observing a result as extreme or more extreme than that observed if the null hypothesis is true.

P2X (P2X3) ATP-gated ion channels (ATP-gated ion channel, subtype 3).

Packaged equipment An assembly of individual pieces or stages of equipment, complete with inter-connecting piping and connections for external piping. The assembly may be mounted on a skid or other structure prior to delivery.

Packaging Identification of the size of the packaging (10, 30, 100 tablets...), usually including drug form (tablets, capsules, suppositories...).

Packaging material Any material intended to protect an intermediate or API (Active Pharmaceutical Ingredient) during storage and transport.

Pain management medicine Pain relief medicine is administered via a pump on a regular basis and is used for hospice patients or patients with chronic pain or post-surgery symptoms.

Pairing A method by which subjects are selected so that two subjects with similar characteristics (for example, weight, smoking habits) are assigned to a set, but one receives Treatment A and the other receives Treatment B.

Palliative or symptomatic therapy Treatment directed only toward relief of the patient's symptoms, toward making the patient feel better without necessarily altering the natural course of the disease. Analgesic agents such as aspirin or morphine have obvious palliative effects.

Pancreas The gland responsible for insulin production.

Pandemic disease An epidemic over an especially wide geographic area.

PAR (proven acceptable range) A range for a critical parameter that has been determined to be achievable and appropriate for the process or processes with which it is associated. It is established by knowledge gained through relevant documentation and actual testing. A process should perform consistently and as intended when all critical parameters are held within the established PARs.

Paracetamol Very valuable for mild to moderate pain.

Parallel trial Volunteers are randomized to one of two differing treatment groups (usually medicine and placebo) and usually receive the assigned treatment during the entire trial. Also called parallel group trial, parallel design trial.

Parameter 1. One of the elements of an experiment which can be varied, but which the experimenter tries to control or maintain constant during the course of a specific experiment, while intentionally altering the independent variable and observing changes in the dependent variable. Parameters in one experiment (stimulus strength, for example) might well be independent variables in another.

2. Terms of an equation that do not vary within the context of an experiment, but may be different under different circumstances. Parameter should be distinguished from the independent and dependent variables. For example, in the equation of a straight line, y = mx + b, x is normally the independent variable (the variable under experimental control), y is the dependent (measured) variable, and the slope m and intercept b are parameters, which are the same for a given line, but may be different for a different line.

Parenteral drug (LVP, SVP) A parenteral drug is defined as one intended for injection through the skin or other external boundary tissue, rather than through the alimentary canal, so that active substances they contain are administered, using gravity or force, directly into a blood vessel, organ, tissue, or lesion. They are infused when administered intravenously (IV), or injected when administered intramuscularly (IM), or subcutaneously into the human body. A large volume parenteral (LVP) is a unit dose container of greater than 100ml that is terminally sterilized by heat. Small volume parenteral (SVP) is a "catch-all" for all non-LVP parenterals products except biologicals.

Parenteral nutrition A method of delivering nutrition directly into the bloodstream through a vein, bypassing the digestive system. The approach is usually a temporary method of getting a patient through a difficult spell of gastroparesis. Fluids given usually include salt (saline), glucose, amino acids, electrolytes, vitamins and medications.

Parkinson's disease Degeneration of nerve cells in certain areas of the brain resulting in motor disturbances like poor mobility and trembling of the limbs in the state of rest and muscle rigidity.

Partial validation Refers to the process of demonstrating that a modification of an already validated bioanalytical method can be incorporated without the need for a complete revalidation of the method. The extent of the partial validation can range from as little as a single analytical run for the determination of intra-assay accuracy and precision to a nearly full, multiple-run validation. Typical changes that fall into this category include method transfer between laboratories or analysts, change in detection method, change in anticoagulant, change in matrix within species, change in species within matrix, change in sample processing, change in calibration range, change in instrument, limited sample volume, selectivity of an analyte in the presence of concomitant medications or specific metabolites, etc.

Participating dentist Is a dentist that is within the DentalGuard Preferred provider network offered by The Guardian Life Insurance Company.

Participating pharmacy A pharmacy that has entered into a contract with a pharmacy benefits plan to fill covered prescriptions for the plan's members.

Particle concentration Number of individual particles per unit volume of air. ISO 14644-1

Particulate Usually a solid particle large enough to be removed by filtration. Nonfilterable solids are usually referred to as colloids.

Particle size The apparent maximum linear dimension of a particle in the plane of observation as seen with a microscope or the equivalent diameter of a particle detected by automatic instrumentation. The equivalent diameter is the diameter of a reference sphere having known properties and producing the same response in the sensing instrument as the particle being measured. ISO 14644-1.

Particle Solid or liquid object which for purposes of classification of air cleanliness, falls within a cumulative distribution that is based upon a threshold (lower limit) size in the range from 0,1 μm to 5 μm. ISO 14644-1.

Passivation A final chemical treatment/cleaning process that removes exogenous iron or iron compounds from the surface of stainless steel piping and equipment by the use of a mild oxidant, such as a nitric acid solution, or by "in-situ electropolishing. The purpose of passivation is to restore and/or enhance the spontaneous formation of the chemically inert surface or protective passive film.

Passive immunity Temporary immunity produced by administration of gamma globulin.

Passive layer A passive oxidized film that forms naturally on a stainless steel surface when exposed to air or similar oxidizing environment thus protecting the underlying base metal from corrosion. Welding disturbs the passive layer by reducing the chromium and increasing the iron, thus altering the chromium/iron ratio (measure of corrosion resistance). Upon completion and approval of the weld, the weld surface and adjacent boundary area must be brought back to a passive state. Additionally, normal operating conditions in typical Water For Injection, reverse osmosis, deionized water, clean steam, Clean In Place, and process piping often lead to formation of the most prevalent form of self catalyzing corrosion called "rouge" (French for red), which is a colloidal form of rust containing iron oxide, chromium and nickel in various forms. This problem is further accentuated by high temperature. The rouge layer acts as a passive layer until it becomes so thick that it "sloughs off" into the process or water stream.

Passivity The state in which a stainless steel exhibits a very low corrosion rate. Also known as passivity, is the loss (or minimizing) of chemical reactivity exhibited by certain metals and alloys under special environmental conditions.

Pasteurization The heating of milk, wines, fruit juices, etc., for about thirty minutes at 68°C (154.4°F) whereby the living bacteria are destroyed, but the flavor or bouquet is preserved; the spores are unaffected, but are kept from developing by immediately cooling the liquid to 10°C (50°F) or lower.

Patent Medically, as opposed to legally, the word means unobstructed or open, e.g., all surgically implanted cannulae must be patent for animals to be used in a study. Usually pronounced with a long "a", i.e.,"PAY-tent".

Pathogen Any microbiological or eukaryotic cell containing sufficient genetic information, which upon expression of such information is capable of producing disease in healthy people, plants, or animals.

Pathogenic Causing or capable of causing disease.

Pathogenic organisms Organisms capable of causing disease, either directly (by infecting) or indirectly (by producing a toxin that causes illness).

Pathway A series of related steps or events along a defined route. In metabolism, the term refers to a sequence of reactions which change one substance into another.

Pathway profiling The process of mapping and identifying additional proteins along a pathway

Patient file Contains demographic, medical, and treatment information about a patient or subject. It may be paper-based or a mixture of computer and paper records.

Patient People with a specific disease or condition, particularly those being treated by a health professional.

Payer The party or group an individual contracts with to cover healthcare services, unless the patient is paying out-of-pocket. This is sometimes referred to as a "third party payer".

PBM PBM is short for pharmacy benefits manager. PBMs are managed care entities that manage or administer pharmacy benefits and programs to promote health to plan sponsors, members and health care providers. Aetna Pharmacy Management is a PBM.

PCI (percutaneous coronary intervention) PCI is the process of using a catheter with a balloon at its tip to open or widen a narrowed blood vessel.

PE (Polyethylene) A thermoplastic material that varies from type to type according to the particular molecular structure of each type, i.e. its crystallinity, molecular weight, and molecular weight distribution. These variations are possible through changes in polymerization conditions used during manufacturing. Low-density polyethylene (LDPE) has a melt point of 221°F (105°C), specific gravity of 0.91 to 0.925 g/cc, increased toughness, stress cracking resistance, clarity, flexibility, and elongation. It also has reduced creep and mold shrinkage. Polyethylene of higher density such as HDPE has better permeation barrier properties, hardness, abrasion resistance, chemical resistance, and surface gloss. It is important to note that photo or light oxidation will occur when natural PE is exposed to UV radiation, usually from the sun.

Penetrance A term indicating the likelihood that a given gene will actually result in disease.

Penicillin An antibiotic containing a ß-lactam ring that inhibits an enzyme responsible for making peptide cross-links in the bacterial cell wall. It is obtained from cultures of the molds Penicillium Notatum or Penicillium Chrysogenum.

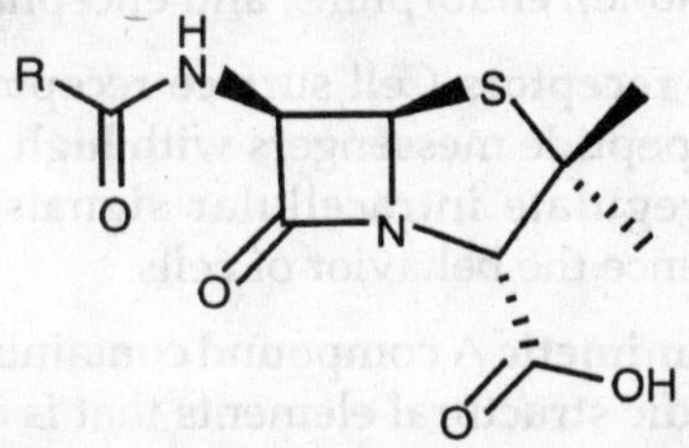

Penicillium The genus of mold causing a zone of inhibition in an agar plate of bacteria. It is the organism, which produces natural penicillin.

Peptide A secondary protein derivative defined as "a definitely characterized combination of two or more amino acids, the carboxyl (COOH) group of one being united with the amino (NH2) group of the other, with the elimination of a molecule of water". They form a peptide bond.

Indications Treatment and prophylaxis of PCP in patients unable to tolerate TMP-SMX or dapsone.

Contraindications: Known hypersensitivity; severe asthma or bronchospasm, active pulmonary tuberculosis (aerosol preparation).

Dosage: Treatment: intravenous 3-4 mg/kg qd for up to three weeks.

Prophylaxis: aerosol 300 mg via Respirgard II nebulizer once a month.

Toxicity: Aerosol: bronchospasm, particularly in patients with history of asthma or chronic obstructive pulmonary disease; pharyngeal irritation; metallic taste.

Intravenous: hypotension, nephrotoxicity, hypoglycemia, hyperglycemia, leukopenia, thrombocytopenia, hypokalemia, hypocalcemia.

Peptide hormones A diverse class of hormones that are synthesized and excreted at various sites within the body. Examples include: insulin, relaxin, glucagons, growth hormone, vasopressin, ACTH (Adrenocorticotropic Hormone), endorphins, and encephalins.

Peptide receptors Cell surface receptors that bind peptide messengers with high affinity and regulate intracellular signals which influence the behavior of cells.

Peptidomimetic A compound containing non-peptidic structural elements that is capable of mimicking or antagonizing the biological action(s) of a natural parent peptide. A peptidomimetic does no longer have classical peptide characteristics such as enzymatically scissille peptidic bonds.

Peptoid A **peptidomimetic** that results from the oligomeric assembly of N-substituted glycines.

Percent recovery In reverse osmosis or ultrafiltration, the ratio of pure water output to feedwater input.

Percent rejection In reverse osmosis or ultrafiltration, the ratio of impurities removed to total impurities in the incoming feedwater. For example, RO membranes typically remove (reject) 90% of the dissolved inorganic contaminants in water.

Performance qualification [PQ] Documented verification that theprocess and/or the total process-related system performs as intendedthroughout all anticipated operating ranges.

Performer Is an employee on the basis of whose services a contributing employer is obligated to contribute to the AFTRA Health and Retirement Funds pursuant to a collective bargaining agreement by and between the employer and AFTRA.

Period effect Designated period during the course of a trial in which subjects are observed and no treatment is administered.

Peripheral arterial occlusive disease Obstruction of the supply of blood to the limbs as a result of arteriosclerosis.

Peristaltic pump A type of positive displacement pump that operates by pulsations of flow caused by passing rollers over flexible tubing. Operating pressure limited by tubing tolerance.

Permeability He ability of a body to pass a fluid under pressure.

Permeate In reverse osmosis, the water that diffuses through the membrane, thereby becoming purified water.

Permissible exposure limit (PEL) The maximum permitted eight-hour time-weighted average concentration of an airborne contaminant. For Permissible Exposure Limits .

Permissions or privileges Security codes that define or restrict which users can read, write, and execute the associated files, directories, or programs. Some departments need to look only at data, some need to input data or run programs, and others may not need to look at the data at all.

Peroxisome Very small membrane-bound particles responsible for photorespiration in plants. Similar to lysosome in structure, but not in function.

Personalized medicine Our core philosophy of delivering the right drugs, directed toward the right molecular targets, to the right patients, at the right time.

Petrolatum White petrolatum is a purified mixture of semi-solid hydrocarbons obtained from petroleum. It is a common base or carrier for ointments. It can be sterile filtered at elevated temperatures.

pH The hydrogen ion concentration of a solution. Numerically the pH is equal to the negative logarithm of hydrogen ion concentration expressed in moles/liter. pH 7 is neutral, above 7 is alkaline and below is acidic.

Phage A virus for which the natural host is a bacterial cell.

Phagocyte A cell that engulfs foreign particles from its surroundings by a process called phagocytosis. The cell releases hydrolytic enzymes from intracellular bodies called lysosomes that partially digest the foreign particle, after which it is further degraded in the phagocyte cytoplasm.

Pharmacare direct PharmaCare's Mail Services Pharmacy.

Pharmaceutical A medicinal drug, or relating to or engaged in pharmacy or the manufacture and sale of pharmaceuticals. A pharmaceutical product is generally one that is made up using available chemical compounds.

Pharmaceutical area A general manufacturing area classification designated by the need for a change of clothing (e.g., Packing Hall).

Pharmacist A professional who fills prescriptions, and in the case of a compounding pharmacist, makes them. Pharmacists are familiar with medication ingredients, interactions, cautions, and hints.

Pharmacodynamic (PD) A study of a pharmacological or clinical effect of the medicine in individuals to describe the relation of the effect to dose or drug concentration. A pharmacodynamic effect can be a potentially adverse effect (anticholinergic effect with a tricyclic), a measure of activity thought related to clinical benefit (various measures of beta-blockade, effect on ECG intervals, inhibition of ACE or of angiotensin I or II response), a short term desired effect, often a surrogate endpoint (blood pressure, cholesterol), or the ultimate intended clinical benefit (effects on pain, depression, sudden death).

Pharmacoeconomics Branch of economics that applies cost-benefit, cost-utility, cost-minimization, and cost-effectiveness analyses to compare the economics of different pharmaceutical products or to compare drug therapy to other treatments. Sometimes referred to as outcomes research.

Pharmacoepigenomics MGMT hypermethylation demonstrates the possibility of pharmacoepigenomics: methylated tumors are more sensitive to the killing effects of alkylating drugs used in chemotherapy.

This review argues that the epigenome, which plays a critical role in controlling gene expression, plays also an important role in drug responsiveness. The epigenome is composed of chromatin and its modifications and DNA methylation. DNA methylation and chromatin structure are dynamic and tightly linked. Alterations in DNA methylation are involved in the pathology of cancer and in normal aging. It is suggested here that pharmacoepigenomics should be recognized as a new field in pharmacology. This field will address the epigenomic basis of issues which were traditionally the focus of pharmacogenetics and pharmacogenomics such as inter-individual differences in drug responsiveness, the impact of drugs on gene expression profiles, identification of unpredicted side effects of drugs at early stages of preclinical development and the discovery of novel drug targets.

Pharmacogenetic test An assay intended to study interindividual variations in DNA sequence related to drug absorption and disposition (pharmacokinetics) or drug action (pharmacodynamics) including polymorphic variation in the genes that encode the functions of transporters, metabolizing enzymes, receptors, and other proteins.

Pharmacogenetics Adverse effects from toxic substances from the environment.

A subset of pharmacogenomics encompassing the study of genetic variation underlying differential response to drugs, particularly genes involved in drug metabolism.

With the implementation of pharmacogenetics, diseases will be evaluated by mechanisms, rather than just symptoms, and early response will be based on prognosis and susceptibility rather than just diagnosis. It will introduce a bottom- up approach to disease, which will be defined in terms of its heterogeneity, and not "averaged out" to conform to a uniform model.

Pharmacogenomic test An assay intended to study interindividual variations in whole genome or candidate gene, single nucleotide polymorphism SNP maps, haplotype markers, or alterations in gene expression or inactivation that may be correlated with pharmacological function and therapeutic response, In some cases the pattern or profile of change is the relevant biomarker, rather than

Pharmacogenomics Comprises the study of variations in targets or target pathways, variation in metabolizing enzymes (pharmacogenetics) or, in the case of infectious organisms, genetic variations in the pathogen.

Pharmacogenomics does not include the use of genetic or genomic techniques for the purposes of biological product characterization or quality control .

Pharmacogenomics technologies The most critical technology is high throughput genotyping (both for large numbers of samples to be genotyped for a few variants, and a smaller number for fuller sequencing of a large number of variants).

Pharmacokinetic pharmacodynamic relationship Quantitative relationship between blood and tissue concentrations of the drug (pharmacokinetics) and the effects (pharmacodynamics) of a drug.

Pharmacokinetics Operationally, the term describes the time course of the variation of a drug's concentration in various body tissues, as well as blood, blood plasma and urine, following dosing. It is the study of ADME, i.e., the absorption (extent and rate from the site of administration), distribution from plasma into tissues (includes binding to plasma proteins and tissue components), metabolism (biotransformation into more readily excretable compounds) and excretion (elimination from the body) of drugs. These factors, combined with dosage, determine the concentration of a drug at its site(s) of action (and the intensity of its effects) as a function of time. Pharmacokinetics frequently utilizes mathematical equations to describe and model the concentration versus time profile of a drug in sampled body fluids such as plasma. Compartmental models are widely used to calculate fundamental parameters from preclinical or clinical experimental data.

Pharmacological Caused by action of the agonist and antagonist at the same site.

In the case of pharmacological antagonisms, the terms competitive and non-competitive antagonism are used with meanings analogous to competitive and non-competitive enzyme inhibition as used in enzymology.

Pharmacology (Gr. Pharmakon - drug, and Logos - word) Is the study of drugs in all their aspects. Pharmacy, although often confused with pharmacology, is, in fact, an independent discipline concerned with the art and science of the preparation, compounding, and dispensing of drugs. Pharmacognosy is a branch of pharmacy that deals with the identification and analysis of the plant and animal tissues from which drugs may be extracted. Pharmacodynamics, which in common usage is usually termed "pharmacology", is concerned with the study of drug effects and how they are produced. The pharmacodynamicist, or pharmacologist, identifies the effects produced by drugs, and determines the sites and mechanisms of their action in the body. The pharmacologist studies the physiological or biochemical mechanisms by which drug actions are produced. The pharmacologist also investigates those factors that modify the effects of drugs, i.e. the routes of administration, influence of rates of absorption, differential distribution, and the body's mechanisms of excretion and detoxification, on the total effect of a drug. Pharmacotherapeutics is the study of the use of drugs in the diagnosis, prevention, and treatment of disease states. Toxicology is the study of drug effects that are inimical to health. The toxicologist may investigate such diverse problems as the effects of overdoses of pharmacotherapeutic agents; the diagnosis, treatment, and prevention of lead poisoning in the paint manufacturing industry; the possibility that criminal poisoning was the cause of an otherwise inexplicable death, etc.

"Experimental pharmacology, in the broadest sense, deals with the reactions of living organisms to chemical agents, or, to put the matter in another way, the behavior of organisms to changes in the chemical environment in which they live. Pharmacology is a part of biology... Of all the vast number of pharmacologic reactions, those that the physician attempts to use for curative purposes are of the greatest interest and most deserved of study. This part of pharmacology, the scientific knowledge of remedial agents, forms the theoretical foundation for therapeutics..."

Pharmacometabonomics The use of metabolomics technologies in all phases of the drug discovery and development process.

Pharmacophore The ensemble of steric and electronic features that is necessary to ensure the optimal supramolecular interactions with a specific biological target structure and to trigger (or to block) its biological response. Does not represent a real molecule or a real association of functional groups, but a purely abstract concept that accounts for the common molecular interaction capacities of a group of compounds towards their target structure. Can be considered as the largest common denominator shared by a set of active molecules. This definition discards a misuse often found in the medicinal chemistry literature which consists of naming as pharmacophores simple chemical functionalities such as guanidines, sulfonamides or dihydroimidazoles (formerly imidazolines), or typical structural skeletons such as flavones, phenothiazines, prostaglandins or steroids. Pharmacophoric descriptors are used to define a pharmacophore, including H- bonding, hydrophobic and electrostatic interaction sites, defined by atoms, ring centers and virtual points.

The ensemble of steric and electronic factors which are necessary to insure supramolecular interactions with a specific biological target structure.

A template of chemical properties for an active site of a protein - representing these properties' spatial relationship to one another - that theoretically defines a ligand that would bind to that site.

Pharmacoproteomics Once you have identified a number of proteins secreted in sera or urine, you can segregate the proteins by which are linked to early disease, the onset of metastasis, who does and does not tolerate treatment, toxic effects, and who is prone to resistance or relapse. Fundamentally, you establish a pharmacoproteomic profile of an individual. Like pharmacogenomics, which allows researchers and clinicians to predict the response of an individual to drug treatment on the basis of his or her genetic profile, the evolving field of pharmacoproteomics allows drug developers and clinicians to further subdivide the treated population.

Pharmacotyping The individualized drug selection and dosage profiling by the health professional, based on patient's genotyping and haplotyping data for genes involved in pharmacodynamic and pharmacokinetic drug actions in the body

Pharmacovigilance The science and activities relating to the detection, assessment, understanding and prevention of adverse effects or any other drug-related problems.

Pharmacy co payment, or co-pay The amount of money a member pays to a participating pharmacy for prescription medications covered by a pharmacy benefits plan.

Pharmacy network This term refers to all of the pharmacies that participate in a particular network. To utilize their prescription coverage, a member must have their prescriptions filled at a network pharmacy.

Phase 1 (clinical trials) The first of three phases of a clinical trial, in which researchers test a new drug or treatment in a small group of people (20-80) for the first time to evaluate its safety, determine a safe dosage range, and identify side effects.

Phase 1 studies. Initial safety trials on a new medicine in which investigators attempt to establish the dose range tolerated by about 20 to 80 healthy volunteers for single and multiple doses. Although usually conducted with healthy volunteers, Phase 1 trials are sometimes conducted with severely ill patients, for example, those with cancer or AIDS. When pharmacokinetic issues are being addressed (for example, metabolism of a new antiepileptic medicine in stable epileptic patients whose microsomal liver enzymes have been induced by other antiepileptic medicines), trials may be conducted in less-ill patients. Pharmacokinetic trials are usually considered Phase 1 trials regardless of when they are conducted during a medicine's development.

Phase 1 unit A facility designed specifically for conducting studies involving normal, healthy volunteers. It may be operated by a sponsor company, a contract research organization (CRO), or a special unit of a hospital.

Phase 2a studies. Pilot clinical trials to evaluate efficacy and safety in selected populations of about 100 to 300 subjects who have the disease or condition to be treated, diagnosed, or prevented. Often involve hospitalized subjects who can be closely monitored. Objectives may focus on dose-response, type of patient, frequency of dosing, or any of a number of other issues involved in safety and efficacy.

Phase 2b studies. Well-controlled trials to evaluate safety and efficacy in subjects who have the disease or condition to be treated, diagnosed, or prevented. These trials usually represent the most rigorous demonstration of a medicine's efficacy. Synonym: pivotal trials.

Phase 3 studies. Multicenter studies in populations of perhaps 1000 to 3000 (or more) subjects for whom the medicine is eventually intended. Phase 3 trials generate additional safety and efficacy data from relatively large numbers of subjectsin both controlled and uncontrolled designs and are used to support a PLA. Trials are also conducted in special groups of patients or under special conditions dictated by the nature of a particular medicine and/or disease. Phase 3 trials often provide much of the information needed for the package insert and labeling of the medicine.

Phase 3b studies. Trials conducted after submission of a new drug application (NDA), but before the product's approval and market launch. Phase 3b trials may supplement or complete earlier trials, or they may seek different kinds of information (for example, quality of life or marketing). Phase 3b is the period between submission for approval and receipt of marketing authorization.

Phase 4 studies. After a medicine is marketed, Phase 4 trials provide additional details about the product's safety and efficacy. They may be used to evaluate formulations, dosages, durations of treatment, medicine interactions, and other factors. Patients from various demographic groups may be studied. An important part of many Phase 4 studies is detecting and defining previously unknown or inadequately quantified adverse reactions and related risk factors. Phase 4 studies that are primarily observational or nonexperimental are frequently called postmarketing surveillance.

Phase 5 studies. Postmarketing surveillance is sometimes referred to as Phase 5.

Phase I The main aim of this phase is to determine drug safety. At this stage, drugs are tested in a small group of healthy volunteers to determine the drug's activity.

Phase I to IV trials The Boehringer Ingelheim definition.

Phase II These trials are aimed at identifying the optimal dose to be used in Phase III trials and, ideally, they identify drugs that will not make it through the next phase of testing. Typically, Phase II trials are double-blinded and have placebo controls.]

Phase III These studies, which take several years, can involve thousands of patients at multiple trial centers. They are aimed at definitively determining the drug's effectiveness and its side- effect profiles. These studies are also typically double-blinded and placebo- controlled.

Phase IIIb Subjects entered on a phase III trial may want to stay on the drug after the study is completed and closed and while the data is being readied for presentation. A Phase IIIB study allows "compassionate" use of the drug during this interim time.

Phase IV/ postmarketing surveillance At this stage, after a drug has been launched, pharmaceutical companies may conduct further studies of its performance, often examining long- term safety.

Phase of a clinical trial Clinical trials are usually conducted in a series of steps, called phases.

Preclinical trials are early experiments performed in the lab prior to being tested in humans. This early research helps to identify potential treatments that are unsafe or ineffective.

Phase I trials are the first step in testing a new approach in humans. In these studies, researchers evaluate what dose is safe, how a new agent should be given (by mouth, injected into a vein, or injected into the muscle, for example), and how often. Researchers watch closely for any harmful side effects. Phase I trials usually enroll a small number of patients and take place at only a few locations.

Phase II trials study the safety and effectiveness of an agent or intervention, and evaluate how it affects the human body. Phase II studies usually focus on a particular medical condition.

Phase III trials compare a new agent or intervention (or new use of a standard one) with the current standard therapy. Participants are randomly assigned to the standard group or the new group, usually by computer. This method, called randomization, helps to avoid bias and ensures that human choices or other factors do not affect the study's results. In most cases, studies move into phase III testing only after they have shown promise in phases I and II. Phase III trials may include hundreds of people across the country.

Phase IV trials are conducted to further evaluate the long-term safety and effectiveness of a treatment. They usually take place after the treatment has been approved for standard use. Several hundred to several thousand people may take part in a phase IV study.

Phase zero, Phase O Phase Zero is a novel preclinical testing service that combines a range of integrated technologies and involves the introduction of human tissue at the earliest stages of drug development. It allows target identification and validation as well as testing the viability of drug leads and candidates in human tissue before entering the clinic. This enables rationalization of the drug development process and improves the outcome at several points along the developmental path.

phases of clinical trials Clinical trials are generally categorized into four (sometimes five) phases. An investigational medicine or product may be evaluated in two or more phases simultaneously in different trials, and some trials may overlap two different phases.

Phencyclidine and analogues Phencyclidine (PCP) was synthesised and tested in the early 1950s and recommended for clinical trials as an anaesthetic in humans in 1957. In 1965, further human clinical investigation of PCP was discontinued and the compound was marketed commercially as a veterinary anaesthetic. .

PCP became available through the drug culture in the late 1960s, referred as "PeaCePill", commonly sold as "angel dust", "crystal" or "hog", on the illicit market in powder, tablet, leaf mixture, and 1 gram "rock" crystal forms, usually taken orally, by smoking, snorting, or intravenous injection.

Phenol An organic acid often used as a disinfectant. Proper strength for a bacteriocidal preparation is 5%. Sometimes dispersed as an aerosol "fog" in manufacturing rooms.

Phenotype standards The characterization of phenotype is important for both the genotype- to- phenotype methods as well as the phenotype - to- genotype methods. Phenotype is difficult to precisely define, but can be thought of as functional features of gene products, ranging in detail from molecular to the individual and population levels.

Phenotype The entire physical, biochemical, and physiological makeup of an individual cell as determined both genetically and environmentally. This is the "outward, physical manifestation" of the organism. These are the physical parts, the sum of the atoms, molecules, macromolecules, cells, structures, metabolism, energy utilization, tissues, organs, reflexes and behaviors; anything that is part of the observable structure, function or behavior of a living organism.

Phenotype to genotype Phenotype- to-genotype approaches take a different approach to pharmacogenomic discovery. Instead of identifying a family of genes in which to characterize genetic variations, investigators search for a phenotypic measure that shows significant variation. This measure can be a clinical measure (such as the rate of clearance of a drug or the peak level of the drug for a given dose), a cellular measure (the rate of cellular uptake of a drug or the profile of gene expression) or a molecular measure (the enzymatic turnover rate of an enzyme or a substrate binding constant).

Phosphorous Related to bone activity and usually follows exact opposite of calcium.

Photo oxidation The mechanism by which ultraviolet light reduces Total Organic Carbon (TOC) to Carbon Dioxide. If halogenated organics are present, both CO2 and mineral acids can be formed.

Phycomycetes Algalike fungi that do not posses chlorophyll and cannot photosynthesize. Aquatic and terrestrial molds belong to this category.

Photoaptamers Aptamers that incorporate a brominated deoxyuridine (BrdU) in place of the thymidine (T) normally found in DNA. A photoaptamer recognizes both the complex shape and charge distribution of its protein target and the presence of specific amino acid residues at specific sites.

Photoautotrophs Facultative autotrophs that obtain their energy from light.

Photoluminescent The property of emitting light as the result of absorption of visible or invisible light, which continues for a length of time after excitation.

Physical barrier Any equipment, facilities, or devices (e.g., fermentors, factories, filters, thermal oxidizers) that are designed to achieve containment.

Physical hazard A classification of a chemical for which there is scientifically valid evidence that it is a combustible liquid, compressed gas, cryogenic, explosive, flammable gas, flammable liquid, flammable solid, organic peroxide, oxidizer, pyrophoric, unstable, (reactive), or water-reactive material.

Physical manipulation A process other than a chemical reaction that may change the purity of the physical properties of the material, including but not limited to, crystallization, recrystallization, gel filtration, chromatography, milling, drying, or blending.

Physical map A map of the locations of identifiable landmarks on DNA (e.g., restriction enzyme cutting sites, genes), regardless of inheritance. Distance is measured in base pairs. For the human genome, the lowest-resolution physical map is the banding patterns on the 24 different chromosomes; the highest resolution map would be the complete nucleotide sequence of the chromosomes.

Physician Means a duly licensed doctor of medicine authorized to perform medical or surgical service within the lawful scope of his or her practice.

Physiological Caused by agonist and antagonist acting at two independent sites and inducing independent, but opposite effects.

Phyto pharmaceuticals Herbal drugs used, for example, to reduce nerve or digestive problems, upper respiratory tract or urinary tract diseases.

Pickle An acid or other chemical solution used as a bath to remove scale and oxides fro the surface of metals before plating or finishing.

Pipe A pressure-tight cylinder used to convey a fluid or to transmit a fluid pressure ordinarily designated "pipe" in applicable material specifications. Materials designated "tube" or "tubing" in the specifications are treated as pipe when intended for pressure service. Types of pipe, according to the method of manufacture, are: 1. Electric resistance-welded pipe (ERW)

2. Furnace butt welded pipe, continuous welded

3. Electric-fusion welded pipe 4. Double submerged-arc welded pipe

5. Seamless pipe

6. Spiral welded pipe.

Pipe size Pipe size is determined by diameter and schedule. For bioprocessing equipment, pipe does not include tube.

Pit A small surface void resulting from a localized loss of base metal by corrosion or etching, or by the removal of surface inclusions during electropolishing or passivation. A pit may or may not be detectable during liquid penetrant inspection.

Pitch To cause to be set at a particular angle or slope. Degree of slope or elevation.

Pituitary gland A gland at the base of the brain. The pituitary secretes several different hormones involved in key metabolic processes.

PKa The pKa is the negative log of the acid ionization constant. The computed quantity is a measure of its apparent pKa , or macroscopic dissociation constant, at equilibrium, normally taken at 25°C. The pKa is the point on the pH scale where the concentration of an acid (AH) and its corresponding conjugate base (A-) are equal. Similarly, it is the point where a conjugate acid (BH+) and its corresponding it base (B) are equal. The degree of ionization at the pKa is 50%.

Placebo (Latin: I will satisfy) "A medicine or preparation with no inherent pertinent pharmacologic activity that is effective only by virtue of the factor of suggestion attendant upon its administration." A placebo is frequently used as a negative control in a blind experiment to prevent results from being confounded by the effect of suggestion.

placebo non responders Non- responders on placebo] define a group that would never improve their condition unless given the drug. They may be a group that, if we could identify them, could be used to reduce clinical trial size. Using this group in a proof-of -concept, it may be possible to test a drug even without a comparative placebo and determine whether it is likely to be active.

Placebo responders Most people think of the placebo response as a true response. But much of it is actually regression to the mean. Clinical trial subjects with more extreme symptoms are often selected because it is desirable to see a dramatic effect upon treatment with the drug.

Plan exclusions and limitations A list of services and prescription drugs contractually excluded from coverage under a benefits plan. For example, drugs used for weight reduction or cosmetic purposes are not covered under many benefits plans. Typically, a medical exception for coverage is not available for such services or drugs.

Plan sponsor The company or organization that assumes financial responsibility for an insured group.

Plankton Those microorganisms that are passively floating or drifting in a body of water.

Plaque A clear zone in a bacterial culture grown on an agar plate caused by localized destruction of bacterial cells by a bacteriophage. Applying the fluid to a culture and counting the number of plaques formed can estimate the concentration of infective virus in a fluid.

Planned change (PMA CSVC) An intentional change to a validated systemfor which the implementation and evaluation program is predetermined.

Plaque Plaque is a deposit of fat or cholesterol that builds up inside a blood vessel which, left untreated, can eventually block the flow of blood through that vessel.

Plasma The liquid portion of blood in which the cellular elements are suspended. As a fresh liquid obtained by centrifugation, plasma is a clear, amber-colored solution containing eight to nine percent solids; of these, 85 percent are proteins while the other components are the lipids, which include the neutral fats, fatty acids, lecithin, and cholesterol. Also present are sodium, chloride and bicarbonate, potassium, calcium and magnesium. A most essential function of plasma is the maintenance of blood pressure and the exchange with tissue of nutrients for waste. Contains fibrinogen.

Plasma cell A cell derived from a B-lymphocyte and solely responsible for the production of antibodies. Each plasma cell forms only one type of antibody and is characterized by an eccentric nucleus, a prominent Golgi zone, bulky basophilic cytoplasm (due to an extensive endoplasmic reticulum) and large numbers of mitochondria.

Plasma membrane The physical barrier that surrounds the cytoplasm of all cells. It is composed of lipid, protein, and carbohydrate and is semi-permeable.

Plasma proteins The proteins found in plasma, usually divided into albumin, globulin and fibrinogen fractions.

Plasma Protein Fraction (PPF)

Plasmid Self-replicating, extrachromosomal circular DNA molecules, distinct from the normal bacterial genome and nonessential for the cell survival under nonselective conditions. Some plasmids are capable of integrating into the host genome. A number of artificially constructed plasmids are used as cloning vectors.

Plastics High molecular weight polymers or copolymers. The wide range in physical properties of polymeric materials allows for utilization as elastomers, fibers, adhesives, rigid castings, composites, and laminates. ASTM D883 defines a plastic as a material that contains as an essential ingredient, one or more organic polymeric substances of large molecular weight, is solid in its finished state, and, at some stage in its manufacture into finished articles, can be shaped by flow. Plastics, or more appropriately polymers, are composed primarily of carbon, hydrogen, oxygen, silicon, chlorine, fluorine, and nitrogen, in various combinations and permutations. Plastics are grouped into two categories: 1. Thermoplastics: can be melted, cooled and remelted without destroying the physical or mechanical characteristics of the polymer. This property permits components to be molded or extruded. Thermoplastic polymers include: Chlorinated Vinyls, Fluorinated plastics, Ketone, Nitrile, Nylon, Polyamide-imide, Polyolefin, Polycarbonate, and Acrylonitrile butadiene styrene (ABS).

2. Thermosets: begin as a liquid or powder that through chemical reaction with a second reactant or through catalyzed polymerization result in anew product with characteristics different from either starting material. Thermoset resins include: Epoxy, Phenolic, Polyurethane, Silicone, Urea and Melamine, Polyester, Vinyl ester, Furan, Bisphenol A fumarate.

PLC (programmable logic controller) An automated system with analog capability as well as binary (discrete). PLCs must be equipped with a digital interface to a "front end" computer for data collection and for programmer interface.

PLC controlled automated system Any automated system using a Programmable Logic Controller as its primary controller.

Plumbing Code

Plena The plural of plenum.

Plenum An enclosure in which air or other gas is at a pressure greater than that outside the enclosure.

Pleural fluid A collection of fluid, which accumulates in the chest cavity in the space surrounding the lung known as the pleural cavity.

Pleuropneumonia A specific infectious disease in cattle characterized by inflammation of the lung and pleura, generally called contagious pleuropneumonia. It is due to a virus.

Pneumocystis carinii pneumonia (PCP): treatment and prophylaxis

PNS Peripheral Nervous System.

PO Literally, through or by the mouth. Refers to the oral route of administration of medications into the gastrointestinal tract—distinct from routes such as buccal or sublingual in which a medication is absorbed through the oral mucosa without being swallowed.

POC Proof of concept.

Poison Any substance which when taken into the body in a single dose of 1.0 gm. or less, is injurious to health or dangerous to life.

Policy (PMA CSVC) A directive usually specifying what is to beaccomplished.

Polished water High purity water after it has undergone a second treatment step. Ultrapure water usually undergoes two or more treatment steps. More economical pretreatment processes (e. g., reverse osmosis) are used to remove all but a very small fraction of the impurities. Highly efficient polishing processes (e. g., mixed-bed deionization) are used to remove the impurities that remain.

Polyalphaolefin (PAO) A synthetic oil used in lieu of DOP for HEPA filter testing.

Polygenic disorder Genetic disorder resulting from the combined action of alleles of more than one gene (e.g., heart disease, diabetes, and some cancers). Although such disorders are inherited, they depend on the simultaneous presence of several alleles; thus the hereditary patterns are usually more complex than those of single gene disorders.

Polymeal The Polymeal diet is based on the ingredients in a traditional "heart-healthy" diet and includes fish, fruits and vegetables, and a small amount of garlic, dark chocolate, and wine.

Polymer A macromolecule (long chain) consisting of five or more repeating units called monomers. Examples include polyethylene, polystyrene, and PTFE (polytetrafluoroethylene).

Polymerase An enzyme that catalyzes production of nucleic acid molecules.

Polymerase chain reaction (PCR) A method for amplifying a DNA base sequence using a heatstable polymerase and two 20-base primers, one complementary to the (+) strand at one end of the sequence to be amplified and the other complementary to the (-) strand at the other end. Because the newly synthesized DNA strands can subsequently serve as additional templates for the same primer sequences, successive rounds of primer annealing, strand elongation, and dissociation produce rapid and highly specific amplification of the desired sequence. PCR also can be used to detect the existence of the defined sequence in a DNA sample.

Polymorphism Difference in DNA sequence among individuals. Genetic variations occurring in more than 1% of a population would be considered useful polymorphisms for genetic linkage analysis.

Polymorphs In ADME, a polymorph is a different crystalline forms of the same drug. The individual crystalline forms within a polymorphic solid dose form may have different chemical and physical properties, the solubility, dissolution rate, stability, and chemical reactivity, which may result in differences in bioavailability. They may, therefore, require individual characterizatin of their physicochemical and absorption properties in order to satisfy regulatory requirements.

Polyolefin The polyolefin polymer is probably one of the most economical and widely used classes of thermoplastics, including such materials as PB, PP, and PE. PB is a semicrystalline polymer based on polybutene, homopolymers, and either polybutene or polyethylene copolymers. The primary use of PB is pipe with hydrostatic pressure rating of 1,000 psi at 73°F. PP is a crystalline polymer that has good resistance to caustics, solvents, acids, and other organic chemicals, but is not resistant to oxidizing-type acids, detergents, alcohols, or chlorinated organic materials. It is suitable for pipe applications. The largest group of polyolefins is linear PE. It includes ULDPE, LLDPE, LDPE, HDPE, HMW-HDPE, and UHMWPE. These density descriptions generally refer to ASTM designations based on unmodified polymers. PE types of higher density have better permeation barrier properties, hardness, abrasion resistance, chemical resistance, and higher surface gloss.

Polypeptide A long chain of amino acids covalently bound by peptide.

Polypill The Polypill is a proposed "cocktail" of six of the drugs known to be effective in treating various kinds of heart and cardiovascular disease, including a statin, three beta blockers, aspirin, and folic acid. It would be taken by everyone over 55 to help prevent CAD and heart disease.

Porcine Of, relating to, or from swine (pigs) such as porcine growth hormone.

Positional cloning A technique used to identify genes, usually those that are associated with diseases, based on their location on a chromosome. This is contrast to the older, "functional cloning" technique that relies on some knowledge of a gene protein product. For most diseases, researchers have no such knowledge.

Positive Cancer Response Clinical benefit from cancer therapy is measured by objective tests: x-ray, blood markers, etc. A positive or favorable response reflects the measurable shrinkage of disease lasting greater than one month.

Positive control drug A drug preparation incorporated into an experiment with the intention that it have effects on the experimental system qualitatively similar to those expected of the independent variable. The positive control drug has two functions in an experiment: 1) to verify that the experimental system is indeed capable of undergoing the changes expected to follow manipulation of the independent variable. If the system fails to respond to the positive control drug, its failure to respond to the independent variable is uninterpretable;

2. to serve as a basis for quantitative estimation of the relative efficacy of the independent variable. In these terms, the positive control drug is a "standard", and the independent variable may be considered the " unknown" in a bioassay.

Positive pressure personnel suit Personnel protection equivalent to that provided by Class III (BSCs). It is a one-piece, ventilated suit worn by the laboratory worker when working with Biosafety Level 3 (BL-3) or Biosafety Level 4 (BL-4) in a "suit area" and using Class I or II Biological Safety Cabinets (BSCs). The personnel suit is maintained under positive pressure with a life-support system to prevent leakage into the suit. In this containment system, the worker is isolated from the work materials. The personnel suit area must be entered through an airlock fitted with airtight doors. A chemical shower is provided as a "dunk tank" to decontaminate the surfaces of the suit as the worker leaves the area. The exhaust air from the suit area is filtered through two HEPA filters installed in series. The entire area must be under negative pressure.

Postmarketing surveillance Ongoing safety monitoring of marketed drugs.

Potable Suitable for drinking.

Potassium A body salt or electrolyte found mostly inside of cells. "Water pills" may lower potassium and increase kidney damage.

Potency A measure of drug activity established by determining the dose of a drug required to produce a standard effect. Potency varies inversely with the magnitude of the dose required to produce a given effect. Thus, if twice the dose of drug "X" is required to produce analgesia equivalent to that produced by a dose of aspirin, it may be said that drug"X" is half as potent as aspirin.

Potent A substance that is "active" in relatively low doses or concentrations.

Potentiation A special case of synergy (q.v.) in which the effect of one drug is increased by another drug that by itself has no effect. For example, although physostigmine has no acetylcholine-like activity of its own, it potentiates the actions of acetylcholine by inhibiting the enzymes responsible for the destruction of acetylcholine. Intensity of effect may be potentiated, duration of effect may be prolonged: potentiation and prolongation are independent phenomena, but frequently occur together.

PP (Polypropylene) A crystalline polymer with a melting point of 330°F (165°C), and heat deflection temperature ranging from 195°F (91°C) to 240°F (116°C) which is higher than other common plastics. Its key properties are high heat resistance (for piping an upper limit of 212°F (100°C)), a specific gravity of 0.91 if unmodified (the lightest of the most common thermoplastics), stiffness, and chemical resistance with respect to handling caustics, solvents, acids, and other organic chemicals. It is not recommended for use with oxidizing type acids, detergents, low boiling hydrocarbons, alcohols, and some chlorinated organic materials. Polypropylene is a relatively inert material and contributes little in the way of contamination to pharmaceutical water.

PPB (Parts per billion) Parts per billion (abbreviated ppb only in the U.S.), or micrograms per liter. One part per billion is like seeing a bottle cap on the earth's equator from an orbiting satellite.

PPF A blood plasma fraction. Identical to NHSA but containing no more than 15% w/w A and ß globulins. Dispensed as a 5% solution.

PPLO Pleuropneumonia Like Organism.

PPM (Parts per million) The most common measure of dissolved ionized impurities in water. It is the same as milligrams per liter. For discussion of ppm as a measure of Total Ionized Solids .

PQ (performance qualification) Documented evidence that a process or system consistently and reproducibly performs as intended and does what it purports to do. This accomplished through extended time studies or process runs with simulated products or conditions.

Pragmatic trial Term used to describe a clinical study designed to examine the benefits of a product under real world conditions.

Pre clinical development Activities prior to testing in humans including pilot manufacture, toxicology and metabolism studies.

Precertification The process of getting certain drugs approved before members can obtain them as a covered benefit.

Precipitate An insoluble reaction product. When a solution reaches saturation, solute will begin to come out of solution, as when water precipitates from the air as rain, or calcium carbonate precipitates out of water to form scale, the chalky white substance deposited on the inside of tea kettles.

Precision The capacity of the system to discriminate between different values of input; the "fineness" with which different values for input can be inferred from measured values of output. The pooled deviation of observed from expected values of output, all divided by the amplification, yields the "index of precision". The square of the reciprocal of the index of precision is the measure of the amount of information that can be delivered by the system.

Specifically, precision is computed in several steps. First, the deviation of each observed value of output from the corresponding predicted value is squared; predicted values are determined from the curve relating input and output for all the data. The squared deviations are summed and divided by N-2, the number of "degrees of freedom"; the square root of the quotient is determined and is a number analogous to the standard deviation. This "root mean square deviation" is then divided by the slope of the input-output curve, i.e., the amplification, to yield the "index of precision "; it is assumed that the input-output relationship is linear.

Preclinical drug development The ability to accurately predict safety earlier the drug development process depends largely on the model that is chosen. Animal models of disease and knowledge of specific pathways provide a means of evaluating and progressing drug candidates. The pressure to accelerate drug discovery and development has increased, driven by technology advancement and strong competitive forces. Numerous opportunities exist to implement innovative paradigms to optimize candidate progression from discovery to early clinical evaluation. Successful development of new translational biomarkers will enable the progression of candidates from preclinical to clinical, and provide a means of predicting success in humans

Preclinical drug evaluations Preclinical testing of drugs in experimental animals or in vitro for their biological and toxic effects and potential clinical applications.

Preclinical investigations Laboratory and animal studies designed to test the mechanisms, safety, and efficacy of an intervention prior to its applications to humans.

Preclinical Literally, "before the clinic". In drug discovery and development, the term refers to in vitro or in vivo (animal) studies that are performed prior to human clinical studies on a compound.

Preclinical research Studies in animals to test drug effectiveness, metabolism and toxicity before the drug is tested in humans.

Preclinical studies Animal studies that support Phase 1 safety and tolerance studies and must comply with good laboratory practice (GLP). Data about a drug's activities and effects in animals help establish boundaries for safe use of the drug in subsequent human testing (clinical studies or trials). Because many animals have much shorter life spans than humans, preclinical studies can provide valuable information about a drug's possible toxic effects over an animal's life cycle and on its offspring.

Preclinical testing Compounds are tested on cell lines (human and animal) for effectiveness. Also, the compounds are tested in live animals for toxicity and to ensure that they maintain their pharmacological properties.

Precommission Preparing the plant for commissioning (start-up). This includes briefly starting (bumping) all pieces of equipment, verifying their shaft rotation is correct, verifying that valves, gauges, and other inline devices are installed in the correct orientation, and performing functionality runs on all equipment and material. This also includes leak tests.

Precursor A chemical that can be converted by the body into another is a precursor of the latter chemical.

Predicate rules A previously published set of rules (such as GLPs, GCP, or cGMPs) that mandate what records must be maintained, the required contents of those records, whether signatures are necessary, and how long the record must be maintained.

Predictive ADME Refers to a process of computational (in silico) pharmacokinetic screening used to predict, for new molecular entities, the ADME parameters that can be expected in vivo. It is valuable tool used to predict the interaction of a compound with the biological system.

Predictive medicine The use of diagnomics and pharmacogenomics to help prescribe the most appropriate course of treatment for a patient.

Predictive pharmacogenomics Various approaches, including pharmacogenomics, that make up the emerging field of predictive medicine. These approaches allow clinicians to predict the risk of disease based on genetic testing, whether a particular therapy will be effective in a particular patient, the risk of an adverse effect, and the risk that a disease will progress in a particular manner. The technologies underlying these new approaches will change drug discovery and development, clinical trials, and diagnosis and treatment of disease.

Predictive toxicogenomics A number of novel approaches to toxicology research that have become available over the past five years that are raising optimism for dramatic improvements in the field. Strategic regulatory, and marketplace issues are driving growth of toxicogenomic and predictive toxicology applications. The ability to predict the toxic effects of potential new drugs is crucial to prioritizing compound pipelines and eliminating costly failures in drug development.

Prednisone A form of steroid therapy very widely used.

Prefilter A filter to trap gross particulates located upstream before a HEPA filter. The efficiency of initial prefilters is usually in the 20% to 30% range by the ASHRAE Atmospheric Dust Spot Efficiency, while intermediate prefilters usually have a collection efficiency of 80% to 90% by the same test.

Pregnenolone The grandmother steroid hormone produced in the mitochondria that is the base "raw-material" for all the steroids and neuro-steroids.

Prescribed drug A drug which has been prescribed by an authorized physician for a patient. A licensed pharmacist must fill the prescription at a pharmacy.

Prescription A physician's order for the preparation and administration of a drug or device for a patient. A prescription has several parts. They include the superscription or heading with the symbol "R" or "Rx", which stands for the word recipe (meaning, in Latin, to take); the inscription, which contains the names and quantities of the ingredients; the subscription or directions for compounding the drug; and the signature which is often preceded by the sign "s" standing for signa (Latin for mark), giving the directions to be marked on the container.

Prescription drugs Are drugs that are obtainable only by a physician's or dentist's written prescription, dispensed by a licensed pharmacist, and approved for their intended use by the United States Food and Drug Administration.

Preservative A bacteriostatic or bacteriocidal agent added to some multiple dose parenterals and most cosmetics. Examples are benzalkonium chloride (BAC), formaldehyde, and thimerosol (merthiolate).

Pressure rating Pressure at which a system is designed to operate, allowing for applicable safety factors.

Pressure vessel A closed vessel designed to operate at pressures above 15 psig (103.4 kPa).

Pretreatment Initial water treatment steps performed prior to final processing to prolong the life of cartridges and filters and to protect downstream elements from premature failure.

Prevention Prevention means to prevent a disease onset.

Primary air Air circulating through HEPA filters used to produce unidirectional flow in critical zones.

Primary Containment The first level of containment, consisting of the inside portion of that container which comes into immediate contact on its inner surface with the material being contained.

Primary site The place where cancer begins. Primary cancer is named after the organ in which it starts. For example, cancer that starts in the kidney is always kidney cancer even if it spreads (metastasizes) to other organs such as bones or lungs.

Primer Short preexisting polynucleotide chain to which DNA polymerase can add new deoxyribonucleotides.

Principle of nonrepudiation The ability to say with confident assurance that only one user entered specific data or performed specific actions on a computer system and that the particular user is identifiable. If more than one user can get into the system in such a way that the audit trail cannot specify who performed what action, the principle of nonrepudiation has been violated.

Prions Virus-like proteinaceous infectious agents. Prions differ from viruses in that they are not known to contain either DNA or RNA.

Probe Single stranded DNA or RNA molecules of specific base sequence, labeled either radioactively or immunologically, that are used to detect the complementary base sequence by hybridization.

Procedures A documented description of the operations to be carried out, the precautions to be taken and measures to be applied directly or indirectly related to the manufacture of an intermediate or API.

Process aids Materials, excluding solvents, used as an aid in the manufacture of an intermediate or API (Active Pharmaceutical Ingredient) which themselves do not participate in a chemical or biological reaction (e.g. filter aid, activated carbon, etc.).

Process efficiency A measure of recovery associated with an analytical method. It is determined by comparing the peak area response ratio of extracted standards prepared in a given matrix vs. standards in solution (typical a mixture of aqueous and organic solvents). Process efficiency is a combination of matrix suppression and extraction efficiency.

Process limits Environmental limits that, if exceeded, may affect product quality adversely.

Process suitability The established capacity of the manufacturing process to produce effective and reproducible results consistently.

Process support systems Systems that do not contact product and are generally engineering systems.

Process system (PMA CSVC) The combination of process equipment,support systems (such as utilities), and procedures used to execute aprocess.

Process validation Establishing, through documented evidence, a high degree of assurance that a specific process will consistently produce a product that meets its predetermined specifications and quality characteristics.

Process validation protocol Documented plan for testing a pharmaceutical product and process to confirm that the production process used to manufacture the product performs as intended. This includes a review of process variables and operational limitations as well as providing the sampling plan under actual use conditions.

Prodrug In politics it means "not opposed to the use of drugs". In ADME the term refers to a pharmacologically inactive form of a drug that is administered and converted to the active moiety in the body. Bioactivation typically involves enzymatic cleavage of an ester or amide bond. Prodrugs are often used when the active drug has extremely poor bioavailability when administered by the preferred route (usually oral) or in order to avoid systemic toxicity in cases where the target tissue expresses higher levels of the activation enzyme(s) than non-target tissues, e.g., anticancer drugs.

Producer Identification of the medicinal preparation producer, usually including the company logo.

Product Any computer system supplied by the supplier to the customeras the result of an agreed contract between the two parties.

Product campaign The production of more than one product in a facility, with strict adherence to accepted cleaning procedures between these products. The products may be run in the same equipment, but not at the same time.

Product contact surface A surface that contacts raw materials, process materials, and/or product.

Product mix The types and number of different products produced in a facility.

Product water The water produced as a result of a treatment process.

Production All operations involved in the preparation of an API (Active Pharmaceutical Ingredient), from receipt of materials, through processing and packaging, to its completion as a finished API.

Progesterone A female hormone preparation, used in breast cancer and uterine treatment.

Progression Disease progression is noted when the tumor size has increased by more than one-quarter or new areas of cancer have been found.

Progression of disease Development of a disease over time.

Prokaryote A unicellular organism having a less complex structure than a eukaryote. It is characterized by the absence of a nucleus and by having the genetic material in the form of simple filaments of DNA. The sizes of most prokaryotes vary from 0.5μm to 3μm in equivalent radius. Different species have different shapes such as spherical or Coccus (for example, Staphylococci), cylindrical or bacillus (E. coli), or spiral or spirillum (Rhodospirillum).

Promiscuous drugs We contend that an ideal drug may be one whose efficacy is based not on the inhibition of a single target, but rather on the rebalancing of the several proteins or events, that contribute to the etiology, pathogeneses, and progression of diseases, i.e., in effect a promiscuous drug.... Corollaries to this argument are that the growing fervor for researching truly selective drugs may be imprudent when considering the totality of responses; and that the expensive screening techniques used to discover these, may be both medically and financially inefficient. Promiscuous drugs compared to selective drugs .

Promiscuous inhibitors Nonspecific, seem to be hits in multiple high- throughput screening (HTS) campaigns, but which turn out to be dead ends when attempts are made to optimise their activity, a key problem in the field of HTS.

Promoter A site on DNA to which RNA polymerase will bind and initiate transcription.

Proof of principle (PoP) Initial experiment to determine feasibility of technology.

Prophylactic surgery Surgery to remove tissue that is in danger of becoming cancerous, before cancer has the chance to develop. Surgery to remove the breasts of women at high risk of developing breast cancer is known as prophylactic mastectomy.

Prophylaxis The prevention of, or protective treatment for disease.

Propylene glycol A common solvent for antibiotics, particularly the tetracyclines. Miscible (soluble) in water, but often filtered as pure propylene glycol prior to combination with the antibiotic. Its high viscosity controls absorption of the dissolved drug.

Prospective study Investigation in which a group of subjects is recruited and monitored in accordance with criteria described in a protocol.

Prospective validation Establishing documented evidence that a system does what it purports to do based on a preplanned protocol.

Prosthetic groups Organic and/or inorganic components other than amino acids, contained in proteins.

Protean ligands The literature contains few examples of ligands that seem to be able to both promote and decrease activity at the same G-protein-coupled receptors. Such 'protean ligands' — so- called after the mythical character Proteus, who could adopt any shape he desired — have been proposed to work by acting as agonists with low efficacy. They thereby increase the activity of receptors that are basically silent under resting conditions, but decrease the activity of receptors that have high levels of ligand-independent, spontaneous (or constitutive) activity. In this model, protean behaviour therefore depends on having two populations of receptors with different levels of spontaneous activity.

Protease A proteolytic enzyme; a protein that can cleave other proteins into smaller fragments.

Proteasome A distinct enzyme complex within cells responsible for breaking down proteins that have been marked for disposal by the attachment of a tag called ubiquitin, including regulatory proteins governing processes such as cell division.

Protein A type of biological compound made up of units called amino acids. Proteins are coded by DNA. They serve many functions and include enzymes, structural elements, hormones and antibodies. They are involved in oxygen transport, muscle contraction and other essential activities throughout the body.

QTc Interval - Used to detect ventricular arrhythmias. Represents the duration of ventricular depolarization and repolarization as measured by an electrocar-diogram (ECG), a clinically important method for examining the electrical activity in the heart.

Protein sequencer An instrument that will determine the sequence of amino acids, which make up a particular protein.

Proteolysis Protein hydrolysis, the decomposition of protein.

Proteolytic enzyme (protease) Any enzyme that takes part in the breaking down of proteins. A system of several such enzymes is necessary to break down proteins to their constituent amino acids.

Proteomics A concept more than a defined technology, it refers to any protein-based approach that has the capacity to provide new information about proteins on a genomewide scale. 75% of the predicted proteins in multicellular organisms have no known cellular function.

Protocol A document that describes the objective(s), design, methodology, statistical considerations, and organization of a trial. The protocol usually also gives the background and rationale for the trial, but these could be provided in other protocol referenced documents. Throughout the ICH good clinical practice (GCP) guideline, the term protocol refers to protocol and protocol amendments.

Protocol amendment A written description of a change(s) to or formal clarification of a protocol.

Protocol Amendment A written description of a change(s) to or formal clarification of a protocol.

Proton The hydrogen ion, H+.

Protoplasm A semifluid, viscous, translucent mixture of water, proteins, lipids, carbohydrates, and inorganic salts found in all plant and animal cells.

Protozoa Nucleated microorganisms, some of which are large enough to be detected with the naked eye. They consist of a single cell and or an aggregation of nondifferentiated cells loosely held together and not forming tissues. The protozoa are divided into four classes: Sarcodina, Mastigophora, Sporozoa, and Infusoria (Ciliata).

Provenacceptable range (PAR) All values of a given control parameter thatfall between proven high and low worst-case conditions.

PSA Abnormal levels in the serum are associated with clinical abnormalities of the prostate, including prostate cancer. Because PSA is found in normal, malignant and benign prostatic tissue, clinical discrimination is based upon its serum level.

Pseudo code (ANSI/IEEE) A combination of programming language and anatural language used for computer program design.

Pseudonomas Diminuta The bacterium used for validation of sterilizing filters. Recognized as the challenge organism for 0.2μm filters, its size is 0.3 x 0.8μm approximately. According to the HIMA (Health Industries Manufacturers Association) standard, filters must be successfully challenged to a titre of 107 per cm² to be validated as sterilizing grade 0.2μm rated.

Psychotropic drugs A group of drugs used to treat mental disorders and diseases.

Psychrometer A hygrometer that uses the difference in readings between two thermometers, one having a wet bulb ventilated to cause evaporation and the other having a dry bulb, as a measure of atmospheric moisture.

Psychrometry Determination of the properties of gas-vapor mixtures. The air-water vapor system is by far the one most commonly encountered.

Psychrophile An organism that requires temperatures below 20°C (68°F) for growth.

PTFE (polytetrafluoroethylene) teflon® A fluoroplastic that is resistant to practically every known chemical or solvent in combination with the highest useful temperature limit of commercially available plastics. PTFE has a melt point of 620°F (327°C), a useful temperature range from -436°F (-260°C) to 500°F (260°C), high impact strength, and exceptionally low coefficient of friction. Usual processing techniques like injection molding are not possible with PTFE due to a very high molecular weight which results in a melt viscosity about 1 million times higher than is acceptable for conventional thermoplastics. PTFE resin is pressed into shapes under high pressure at room temperature and then heated to 700°F (371°C) to complete the molding (sintering process) and adjust the crystalline content.

Public key certificate (PKC) A data file issued by a certified authority to a person or company that acquires a digital signature service. The certificate includes information identifying the subject, the issuing authority, and the period of validity, and it provides the related public key. The certified authority signs the PKC digitally.

Pure culture A culture containing only one species of microorganism.

Pure steam Steam that is produced by a steam generator which, when condensed, meets requirements for WFI.

Purification The removal of impurities of concern. The term has one meaning when applied to the preparation of drinking water, another when applied to reagent grade water for the laboratory, and still another when applied to water used to rinse ICs (Integrated Circuit devices).

Purified water, U.S.P. Water rendered suitable for pharmaceutical purposes by processes such as distillation, ion-exchange treatment (deionization or demineralization), or reverse osmosis. Cannot be used as raw material for parenterals. Common uses are: a rinse for equipment, vials, and ampoules, and as make up for cosmetics, bulk chemicals, and oral products. For acceptance, purified water must contain less than 0.5 mg/l of TOC (Total Organic Carbon), and less than 100 CFU (Colony Forming Units).

Purine A nitrogen-containing, double-ring, basic compound that occurs in nucleic acids. The purines in DNA and RNA are adenine and guanine.

Purity The ratio of desirable to undesirable components in a liquid as determined on a weight basis per unit volume of sample.

PVC (polyvinyl chloride) The largest volume of the vinyl family of plastics. Overall it has excellent basic properties, may be easily processed and welded, and is exceptionally economical in cost. Homopolymers grades of PVC comprise over 80% of all PVC used, and contain 56.8% chlorine by weight. When the chlorine content is increased to about 67% its heat deflection temperature at 264 psi increases from 155°F (68°C) to 218°F (103°C). Because PVC is a thermally sensitive thermoplastic compounding ingredients such as heat stabilizers, lubricants, fillers, plasticizers, impact modifiers, pigments, and processing aids must be added to make it processible. PVC is prone to produce extractables during start-up in high purity water.

PVDF (polyvinylidene fluoride) kynar®, sygef®, solef® A thermoplastic fluoropolymer with a melt point of 352°F (178°C), and a wide service range from -40°F (-40°C) to 284°F (140°C). It has a very linear chemical structure, and is similar to PTFE with the exception of not being fully fluorinated, i.e. having 3% hydrogen by weight. Its drawbacks in the area of chemical resistance include unsuitability with strong alkalis, fuming acids, polar solvents, amines, ketones, and esters. It has a high tensile strength as well as a high heat deflection temperature. It is readily weldable, offers high purity qualities, and is resistant to permeation of gases. PVDF is a relatively inert material and contributes little in the way of contamination to pharmaceutical water.

Pyrazinamide (PZA) Indications: Treatment of TB in combination with other agents.

Contraindications: Known hypersensitivity, significant hepatic disease.

Dosage: 25 mg/kg po qd.

Toxicity: Abnormal liver function tests, hyperuricemia, rash.

Pyrimidine A nitrogen-containing, single ring, basic compound that occurs in nucleic acids. The pyrimidines in DNA are cytosine and thymine, in RNA, cytosine, and uracil.

Pyrogen A foreign substance that produces a fever response in humans and animals, hence the name pyrogen (heat producing). Chemically, the lipopolysaccharide outer layer of gram-negative bacteria. Bacterial pyrogens were at one time believed to be toxic substances released when bacterial cells disintegrate and are therefore still referred to as endotoxins. Parenteral drugs must be essentially pyrogen free. Pyrophoric A chemical that will spontaneously ignite in air at or below a temperature of 130°F (54.5°C).

Pyrogens Substances which cause fever if they are present in an injection. Most of them are bacterial endotoxins (lipid constituents of the cell walls of Gram-negative bacteria). The standard pyrogen test measures temperature increases in 3 rabbits.

Q

QA (quality assurance) The sum total of the organized arrangements made to ensure that all APIs (Active Pharmaceutical Ingredients) are of the quality required for their intended use and that quality systems are maintained.

QC (quality control) Checking or testing, that specifications are met, or the regulatory process through which the industry measures actual quality performance, compares it with standards, and acts on the difference.

Qualification Action of providing that equipment or ancillary systems are properly installed, work correctly, and actually lead to the expected results. Qualification is part of validation, but the individual qualification steps alone do not constitute process validation.

Qualification protocol A prospective experimental plan that whenexecuted is intended to produce documented evidence that a system orsubsystem has been properly qualified.

Qualifying year Refers to eligibility for coverage under the Senior Citizen or Early Retiree Program. It is a Base Year during which an individual had covered earnings equal to the greater of:

The amount required as of the last day of such Base Year to qualify for a year of eligibility under the AFTRA Individual Health Plan or $2,000.

Qualitative variable One that cannot be measured numerically (race or sex, for example).

Quality assurance (QA) All those planned and systematic actions that are established to ensure that the trial is performed and the data are generated, documented (recorded), and reported in compliance with good clinical practice (GCP) and the applicable regulatory requirement(s).

Quality control (QC) The operational techniques and activities undertaken within the quality assurance system to verify that the requirements for quality of the trial related activities have been fulfilled.

Quality function The entire collection of activities from which the industry achieves fitness for use, no matter where these activities are performed.

Quality of life When used as a clinical trial endpoint, quality of life refers to the effect of treatment on a patient's ability to cope with daily life. For example, a treatment that is painful, disturbs sleep or affects mobility will have an adverse effect on a patient's quality of life.

Quality plan A plan created by the supplier to define actions,deliverables, responsibilities and procedures to satisfy the customerquality and validation requirements.

Quality system The organisational structure, responsibilities,procedures, processes and resources for implementing qualitymanagement.

Quality unit(s) An organizational unit independent of production that fulfills both Quality Assurance and Quality Control responsibilities. This may be in the form of separate QA and QC units, a single individual (or group), depending upon the size and structure of the organization.

Quantitative variable One that can be measured (blood pressure, for example).

Quantity limits Coverage limits on certain medications that exceed department of health dosage guidelines.

Quarantine The status of materials isolated physically or by other effective means pending a decision on their subsequent approval or rejection.

Quick stop DNA mutants of E. coli cease replication immediately when the temperature is increased to 42°C.

Quinine The original antimalarial agent, quinine took its name from the Peruvian Indian word "kina" meaning "bark of the tree" referring to the cinchona tree. From this tree, quinine was first obtained. The Peruvian Indians called it "the fever tree."

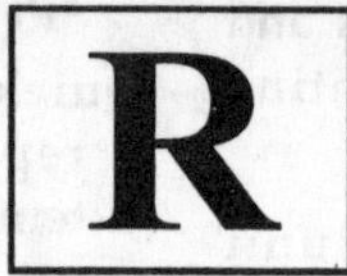

R&D Research and development

Racemate An equimolar mixture of a pair of enantiomers. It does not exhibit optical activity. The chemical name or formula of a racemate is distinguished from those of the enantiomers by the prefix (±)- or rac- (or racem-) or by the symbols RS and SR.

Radiation Cancer therapy which refers to beam and non-beam therapy; non-beam therapy includes implants and radioactive isotopes.

Radiation sterilization Sterilization using gamma radiation emitted from radioactive materials such as cobalt-60, or cesium 137. If proper dosage of nuclear radiation can be documented, sterility testing is not required.

Radio immunoassay (RIA) A highly sensitive method of detecting and measuring the concentration of biological compounds in vivo.

Radioactive material A material or combination of materials that spontaneously emits ionizing radiation.

Radiofrequency A procedure used to treat some types of rapid heart beating. Radiofrequency-based procedures cure atrial fibrillation in 70% to 80% of patients.

Radiotherapy Treatment using X-rays, cobalt-60, radium, neutrons, or other types of cell-destroying radiation.

Random allocation Assignment of subjects to treatment (or control) groups in an unpredictable way. Assignment sequences are concealed, but available for disclosure in the event a subject has an adverse experience.

Random number table Table of numbers with no apparent pattern used in the selection of random samples for clinical trials.

Random sample Members of a population selected by a method designed to ensure that each person in the target group has an equal chance of selection.

Randomised clinical trial A study in which patients with one or more similar traits (eg, tumor type, gender, age, extent of disease, prior treatment, history, etc) are arbitrarily distributed into separate groups, each receiving a different treatment regimen. Because the distribution of patients is arbitrary, or random, there is no risk of selection bias. The treatment groups can therefore be considered comparable and the results of the different treatments used in different groups directly compared.

Randomization The process of assigning trial subjects to treatment or control groups using an element of chance to determine the assignments in order to reduce bias.

Randomized clinical trials RCTs The gold standard for evaluating drugs intended to prevent or treat disease. Given this credibility, a poorly designed or conducted RCT, yielding misleading results, can actually hinder the overall research effort. Indeed, it may not be possible to overcome research mistakes rapidly, either because the treatments become widely accepted or because another trial would be too costly.

Range In the context of an assay or analytical method, the range is the concentrations of analyte or assay values between the low and high limits of quantitation. Within the range specified in the protocol for a validated method, linearity, accuracy and precision are acceptable.

Range testing Checking each input output loop across its intendedoperating range.

RAST An abbreviation for RadioAllergo Sorbent Test, a trademark of Pharmacia Diagnostics, which originated the test. RAST is a laboratory test used to detect IgE antibodies to specific allergens.

Rate limiting step This is slowest point in a series of reactions (ie. uptake of choline into the nerve terminal in the synthesis of Ach) or where the enzyme involved is subject to regulatory control (ie. Tyrosine hydroxlase involved in NA systhesis)

Raw data The department of health defines Raw data as: [the] "means any laboratory worksheets, records, memoranda, notes, or exact copies thereof, that are the result of original observations and activities of a nonclinical laboratory study and are necessary for the reconstruction and evaluation of the report of that study. In the event that exact transcripts of raw data have been prepared, e.g., tapes which have been transcribed verbatim, dated, and verified accurate by signature, the exact copy or exact transcript may be substituted for the original source as raw data. Raw data may include photographs, microfilm or microfiche copies, computer printouts, magnetic media, including dictated observations, and recorded data from automated instruments."

Raw material A general term used to denote starting materials, reagents, intermediates, process aids, and solvents intended for use in the production of intermediates or APIs (Active Pharmaceutical Ingredients).

Raynaud's syndrome Condition in which small arteries, most commonly in the fingers and toes, spasm and cause the skin to turn pale or a patchy red to blue on exposure to cold or even the thought of cold. Although Raynaud's is usually a mild condition, it can have serious direct consequences, such as gangrene serious enough to warrant amputation.Treatment: Treatment: simple exercise may suffice (ie. swinging your arms around like a windmill), however if attacks are frequent or severe, dilating agents, such as nifedipine, calcium channel blocker may be prescribed.

rDNA (Recombinant DNA) The hybrid DNA produced by joining pieces of DNA from different sources.

Re qualification (PMA CSVC) Repetition of the qualification or aportion thereof.

Reaction phenotyping A means of establishing, through the use of in vitro assays, which, if any, human CYP enzyme(s) participate in the metabolism of a drug and the extent of involvement of each enzyme. Reaction phenotyping studies generally include metabolism of the test compound by recombinant CYP enzymes, chemical and/or antibody inhibition, and correlation analysis—metabolism by a panel of human liver microsomes with known CYP phenotypes. The output from a reaction phenotyping study may include the Km and Vmax values for metabolite formation if authentic standards for metabolites are available.

Reagent A substance used (as in detecting or measuring a component, in preparing a product, or in developing photographs) because of its chemical or biological activity.

Reagent grade water Water suitable for use in making up reagents or for use in sensitive analytical procedures. There are several grades of reagent grade water as defined by various professional organizations, such as ASTM, CAP, NCCLS, and ACS: 1. Type I: Used for procedures requiring maximum accuracy and precision, such as atomic spectrometry, flame photometry, enzymology, blood gas, pH and specific ion determinations; reference buffer solutions; and reconstitution of lyophilized materials used as standards. ASTM to produce Type I water specifies distillation pretreatment of feedwater.

2. Type II: Recommended for most analytical or general laboratory testing such as hematological, seralogical, and microbiological procedures as well as chemical methods not specifically stated or proven to require Type I quality. ASTM specifies preparation of Type II by distillation and recommends it whenever freedom from organic impurities is important.

3. Type III: Satisfactory for some general laboratory tests; for most qualitative analyses such as urinalysis, parasitology, and histological procedures; for rinsing of analytical samples; preparation of stock solutions; and for washing or rinsing of glassware (final glassware rinsing should be performed with the water type specified for the procedure performed). Distillation, mixed-bed deionization, and reverse osmosis (with high quality feedwater) can be used to generate Type III.

Rebound effects Discontinuation of an agent my cause exacerbation of previous symptoms to a level which is greater than before, and than that which would have been expected. ie. sudden discontinuation of clonidine leads to rebound hypertension, tachycardia and angina.

Recalcification A technique producing serum from anticoagulated plasma. Citrate and oxalate act as anticoagulants because they are Ca++ (Calcium Ion) chelating agents; Ca++ as calcium chloride is added in excess (1/40 Molar). Ca++ is a coagulation co-factor (catalyst) and promotes clot formation.

Receptor A protein or a protein complex in or on a cell that specifically recognizes and binds to a compound acting as a molecular messenger (neurotransmitter, hormone, lymphokine, lectin, drug, etc.). In a broader sense, the term receptor is often used as a synonym for any specific (as opposed to non-specific such as binding to plasma proteins) drug binding site, also including nucleic acids such as DNA.

Recessive allele A gene that is expressed only when its counterpart allele on the matching chromosome is also recessive (not dominant). Autosomal recessive disorders develop in persons who receive two copies of the mutant gene, one from each parent who is a carrier.

Recirculation Continuous recirculation may be necessary to maintain uniformly high purity in larger water systems. Water is continuously recirculated and reprocessed to prevent stagnation and to rinse out residual impurities in the system. Bacteria flourish in stagnant water, especially if temperature is conducive to growth.

Recombinant Pertaining to the recombining of generic material from one species into alternate sequences. Plasmids may then be used to incorporate the genetic material into other organisms such as E. coli bacteria.

Recombinant clone Clone containing recombinant DNA molecules.

Recombinant DNA (rDNA) The hybrid DNA produced by joining pieces of DNA from different sources.

Recombinant DNA molecules In the context of the NIH Guidelines, recombinant DNA molecules are those constructed outside living cells by joining natural or synthetic DNA segments to DNA molecules that can replicate in a living cell, or molecules that result from the replication of those described above.

Recombinant DNA technology Procedure used to join together DNA segments in a cell-free system (an environment outside a cell or organism). Under appropriate conditions, a recombinant DNA molecule can enter a cell and replicate there, either autonomously or after it has become integrated into a cellular chromosome.

Recovery The extraction efficiency of an analytical process, reported as a percentage of the known amount of an analyte carried through the sample extraction and processing steps of the method. Recovery is most valid when an internal standard is carried through the process along with the analyte of interest. In some applications, low recovery is not a problem because the observed amount of analyte can simply be normalized to the recovery of the internal standard. In other cases, like in a Caco-2 cell based permeability study, low recovery is indicative of a high degree of non-specific binding and can confound the interpretation of the observed results.

Recovery time The time after an upset in a room's HVAC environmental parameters for the room to return to "normal" conditions, such as a return to acceptable humidity levels after a room wash down. This occurs within a certain number of air changes after the upset source is removed, minimally six to ten, depending on the severity of the upset, the quality of the air supply, and the degree of mixing of room air.

Recruitment (subjects) Process used by investigators to enroll appropriate subjects into a clinical study, i.e, those selected on the basis of the protocol's inclusion and exclusion criteria.

Recruitment period Time period during which investigators must complete enrollment of their quota of subjects for a trial.

Recruitment target Number of subjects that must be recruited into a study to meet the requirements of the study protocol. In multicenter studies, each investigator has a recruitment target.

Recurrent Cancer that returns after remission.

Reference Standard A drug, chemical, or dosage form, etc., of specified properties used as the basis for quantitative comparison with other materials of qualitatively similar properties. The purpose of such a comparison is to express the amount or degree of the designated property in the "other" material as a fraction or multiple of the amount or degree of the property contained in the standard. The reference standard serves as a unit of measurement for the properties of the other, or "unknown," material.

Even physical systems of measurement are based on reference standards. The use of reference standards is of particularly great importance to the design and interpretation of biological experiments. In biological experiments, particularly, variability and instability of the biological test system can markedly influence the apparent effects and effectiveness of substances being tested.

Referential integrity Relationship between records that ensures data integrity by maintaining unbreakable links between related electronic records. It ensures confidence that a specific record (such as a calculated chromatographic result) is unmodified, unmanipulated, and otherwise uncorrupted after its creation and that still carries the references to the other electronic records that were used to generate it.

Reflux esophagitis Inflammation of the esophagus caused by reflow of gastric juice.

Refrigerants Fluids used for heat transfer in a refrigerating system; the refrigerant absorbs heat and transfers it at a higher temperature and higher pressure, usually with a change of state. Refrigerants can be: 1. Primary refrigerants. Liquids with low boiling points that change from a liquid to a gas after absorbing heat.

2. Secondary refrigerants. Substances that act only as heat carriers, such as brine, air, and water.

Regenerate Restore ion exchange of resins by reversing the process. An acid rinse is used to restore cation resin capacity and a sodium hydroxide rinse is used to restore anion resin capacity.

Regeneration The regrowth of cells, tissues, organs or limbs.

Regional absorption In the context of ADME, the term refers to drug absorption that is confined primarily or exclusively to a discrete region of the gastrointestinal tract—the duodenum, jejunum or ileum—due to regionally specific expression of a particular transporter, like PepT1 in the duodenum and jejunum, anatomical features like tight intercellular junctions, as in the colon or physicochemical properties like pH, which increases gradually but significantly from the duodenum to the colon. Regional absorption can profoundly affect the pharmacokinetics of some drugs; it may result in poor oral bioavailability for compounds that dissolve slowly and are absorbed mainly in the duodenum. It may also confound attempts to develop an extended-release formulation of a drug.

Registration number A special code under which the preparation is approved (registered).

Regression Describes the shrinkage or disappearance of a cancer.

Regulatory affairs Drug companies must show that their products consistently meet standards set by government agencies. Regulatory affairs departments document those activities, submit proposals, and follow those proposals through completion or approval.

Regulatory authorities Bodies having the power to regulate. In the ICH good clinical practice (GCP) guideline, the expression "Regulatory Authorities" includes the authorities that review submitted clinical data and those that conduct inspections. These bodies are sometimes referred to as competent authorities.

Regulatory region or sequence A DNA base sequence that controls gene expression.

Reject stream In reverse osmosis and ultrafiltration, those impurities not able to permeate the membrane are said to be rejected (removed). They are flushed away in the reject (waste) stream.

Relapse A return of disease symptoms after recovery had apparently been achieved. In cancer patients, this means cancer cells have returned after initial success in eradicating those cells with treatment.

Related employee Is an employee (other than a temporary employee) of AFTRA or the AFTRA Health and Retirement Funds.

Relational database management system (RDBMS) A type of database system that stores data in related tables. A relational database is powerful because it does not assume how data are related or how they will be extracted from the database. As a result, the same database can be viewed in many different ways.

Relative humidity (% RH) The ratio (measured in percent) of actual water vapor pressure in air to the pressure of saturated water vapor in air at the same temperature and pressure.

Release The discharge of a microbiological agent or eukaryotic cell from a containment system.

Remission The decrease or disappearance of evidence of a disease; also the period during which this occurs.

Renal clearance Renal plasma (or blood) clearance ClR is the volume of plasma (or blood) freed of a substance by only renal mechanisms, per unit time. The amount of drug (AU) excreted in the urine during the time interval t - t′ is determined; the plasma (or blood) concentration at the mid-point of the interval (Cp) is found by interpolation on the line relating log C and t. The urinary excretion rate of the drug,

AU/(t - t′), divided by Cp is the renal clearance.

Renal plasma clearance will vary with such factors as age, weight, and sex of subject, the state of cardiovascular and renal function, the nature of the material being excreted, species, etc. Renal clearance by only glomerular filtration is defined and measured as the clearance of the sugar inulin, which is eliminated from the body by no route other than glomerular filtration. Total renal clearance is defined and measured by clearance of para-amino-hippurate (PAH), a substance that is eliminated by both glomerular filtration and tubular excretion (at the maximum rate of which the tubular mass is capable). Neither inulin nor PAH undergoes reabsorption by the tubules as some materials do. (N.B.: Blood and plasma are completely cleared of PAH by a single "pass" through the kidney; PAH clearance is therefore, the standard measure of renal plasma, or blood, flow).

In normal adult human males, plasma clearance of inulin is about 130 ml plasma/min; of PAH, about 700 ml plasma/min. In normal adult human females, clearance of inulin is about 115 ml plasma/min; of PAH, about 600 ml plasma/min. The relationship between clearance of blood and clearance of plasma is given by the relationship ClR (blood) = ClR (plasma)/(1-Hct), where "Hct" is the hematocrit, the proportion, as a fraction - of the blood which consists of cells, not plasma; on the average, normal adult human subjects can be assumed to have a hematocrit of about 0.45.

Renaturation The restoration of biological activity to a denatured protein or nucleic acid. The strands of a DNA duplex, for example, are denatured at high temperatures but can be correctly reformed by a slow cooling.

Renewal The term used when a prescription has exhausted all of its refills and requires the physician to write a new prescription. This is considered renewing a prescription.

Rennin A protease released by the kidney that cleaves angiotensinogen to angiotensin I. Angiotensin I breakdown products mediate responses that elevate blood volume and pressure. Renin release is stimulated by:

sympathetic tone

low blood flow and pressure in the kidney

low sodium in the urine.

Repeatability Repeatability is the within-run, or intra-batch, precision of an assay and typically refers to a set of results obtained on the same day. It is the variability of the measurements obtained by one person while making the same measurement repeatedly.

Representative sample A sample that consists of a number of units that are drawn based on rational criteria such as random sampling and intended to assure that the sample accurately portraits the material being sampled.

Reprocessing (ICH API definition) Introducing an intermediate or API, including that which does not conform to standards or specifications, back into the process and repeating a crystallization step or other appropriate chemical or physical manipulation steps (e.g., distillation, filtration, chromatography, milling, etc.) that are part of the established manufacturing process. Continuation of a chemical reaction after an in-process control test shows the reaction to be incomplete is considered to be part of the normal process, and not reprocessing.

Reproducibility Reproducibility is the between-run, or inter-batch, precision of an assay. It typically refers to sets of results obtained with the same test material on different days, by different operators, using different analytical instruments, in different laboratories, etc. It can be viewed as the variation in measurements obtained when two or more people perform the same assay on identical test articles.

Reproductive toxicology Studies of whether exposure affects male or female fertility.

Requirement (ANSI/IEEE) .

A condition or capability needed by a user to solve a problem orachieve an objective.

A condition or capability that must be met or possessed by a systemor system component to satisfy a contract, standard, specification, orother formally imposed document. The set of all requirements forms thebasis for subsequent development of the system or system component.

Research hypothesis The research hypothesis is the conclusion a study sets out to support (or disprove); for example, "blood pressure will be lowered by [specific endpoint] in subjects who receive the test product."

Resin Ion exchange resins are usually bead-like spherical materials with an affinity for particular ions. Cation exchange resins made of styrene and divinylbenzene containing sulfonic acid groups will exchange hydrogen ions for any cations they encounter. Similarly, anion exchange resins made of styrene and divinylbenzene containing quaternary ammonium groups will exchange a hydroxyl ion for any anions.

Resistance (Filter) The pressure drop across a filter at a stated flow and under given conditions; generally expressed in millimeters water gauge or PSI, or in SI units as N/m^2 or Pascals.

Resistivity The reciprocal of conductivity (R=1/C). A measure of specific resistance to the flow of electricity. In water, provides an easy mean of continuously measuring the purity of very low Total Dissolved Solids (TDS), or ionic concentration. The fewer the dissolved ions in water, the higher its resistivity. Resistivity is normally expressed in Megohm-cm and is equivalent to one million ohms of resistance measured between two electrodes one centimeter apart. The theoretical maximum ionic purity of water is 18.3 Megohm-cm at 25°C.

Resistance The ability of tumor cells to withstand the effects of a chemotherapeutic drug that should normally kill them.

Resolution Degree of molecular detail on a physical map of DNA, ranging from low to high.

Restriction Enzyme, Endonuclease A protein that recognizes specific, short nucleotide sequences and cuts DNA at those sites. Bacteria contain over 400 such enzymes that recognize and cut over 100 different DNA sequences.

Respiratory system The respiratory system is the group of organs responsible for carrying oxygen from the air to the bloodstream and for expelling the waste product carbon dioxide.

Response rate A determination of the effectiveness of treatment that usually requires a measurable amount of cancer. A complete clinical response means that a previously measurable cancer has gone away with treatment. It cannot be detected by examination, x-ray or scan. A complete surgical response means that even with a surgical exploration there is no trace of a cancer previously known to be present. A partial response means that the measurable amount of cancer has substantially decreased.

Restorative therapy Therapy directed at rapid restoration of health, usually regardless of the nature of the original disease; restorative therapy is most frequently given during convalescence. Vitamin supplements or sex hormones used for their anabolic effects might be considered as providing restorative therapy.

A single drug may have two or more therapeutic effects in the same patient at the same or different times, or in different patients. A patient may require more than one kind of therapy at a given time, or in the course of his/her disease.

Drugs may be used prophylactically to prevent disease or to diminish the severity of a disease should it occur subsequent to or during treatment; with a fine disregard for precision of definition, such a use of drugs is commonly called "prophylactic therapy". Drugs are sometimes used to measure bodily function and contribute toward the diagnosis of disease; such diagnostic agents have not yet been accused of participating in "diagnostic therapy".

Restriction enzyme cutting site A specific nucleotide sequence of DNA at which a particular restriction enzyme cuts the DNA. Some sites occur frequently in DNA (e.g., every several hundred base pairs), others much less frequently (rarecutter; e.g., every 10,000 base pairs).

Restriction fragment length polymorphism (RFLP) Variation between individuals in DNA fragments sizes cut by specific restriction enzymes; polymorphic sequences that result in RFLPs are used as markers on both physical maps and genetic linkage maps. RFLPs are usually caused by mutation at a cutting site.

Retest date The date when samples of the API (Active Pharmaceutical Ingredient)a material should be re-examined to ensure that material is still suitable for use.

Retinoblastoma An eye cancer caused by the loss of a pair of tumor-suppressor genes; the inherited form typically appears in childhood, since one gene is missing from the time of birth.

Retrometabolic drug design An approach to drug design that begins with the identification of a non-toxic, easily excreted end-product, which is then reverse engineered to a new drug candidate.

Retrospective validation Establishing documented evidence that a system does what it purports to do based on review and analysis of historic information.

Retrovirus An oncogenic, RNA-containing virus, which replicates through a double-stranded DNA intermediate necessitating the presence of an RNA-dependent DNA polymerase.

Revalidation Extent of validation necessary to assure that changes made to qualified or validated equipment, utilities, systems and process do not adversely affect the finished product. Implemented changes should be tracked and evaluated through a thorough, dynamic, change control program.

Reverse osmosis (RO) RO is one of two acceptable techniques for producing Water For injection (WFI), U.S.P. Procedure involves passing purified water across a semipermeable membrane against an osmotic gradient. R.O. is an excellent pretreatment for deionized water that will be subsequently filtered, because silt and colloids are removed. Usual performance of R.O. is removal of organics, multi-valent ions, and 90% of mono-valent ions.

Reworking Subjecting an intermediate or API (Active Pharmaceutical Ingredient) that does not conform to standards or specifications, to one or more processing steps that are different from the established manufacturing process so that its quality may be made acceptable (e.g., recrystallizing with a different solvent).

A molecule consisting of a number of ribonucleotides attached together to form a long strand one nucleotide thick. Each nucleotide contains the sugar, ribose, and one of four different bases: cytosine, adenine and guanine (as in DNA) and uracil (as opposed to thymine in DNA). The major portion of cellular RNA occurs as ribosomal RNA (rRNA), to a lesser extent as transfer RNA (tRNA) and less still as messenger RNA (mRNA), all three forms being concerned with transformation of the DNA sequence into the complementary protein sequence. It also occurs in some viruses where it acts as the hereditary material.

Rheumatic heart disease A condition in which the heart valves are damaged by rheumatic fever, an inflammatory disease which begins with a throat infection and can affect many of the body's connective tissues, especially those of the heart, joints, brain or skin.

Rhinitis Rhinitis is an inflammation of the mucous membrane that lines the nose, often due to an allergy to pollen, dust or other airborne substances. Seasonal allergic rhinitis also is known as "hay fever," a disorder which causes sneezing, itching, a runny nose and nasal congestion.

Ribonucleotides Building blocs of RNA.

Ribosomal RNA (rRNA) A class of RNA found in the ribosomes of cells.

Ribosomes Small cellular components composed of specialized ribosomal RNA and protein; site of protein synthesis.

Rickettsias Gram-negative microorganisms that are often carried by arthropod vectors and may infect humans and other mammals. Generally smaller than other bacteria, they require living cells for growth.

Rifabutin (Mycobutin) Indications: Treatment of MAC infection in combination with other agents; treatment of TB in combination with other agents; prophylaxis of MAC infection in patients unable to tolerate clarithromycin or azithromycin.

Contraindications: Known hypersensitivity.

Dosage: Treatment and prophylaxis: 300 mg po qd (or 600 mg 2-3 times a week [DOT]). There are many potential drug interactions, some of which require dosage modification

Toxicity: Orange discoloration of body secretions, gastrointestinal intolerance, abnormal liver function tests. Acute uveitis has been reported when used in association with clarithromycin.

Rifampin

Indications: Treatment of TB in combination with other agents.

Contraindications: Known hypersensitivity.

Dosage: 600 mg po qd. There are many potential drug interactions, some of which require dosage modification

Toxicity: Orange discoloration of body secretions, gastrointestinal intolerance, abnormal liver function tests, rash.

Rinse The operation that follows regeneration, a flushing out of excess regenerant solution.

Risk The likelihood that harm will result from exposure to a hazard. More generally, the probability that an event has occurred, or will occur, in members of a population under specified conditions, e.g., of exposure to a hazardous chemical; the "population at risk" consists of the subjects who could experience the event, e.g., who were exposed to the chemical. Risk is calculated by dividing the number of subjects who experience an event by the number of subjects in the population at risk. The risk, so calculated, is one of the bases used to estimate the likelihood that the event will occur in the future, the predicted risk. Risk, calculated as described, also indicates the probability that any individual subject in the population at risk experienced the event. (Formally, the idea of "risk" is applicable to the study of both desirable and undesirable events.)

For a meaningful estimate of risk (following exposure of subjects to some hazard), it is necessary to have carefully defined the harm that was done, to have characterized the population at risk, and to have specified the conditions of exposure. Interpreting an estimate of risk requires comparing the data with those from a "control" population, ideally one never exposed to the hazard. The statistical techniques used to estimate risks and to compare them are, generally, the techniques used in epidemiology.

Perceived risk is the subjective assessment of the importance of a hazard to individuals or to groups of individuals, For example, hazards that affect children generally have higher perceived risks than those that tend to affect adults. Hazards viewed as under a person's control (e.g., driving a car) generally have lower perceived risks than those viewed as not under such control (e.g., riding in a aircraft piloted by someone else). Hazards that produce fatalities grouped in time and space (e.g., airplane crashes) generally have higher perceived risks than those which produce fatalities scattered in time and space (e.g., automobile accidents), etc. Perceived risks are not necessarily correlated with the risks, for the same hazards, measures by epidemiologic techniques.

Risk management is the effort to reduce the likelihood that a hazard will produce harm. Risk management may involve decreasing the size of the population at risk (e.g., by prohibiting the use of a chemical as a food additive), altering the conditions of exposure (e.g., requiring adequate ventilation in an industrial environment), developing and using therapeutic regimens to minimize the consequences of exposure, etc.

Risk ratio The ratio of risk in the treated group (EER) to the risk in the control group (CER). This is used in randomised trials and cohort studies and is calculated as EER/CER.

Ritonavir (Norvir) Indications: Treatment of HIV infection in combination with other agents.

Contraindications: Known hypersensitivity.

Dosage: 600 mg po q12h with food following two week dose escalation regimen (day 1 and 2: 300 mg po bid; days 3-5: 400 mg po bid; days 6-13: 500 mg po bid). When coadministered as pharmacologic booster with other protease inhibitors, dosage is reduced. There are many potential drug interactions, some of which require dosage modification

Toxicity: Gastrointestinal intolerance, circumoral paresthesias, abnormal liver function tests.

S N N S H_3C—N O O O HN HN OH H N

RLS Restless Legs Syndrome

Painful hyperkinesia and convulsions of the legs mainly in the evenings and at night.

RNA (ribonucleic acid) A nucleic acid that transmits genetic information from DNA to the cytoplasm of a cell. Like DNA (deoxyribonucleic acid), it consists of long chains of four nucleotides, A, C, G, and U (rather than the "T" found in DNA).

RNA Ribonucleic acid, which carries instructions from DNA in the nucleus to cell polyribosomes, where proteins are, made according to the RNA instructions.

Robustness A measure of the capacity of an assay to remain unaffected by small changes in test conditions. Robustness provides an indication of the ability of an assay to perform under normal usage. Studies of the robustness of an assay measure the effect on the assay ouput of deliberate changes in assay inputs (incubation time, temperature, sample preparation, buffer pH) that can be controlled through specifications in the assay protocol.

Robustness Lack of effect of deliberate variations in the analytical procedure on the result

Roller bottles Small cylindrical bottles often used as bioreactors in the production of products by cell culture. The bottles are kept on a device that rotates them slowly to help assure proper growth. Automated systems may also be used for large arrays of roller bottles introducing sterile media and harvesting finished product automatically.

Rouge Form of surface corrosion that occurs in some stainless steel piping systems.

Roughness Consists of the finer irregularities of the surface texture, usually including those irregularities that result from the manufacturing process. These are considered to include traverse feed marks and other irregularities within the limits of the roughness sampling length.

RS Reference standard (typically a substance carefully prepared by (or for) the US Pharmacopeial Convention)

Ruggedness The reproducibility of an assay under a variety of normal, but variable, test conditions. Variable conditions might include different instruments, operators, reagent lots, etc. Ruggedness provides an estimate of experimental reproducibility with unavoidable error. In the process of developing an assay, it is necessary to consider the effect of environmental factors on the output of the assay. If this effect is not considered, the results of the assay in actual use may not be as accurate as expected. The purpose of a ruggedness test is to identify the variables (experimental factors) that strongly influence the measurements provided by the assay, and to determine how closely these variables need to be controlled. Ruggedness tests do NOT determine the optimal conditions for the assay.

S

S If followed by a number, a chromatographic support. E. g., S7 is graphitized carbon with a nominal surface area of 12 m^2/g. (Defined in USP/NF.)

S9 The S9 fraction (post-mitochondrial supernatant fraction) is a mixture of microsomes and cytosol. Accordingly, it contains a wide variety of phase I and phase II enzymes including P450 enzymes, flavin-monooxygenases, carboxylesterases, epoxide hydrolase, UDP-glucuronosyltransferases, sulfotransferases, methyltransferases, acetyltransferases, glutathione S-transferases and other drug-metabolizing enzymes.

Saccharomyces cerevisiae Better known as beer yeast, ordinary yeast. Yeast used in rDNA research.

Safe harbor Implementation of new microbiological methods poses significant problems and risks. These include validation of methods that will not yield results equal to traditional methods. Additionally, comparative parallel testing is not always informative. Experimental designs for validating the methods can be developed, but may not be a perfect solution. Therefore, some risk is involved and there is a need to create a "safe harbor" for firms willing to undertake new microbiological tests. The safe harbor concept for sterility testing using new/rapid microbiological test methods (a specification change using the ICH definition of specification) may be limited because the test is qualitative and the established release test requirement is a critical parameter. For a critical parameter, the batch cannot be released if the parameter is not met. The safe harbor concept for sterility testing may not afford much latitude because a failed criterion prohibits retesting by the same method or even a compendial method. The batch must be rejected. Otherwise, the batch is "tested into compliance."

Safety Relative freedom from harm; in clinical trials, this refers to an absence of harmful side effects resulting from use of the product and may be assessed by laboratory testing of biological samples, special tests and procedures, psychiatric evaluation, and/or physical examination of subjects.

Safranin A base, obtained from aniline; aniline pink; used as a stain in histology.

Salinity The concentration of soluble minerals (mainly salts of the alkali metals or of magnesium) in water.

Salmonella A large genus of the tribe Salmonellae, family Enterobacteriaceae, containing motile, gram-negative, rod-shaped organisms that ferment dextrose, forming acid and usually gas. Several species occur as intestinal pathogens in acute inflammations in humans and domestic animals. Salmonella typhimurium causes food poisoning in humans.

Salt A compound formed by the interaction of an acid and a base, the hydrogen atoms of the acid being replaced by another positive ion derived from the base.

Salt rejection In reverse osmosis, the ratio of salts removed (rejected) to the original salt concentration.

Sanitization That part of decontamination that reduces viable microorganisms to a defined acceptance level, normally achieved by using a chemical agent or heat.

Saponification Alkaline hydrolysis of triacyl glycerols to yield fatty acids as soaps.

Saquinavir (Invirase, fortovase) Indications: Treatment of HIV infection in combination with other agents. Fortovase (soft gel cap formulation) is preferred to Invirase (hard gel cap) because of its enhanced absorption and bioavailability.

Contraindications: Known hypersensitivity.

Dosage: 1200 mg po tid with food. When coadministered with ritonavir (400 mg po bid) as pharmacologic booster, dose is 400 mg po bid. There are many potential drug interactions, some of which require dosage modification

Toxicity: Gastrointestinal intolerance, abnormal liver function tests.

Sarcomas Cancers arising from cells found in the supporting tissues of the body such as bone, cartilage, fat, connective tissue, and muscle.

Saturated air When there is a state of mutual equilibrium between the moist air and the liquid or solid phases of water. Saturated air holds as much water vapor as it can for a given temperature and pressure.

Saturated fatty acids Fatty acids containing fully saturated alkyl chains.

Saturation humidity The air is saturated when the partial pressure of water vapor in the air at a given temperature equals the vapor pressure of water at the same temperature.

Saturation index The relation of calcium carbonate to the pH, alkalinity, and hardness of water to determine its scale-forming tendency.

SCADA Supervisory Control And Data Acquisition.

Scale The mineral deposit that can coat the insides of boilers or the surfaces of RO membranes. It consists mainly of calcium carbonate that precipitates out of solution under certain conditions of pH, alkalinity, and hardness.

Scale up To take a biopharmaceutical manufacturing process from the laboratory scale to a scale at which it is commercially feasible.

Scheduled allowance Is the maximum dollar amount of a medical provider's fee for a particular service in a particular geographic area, which will be taken into account (prior to application of any deductible, co-insurance or maximum) in determining benefits under the Plan. In the case of a fee billed by a Network Provider, the scheduled allowance shall be deemed equal to the discount fee. For Major Medical benefits, in the case of a fee billed by a Non-Network Provider, the scheduled allowance will be based on the highest amount charged for the specific service by 70% of medical providers in the geographic area.

Scratch An elongated mar in the metal's surface not associated with the predominant surface texture pattern, which is visible to the unaided eye.

Script A program or a sequence of instructions that are interpreted or carried out by another program.

Search engine An online service that compares your search criteria with its database of information about the Internet and displays the results.

Second line therapy Treatment when a patient has failed to respond to first-line therapy.

Secondary containment Level of containment that is external to and separate from primary containment.

Secure retention The ability to generate accurate and complete copies of records in both human-readable and electronic form suitable for inspection, review, and copying by department of health. Records must be protected to enable their accurate and ready retrieval through the records retention period.

Security (IEEE) The protection of computer hardware and software fromaccidental or malicious access, use, modification, destruction, ordisclosure. Security also pertains to personnel, data, communications,and the physical protection of computer installations.

Sedimentation A primary step in municipal water treatment. Water is allowed to stand long enough for solids to settle by gravity. Also called settling.

Sedimenters For sedimentation, batch and continuous centrifuges are available. There are three types of centrifuges for continuous sedimentation. a) Disc - constructed on the vertical axis, disc centrifuges are solid-bowl units. All are capable of separating liquids from solids, solids from two immiscible liquids and two immiscible liquids. Disc-stack centrifuges differ in their ability to handle different volumes of solids in the feed stream, and in the way that the separated solids are removed from the separation vessel: solids-retaining, solids-ejecting, and nozzle-bowl separators. b) Decanters - consists of a cylindrical settling section with a tapered end. Inside the bowl is a scroll conveyor that is driven usually at a slightly faster rate than the bowl and can be controlled by a differential speed device or back drive. c) Tubular - a vertical solid-wall cylinder provided with caps on both ends; a tubular centrifuge generally has a bottom feed inlet. When two liquids of different specific gravities are fed, the heavier phase is concentrated against the wall, while the lighter phase "floats" on the heavier phase.

Seed lot system A seed lot system is a system according to which successive batches of a product are derived from the same master seed lot at a given passage level. For routine production, a working seed lot is prepared from the master seed lot. The final product is derived from the working seed lot and has not undergone more passages from the master seed lot than the vaccine shown in clinical studies to be satisfactory with respect to safety and efficacy. The origin and the passage history of the master seed lot and the working seed lot are recorded.

Seed stock The initial inoculum, or the cells placed in growth medium from which other cells will grow.

Seed Tank Industrial fermentations are generally started in tanks smaller than a 1,000 to 50,000 gallon main fermenter. This small "seed" tank may be up to 100 gallons and propagate enough organisms to "kick-off" the main fermentation. Often, a seed tank may be large enough to require its own seed tank.

Segregated Storage in the same room or inside area, but physically separated by distance from incompatible materials.

Selectivity The capacity or propensity of a drug to affect one cell population in preference to others, i.e., the ability of a drug to affect one kind of cell, and produce effects, in doses lower than those required to affect other cells. Selectivity can be measured or described by means of such numbers as the Therapeutic Index, or the Standardized

Safety Margin: not infrequently one wishes to express selectivity of drug action with respect to two potentially beneficial effects, or two potentially toxic doses, or two toxic doses, instead of one each.

"Selectivity" is not to be confused with " potency"; a potent drug may be non-selective or a selective drug may be impotent. "Selectivity" is however, a measure of the relative potency of a drug in producing different effects.

Selectivity is generally a desirable property in a drug, e.g., it is desirable that an antibacterial agent affect parasites in doses too small to affect host cells. Sometimes, selectivity of action is virtually precluded by the nature of the drug, e.g., in the case of analogs of hormones that have many target cells or tissues. Sometimes selectivity of action for cells within an organism is not necessarily desirable, as in the case of certain economic poisons, i.e., pesticides, herbicides, rodenticides; even in this case, however, it is desirable to have a drug selective for cells of a particular species, and this criterion can most easily be met by drugs selective for certain cell types in the organisms of the target species.

"Selectivity" and "specificity" are, unfortunately, frequently used as synonyms for each other. They describe separate phenomena, each of which deserves an unambiguous name.

Self draining Capable of elimination of all fluid from the system due to the force of gravity alone.

Self insurance A type of insurance in which employers, usually with 100 employees or more, decide to retain the cost risk component of providing health insurance to their own employees rather than contract with an insurance company. Usually, these employers hire a third-party administrator to set up and administer the program.

SEM (Scanning electron microscopy) Utilizes an electron beam to produce images over a very broad magnification range of 10X to 105X. The technique is somewhat limited by the conductivity of the material but works very well to inspect 316L stainless steel. Typical magnification levels for surface defect evaluation are from 100 to 4,000.

Semiautomatic arc welding Arc welding with equipment that controls only the filler metal feed. The advance of the welding is manually controlled.

Semipermeable Membranes that do not have measurable pores but through which smaller molecules can pass.

Semi synthetic drugs Are products from natural sources, they have to undergo a chemical process (heroin, LSD).

Senility The aging related loss of mental faculties.

Senscequence The reduction and decline of a gland's output over age.

Sensible heat (SH) Heat that causes a change of temperature without causing a change of state.

Sensible heat ratio The ratio of room sensible heat to room total heat as expressed in the formula: Sensible Heat ratio (SHR) = Room Sensible Heat (SH)/Room Total Heat (TH).

Sensitivity The ability of a population, an individual or a tissue, relative to the abilities of others, to respond in a qualitatively normal fashion to a particular drug dose. The smaller the dose required to produce an effect, the more sensitive is the responding system. A patient would be considered abnormally sensitive to aspirin if a small fraction of the normal analgesic dose gave adequate pain relief; or, were an abnormally large dose of aspirin required to afford pain relief, the subject would be said to be "insensitive" to aspirin. Conversely, the drug would appear to be extraordinarily potent or impotent in such a patient. If a patient manifested an allergic response after raking aspirin, he would be considered hypersensitive to aspirin, regardless of whether the aspirin afforded him relief from pain, and regardless of the size of the dose required to elicit the allergic response. Such a patient might be simultaneously hypersensitive to aspirin, and insensitive to aspirin, acting as an analgesic agent.

Every subject is sensitive to a drug; the question of importance is "how sensitive?" In any event sensitivity is a property ascribed to the organism; potency is a property ascribed to the drug. Hypersensitivity is a property ascribed to a subject in a particular immunologic state.

Sensitivity may be measured or described quantitatively in terms of the point of intersection of a dose-effect curve with the axis of abscissal values or a line parallel to it; such a point corresponds to the dose just required to produce a given degree of effect In analogy to this, the "sensitivity" of a measuring system is defined as the lowest input (smallest dose) required to produce a given degree of output (effect).

Sensitivity tests Generally refers to the laboratory methodologies applied to measure sensitivity or resistance of cancer cells to drugs.

Sensitizer A chemical that causes a substantial proportion of exposed people or animals to develop an allergic reaction in normal tissue after repeated exposure to the chemical.

Sepsis The presence of various pus-forming and other pathogenic organisms or their toxins in the blood or tissues; septicemia.

Septic shock Serious condition that occurs when an overwhelming infection leads to low BP and low blood flow. Vital organs, such as the brain, heart, kidneys, and liver may not function properly or may fail. Treatment: Dopamine (iv) is the drug of choice.

Sequence The order of nucleotides in a DNA or RNA molecule, or the order of amino acids in a protein molecule

Sequence tagged site (STS) Short (200 to 500 base pairs) DNA sequence that has a single occurrence in the human genome and whose location and base sequence are known. Detectable by polymerase chain reaction, STSs are useful for localizing and orienting the mapping and sequence data reported from many different laboratories and serve as landmarks on the developing physical map of the human genome. Expressed sequence tags (ESTs) are STSs derived from cDNAs.

Sequencing (of DNA or RNA) Determination of the order of nucleotides (base sequences) in a DNA or RNA molecule or the order of amino acids in a protein.

Sera One of the plural forms of serum.

Serious Adverse Event (SAE) or Serious Adverse Drug Reaction (Serious ADR) Any untoward medical occurrence that at any dose:- results in death,- is life-threatening,- requires inpatient hospitalization or prolongation of existing hospitalization,- results in persistent or significant disability/ incapacity, or- is a congenital anomaly/birth defect.

Serious adverse experience The Nordic Guidelines for Good Clinical Trial Practice define a serious AE as "Any experience that suggests a significant hazard, contra-indication, side effect or precaution."

Serotonin An inhibitory neurotransmitter required for sleep.

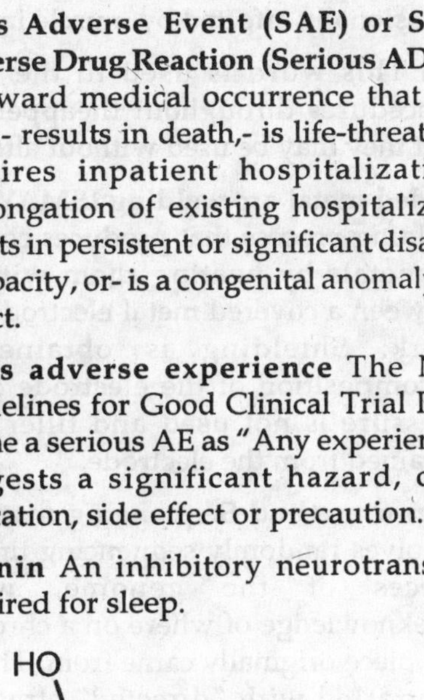

Serratia marcescens They are minute, rod-shaped or coccoid, aerobic, gram-negative organisms, found on various foodstuffs as a pink or reddish growth, nonpathogenic. Used to validate 0.45μm removal rated filters.

Serum The liquid portion remaining after clotting whole blood or plasma.

Server A computer program that provides services to other computer programs in the same or other computers.

Service life The life expectancy or number of cycles for which a processing unit will maintain its performance.

Sex chromosomes Those whose content is different in the two sexes - usually labeled X and Y (or W and Z), female sex has XX (or WW), male is XY (or WZ).

SGOT, SGPT Two measures of liver function; occasionally affected by muscle injury.

Shall This word is used in the example procedures throughout theappendices so that they may be used without alteration.

Shielded metal arc welding (SMAW) An arc welding process that produces coalescence of metals by heating them with an arc between a covered metal electrode and the work. Shielding is obtained from decomposition of the electrode covering. Pressure is not used and filler metal is obtained from the electrode.

Shotgun method Sequencing method that involves randomly sequencing tiny cloned pieces of the genome, with no foreknowledge of where on a chromosome the piece originally came from. This can be contrasted with "directed" strategies, in which pieces of DNA from adjacent stretches of a chromosome are sequenced. Direct strategies eliminate the need for complex reassembly techniques. Because there are advantages to both strategies, researchers expect to use both random (or shotgun) and directed strategies in combination to sequence the human genome.

Should The stated requirement is strongly recommended.

Sickle cell anemia An inherited, potentially lethal disease in which a defect in hemoglobin, the oxygen-carrying pigment in the blood, causes distortion (sickling) and loss of red blood cells, producing damage to organs throughout the body.

Side effects Drug effects which are not desirable or are not part of a therapeutic effect; effects other than those intended. For instance, in the treatment of peptic ulcer with atropine, dryness of the mouth is a side effect and decreased gastric secretion is the desired drug effect. If the same drug were being used to inhibit salivation, dryness of the mouth would be the therapeutic effect and decreased gastric secretion would be a side effect.

Pharmacological side effects are true drug effects. With increasing doses of a drug, the intensity of pharmacological side effects in individuals, and/or the frequency with which a pharmacological side effect is observed in a population is increased.

Signed (signature) (ICH API definition) The record of who performed a particular action or review. This record may be initials, full handwritten signature, personal seal, or authenticated and secure electronic signature.

Silica silicon Dioxide (SiO2) and its hydrated forms are classified as reactive and nonreactive. Generally, reactive Silica is removed by the anion exchange resin. Reactive Silica is only slightly ionized and is held lightly by the anion resin. It is for this reason that Silica is the first thing to break through when the resin nears exhaustion. Nonreactive Silica is generally considered to be particulate (colloidal) in nature.

Simulation (ANSI/IEEE/ISO) The representation of selectedcharacteristics of the behaviour of one physical or abstract system byanother system. In a digital computer system, simulation is done bysoftware; for example, (a) the representation of physical phenomena bymeans of operations performed by a computer system, (b) therepresentation of operations of a computer system by those of anothercomputer system.

Single controlled trial SCT Since 1998, the department of health has allowed drug developers to use what is known as the single controlled trial (SCT) to support their drug approval applications. The SCT provision allows applicants to prove the effectiveness of new drugs by submitting data from only one controlled clinical study instead of multiple studies.

Single gene disorder Hereditary disorder caused by a mutant allele of a single gene (e.g., Duchenne muscular dystrophy, retinoblastoma, sickle cell disease).

Single nucleotide polymorphism (SNP) A single erroneous "letter" substitution in a string of DNA. SNPs can serve as unique genetic markers, but they may also form the basis for an individual's susceptibility to a disease or lack of response to a given drug.

Single blind study One in which subjects do not know whether they are receiving the active drug or a placebo.

Sinus The sinuses (paranasal sinuses) are air cavities within the facial bones. They are lined by mucous membranes similar to those in other parts of the airways.

Sinusitis Sinusitis is inflammation of the membrane lining the facial sinuses, often caused by bacterial or viral infection.

SIP (Steam in place) The introduction of steam to sanitize or sterilize a piece of equipment without relocating the equipment.

SiRNA Short interference RNA: short double stranded (19 to 21 nucleotides in length) RNAi molecule

Slope An incline or deviation from the horizontal. A tube or pipe installed in the horizontal plane is said to slope if one end is positioned higher than the other.

Small molecule Chemical entity used for screening against drug targets.

Small molecule drug One or more active chemical compounds, typically formulated as an orally available pill, that interact with a specific biological target, such as a receptor, enzyme or ion channel, to provide a curative effect.

Smoke control The use of physical barriers and mechanical ventilation to control the spread of smoke from a fire.

Smoke purge The use of mechanical ventilation to remove smoke resulting from fire.

Smoke test Visualization of airflow streams in a clean space using artificially generated smoke, such as Titanium smoke, CO_2, or glycol fog.

Smooth muscle disorder A disease that affects the muscle tissue responsible for the contractility of hollow organs, such as blood vessels, the gastrointestinal tract, the bladder, or the uterus. Smooth muscle disorders are a major cause of gastroparesis. Examples include irritable bowel syndrome, scleroderma (hardening of the skin), and arteriosclerosis (hardening of the arteries).

SNSR Sensory neuron-specific G protein-coupled receptor.

Sodium A body salt, also termed electrolyte. Kidney disease and some diseases of the adrenal gland and dehydration can cause abnormal results.

Soft drug A compound that is quickly broken down in the body to predictable non-toxic and inactive metabolites after having achieved its therapeutic role.

Softener Water treatment equipment that uses a sodium-based ion-exchange resin, principally to remove cations.

Softening A pretreatment process which uses cation exchange resin to remove hardness elements (calcium and magnesium) from water. The cation resin is regenerated with Sodium Chloride (NaCl) and during the exchange process, the calcium and magnesium are removed from the water and replaced with sodium ions (Na+). The resulting sodium salts are much more soluble and do not precipitate, which provides better feed water to the RO system.

Software (PMA CSVC) A collection of programs, routines, andsubroutines that controls the operation of a computer or a computerisedsystem.

Software life cycle (ANSI/IEEE) The period of time that starts when asoftware product is conceived and ends when the product is no longeravailable for use. The software life cycle typically includes arequirements phase, test phase, installation and checkout phase, andoperation and maintenance phase.

Soldering A metal joining process wherein coalescence is produced by heating to suitable temperatures and by using a nonferrous alloy fusible at temperatures below 427°C (800°F) and having a melting point below that of the base metals being joined. The filler metal is distributed between closely fitted surfaces of the joint by capillary attraction. In general, solders are lead-tin alloys and may contain antimony, bismuth, and other elements.

Solid phase extraction Is an extraction method that uses a solid phase and a liquid phase to isolate test article(s) from a sample or specimen. It is usually used to clean up a sample before using a chromatographic or other analytical method to quantitate the test artcile(s). The general procedure is to load a solution onto the SPE phase, wash away matrix interferences, and then elute the desired analytes.

Solid tumor An abnormal mass of tissue that usually does not contain cysts or liquid areas. Solid tumors may be benign (not cancerous), or malignant (cancerous). Different types of solid tumors are named for the type of cells that form them. Examples of solid tumors are sarcomas, carcinomas, and lymphomas. Leukemias (cancers of the blood) generally do not form solid tumors.

Solubility The analytical composition of a saturated solution, expressed in terms of the proportion of a designed solute in a designated solvent is the solubility of that solute. The solubility may be expressed as a concentration, **molality**, mole fraction, mole ratio, etc.

Soluble antigen Generally used in reference to vaccine production. As opposed to a whole live or attenuated virus, a soluble antigen is a fragment of the virus that produces immunity. Also refers to large molecular weight polysaccharides from some bacteria which can act as vaccines.

Solute The substance that dissolves to form ions in solution.

Solutions w/w: percent by weight: grams per 100 g of solution

w/v: percent by volume: grams per 100 ml of solution

v/v: percent by volume in volume; ml per 100 ml of solution. Solvent An inorganic or organic liquid used as a vehicle for the preparation of solutions or suspensions in the manufacture of an intermediate or API (Active Pharmaceutical Ingredient).

Somatic cell Any cell in the body except gametes and their precursors.

Somatic nervous system Controls all voluntary systems within the body with the exception of reflex arcs. This system is comprised of the afferent nerve network, which include all sensory nerves leading to the brain, and the efferent nerve network, which includes all motor nerves leading from the brain to the muscles (NMJ). The somatic system is generally associated with all body movement and is not part of the Autonomic NS (involuntary).

Somoclonal variation Genetic variation produced from the culture of plant cells from a pure breeding strain; the source of the variation is not known.

SOP (Standard operating procedures) The description of necessary activities to respond to normal and abnormal situations in an operating system. The SOP may include a troubleshooting checklist, list of personnel to contact, etc. SOPs should also describe normal operation, maintenance, and cleaning of the system, and normal operating parameters. An SOP may be created for any system but an SOP must be created for each system requiring qualification.

Source code (PMA CSVC) An original computer program expressed inhuman-readable form (programming language), which must be translatedinto machine-readable form before it can be executed by the computer.

Source data All information in original records and certified copies of original records of clinical findings, observations, or other activities in a clinical trial necessary for the reconstruction and evaluation of the trial. Source data are contained in source documents (original records or certified copies).

Source documents Original documents, data, and records (e.g., hospital records, clinical and office charts, laboratory notes, memoranda, subjects' diaries or evaluation checklists, pharmacy dispensing records, recorded data from automated instruments, copies or transcriptions certified after verification as being accurate and complete, microfiches, photographic negatives, microfilm or magnetic media, x-rays, subject files, and records kept at the pharmacy, at the laboratories, and at medico-technical departments involved in the clinical trial).

Southern blotting Transfer by absorption of DNA fragments separated in electrophoretic gels to membrane filters for detection of specific base sequences by radiolabeled complementary probes.

Spare receptors A pharmacological system has spare receptors (a receptor reserve), if an agonist can induce a maximum response when occupying less than 100% of the available receptors. The existence of spare receptors reflects a circumstance in which the maximum effect produced by an agonist is limited by some factor other than the number of activated receptors. Whether or not a system has spare receptors depends upon the nature of the receptor and its coupling to the measured response, the number of receptors, and the intrinsic activity of the agonist.

Sparger A device used to agitate, oxygenate, aerate, or add a chemical to a liquid by means of compressed air or gas entering through small holes in a pipe below the liquid surface.

Spasmolytics Drugs eliminating muscular spasms of internal hollow organs, such as intestines, biliary and urinary tracts, female sexual organs; they are administered for colics and pain stemming from the aforementioned organs, also for certain forms of migraine, etc.

Specific conductance The reciprocal of specific resistance usually expressed in micromhos/cm.

Specific humidity Also known as Humidity Ratio, and Absolute Humidity, is the weight of water vapor in each pound of dry air expressed in grains of moisture per pound of dry air, or pounds of moisture per pound of dry air. NOTE: 7,000 grains = 1.0 pound.

Humidity of air mixtures is normally discussed in terms of grains of moisture per pound rather than the more common term of relative humidity because the grains of moisture in an air stream do not change when it is heated or cooled, unless condensation takes place.

Specific ion determinations Electrochemical measurement of trace ion levels in solution.

Specific resistance The resistance of a one-centimeter cube of water to the passage of electricity under standard conditions, expressed in ohms/cm. A measure of the Total Ionized Solids concentration.

Specific volume In Psychrometry, the cubic feet of the mixture per pound of dry air.

Specification A list of testes, references to analytical procedures, and appropriate acceptance criteria that are numerical limits, ranges, or other criteria for the test described. It establishes the set of criteria to which an intermediate or API (Active Pharmaceutical Ingredient) should conform to be considered acceptable for its intended use. "Conformance to Specifications" means that the intermediate or API, when tested according to the listed analytical procedures, will meet the listed acceptance criteria.

Specification qualification A documented evaluation of the detailedspecification, carried out for the purpose of confirming compliancewith the User Requirement and Functional Specifications and providingthe detailed design documentation required for subsequent stages ofvalidation (eg Installation and Operational Qualification) and ongoingoperation of the facility or system in compliance with regulatoryrequirements related to product quality.

Specificity The capacity of a drug to manifest only one kind of action. A drug of perfect specificity of action might increase, or decrease, a specific function of a given cell type, but it would not do both. Nicotine is not specific in its actions in autonomic ganglia; it both stimulates and depresses ganglionic function by a number of means. Atropine is quite specific in only blocking the actions of acetylcholine at certain receptors; in general atropine does not stimulate cellular activity when it combines with receptors, nor does it block interaction with receptors of agonists other than acetylcholine. In affecting exocrine glands, acetylcholine itself is very specific, in that it causes only stimulation or secretion; acetylcholine, at the same time, is non-selective in its action, in that stimulation of all exocrine glands is produced by about the same dose of acetylcholine.

Selectivity is concerned with site of action; specificity, with the kinds of action at a site.

Spinner flasks Small laboratory bioreactors used for the initial growth of mammalian cells lines.

Sponsor An individual, company, institution, or organization that takes responsibility for the initiation, management, and/or financing of a clinical trial.

Sponsor investigator An individual who both initiates and conducts, alone or with others, a clinical trial, and under whose immediate direction the investigational product is administered to, dispensed to, or used by a subject. The term does not include any person other than an individual (e.g., it does not include a corporation or an agency). The obligations of a sponsor-investigator include both those of a sponsor and those of an investigator.

Spore, bacterial A bacterial spore is a resistant body formed as part of the life cycle of some bacteria. Bacterial spores are able to withstand severe environmental conditions (e.g., heat, drying, chemicals) for many years. When conditions are favorable, spores germinate into vegetative bacterial cells capable of replication.

Sporicide An agent that destroys bacterial and fungal spores.

Spray drying Process by which a material in suspension is converted into droplets that may be coated by a substance, either melted or dissolved in the droplet's media. The action in spray drying is primarily that of evaporation, energy is applied to the droplet forcing evaporation of the media with both energy and mass transfer through the droplet. Examples of this technology include, pharmaceutical tablet granulation, and rapid drying which results in free-flowing powders on a continuous basis. Spray drying process consists of the following steps: 1. Formation of a slurry to be sprayed; this slurry may be a simple concentrated solution or the dispersion of an insoluble material in a solution.

2. Liquid atomization into droplets; this action is critical as the droplet size will dictate the equipment size as well as the final product size. There are four types of atomization devices: air, airless, disk (or rotary) spray, and ultrasonic.

3. Exposure of the droplet to a heated gas flow; this gas (normally air) supplies the energy required to vaporize the solvent. Collection of the dry free-flowing powder or encapsulated liquid or solid.

Stability Generally, stability refers to the physico-chemical condition of a parenteral, biological, or shelf life of labile drugs. Certain drugs must pass U.S.P. stability tests. For example, human serum albumin must pass certain limits of nephelometric turbidity. Also manufacturers must have documentation of potency of labile products under labeled storage conditions.

Stability index An empirical modification of the saturation index used to predict scaling or corrosive tendencies in water systems.

Stability testing Determination of the period over which a product continues to meet the USP specifications, generally by long-term 'real time' tests at room temperature and about 65% relative humidity. Accelerated tests (40 °C, 75% RH) are used to determine tentative stability periods for new formulations.

Stabilizer A stabilizer is an additive ensuring the stability of a drug, i.e. the capacity of a drug to maintain certain qualitative features at specified limits for a certain period of time and under specified conditions.

Staff performer A performer who is a full-time employee of a radio or television station or network.

Staging The process of determining whether cancer has spread and, if so, how far. There is more than one system for staging.

Stainless steel There are more than 70 standard types of stainless steel and many special alloys. These steels are produced in the wrought form (AISI types) and as cast alloys (ACI types). Generally, all are iron based, with 12 to 30 percent chromium, 0 to 22 percent nickel, and minor amounts of carbon, columbium, copper, molybdenum, selenium, tantalum, and titanium. There are three groups of wrought stainless steels:

1. Martensitic Alloys: characteristically magnetic and hardenable by heat treatment are oxidation resistant. They are exemplified by Type 410 (UNS S41000). Contain 12 to 20 percent chromium with controlled amount of carbon and other additives. Their corrosion resistance is inferior to austenitic stainless steels, and is generally used in mildly corrosive environments and for cutlery, turbine blades, and high-temperature parts.

2. Ferritic Stainless: characteristically magnetic but not hardenable by heat treatment. Contain 15 to as much as 30 percent Cr with low carbon content (0.1 percent). The higher chromium content improves its corrosive resistance. Type 430 (UNS S43000) widely used in nitric acid plants is a typical example. Corrosion resistance is rated good, although ferritic alloys are not good against reducing acids such as HCl.

3. Austenitic Stainless: widely used in bioprocessing, are characteristically non-magnetic, not hardenable by heat treatment, and are the most corrosion resistant of the three groups. These steels contain 16 to 26 percent chromium, 6 to 22 percent nickel. Carbon is kept low (0.08 percent) to minimize carbide precipitation. To avoid precipitation, special stainless steels stabilized with titanium, columbium, or tantalum, have been developed (types 321, 347, 348). Another approach to the problem is the use of low-carbon steels such as 304L and 316L, with 0.03 percent maximum carbon. Type 302 is the basic alloy of this group. Types 304 (UNS S30400) and 304L are low-carbon versions of 302. Types 316 (UNS S31600), 316L, and 317 (UNS S31700), with 2.5 to 3.5 percent molybdenum, are the most corrosion resistance.

Cast Stainless Alloys: are widely used in pumps, valves, and fittings. All corrosion resistant alloys have the letter C plus a second letter (A to N) denoting increasing nickel content. Numerals indicate maximum carbon. Typical members of this group are CF-8, similar to 304 stainless, CF-8M, similar to 316, and CD-4M Cu, which has improved resistance to nitric, sulfuric, and phosphoric acids.

Standalone system A self-contained computer system which provides dataprocessing, monitoring or control functions but which is not embeddedwithin automated equipment. This is contrasted with an embedded system,the sole purpose of which is to control a particular piece of automatedequipment.

Standard atmospheric conditions At sea level these conditions are: 1. Temperature - 59°F.

2. Pressure - 29.921 Inches of mercury

3. Density - 0.0765 lbs dry air/cubic foot.

Standard deviation Indicator of the relative variability of a variable around its mean; the square root of the variance. (statistics).

Standard dimensional ratio (SDR) The most commonly accepted means for providing a pipe wall thickness category and constant mechanical properties for many plastic materials. Used for solid, homogeneous pipe, the SDR is found by dividing the average outside diameter of a pipe by the wall thickness.

Standard Operating Procedures (SOPs) Detailed, written instructions to achieve uniformity of the performance of a specific function.

Standard report A Standard Report contains:

a cover page,

a description of the each assay specified in the proposal or change order

the table of results for each assay specified in the project or study,

a list of specifications for the results,

if relevant, any observation about how test system, i.e., cell monolayers, animals, etc., reacted to the test compound(s),

if relevant, any observations about analytical method,

if relevant, an appendix containing the animal observation records,

if relevant, an appendix with an overview of the analytical assay conditions,

A standard report is by default sent to the customer in both a doc and a pdf format. A customer can specify that only one of these formats be used. The customer can also specify whether the reports are password protected.

Standard treatment A treatment or other intervention currently being used and considered to be of proven effectiveness based on past studies.

Standardized safety margin A number, LD1-ED99/ED99 x 100%, which is a measure of the selectivity of action or relative "safety" of a drug. The standardized safety margin indicates by what percentage of itself a dose effective in virtually all (99%) of a population must be exceeded in order to produce a lethal effect in a minimum number (1%) in the population. The therapeutic index (q.v.) measures by what factor an effective dose must be increased to produce a standard lethal effect in a population. Clinically, the standardized safety margin probably has greater practical meaning than does the therapeutic index, and, unlike the therapeutic index, the meaningfulness of the standardized safety margin does not depend on the parallelism of the dose effect curves from which the LD1 and ED99 are inferred. The standardized safety margin (more frequently than the therapeutic index) can sometimes be computed from clinical data not involving lethal effects, e.g., the ED99 for control of epileptic seizures and the ED1 for the production of drowsiness or ataxia, in a population of patients with epilepsy.

Standpipe system A wet or dry system of piping, valves, outlets, and related equipment designed to provide water at specified pressures and installed exclusively for the fighting of fires.

Start up The initial operation of equipment to prove that it is installed properly and operates as intended. Start-Up is considered complete when the selected equipment will adequately process product as specified.

State institute of drug control, sÚKL This institution is controlled by the Ministry of Health whose mission is to ensure that in the Czech Republic only safe, effective and high-level quality drugs are available. The Institute provides surveillance over the properties of drugs and medical devices used in human medicine.

State of control A condition in which all operating variables that affect performance remain within such ranges that the system or process performs consistently and as intended.

Statins Statins are a class of drugs that help lower cholesterol levels in the blood.

Statins are a class of LDL-cholesterol lowering drugs that has been found to be highly effective.

Statistical process control (SPC) A process control method to demonstrate mathematically that a process or system is operating within the limitations established for the parameter(s) in question.

Statistical significance State that applies when a hypothesis is rejected. Whether or not a given result is significant depends on the significance level adopted. For example, one may say "significant at the 5% level". This implies that a level of significance has been applied such that when the null hypothesis is true there is only a 1 in 20 chance of rejecting it or that the observed result has led to rejection of the null hypothesis.

Stavudine (d4T, Zerit) Indications: Treatment of HIV infection in combination with other agents.

Contraindications: Known hypersensitivity, concurrent ZDV use because of pharmacologic antagonism.

Dosage: Based on weight: > 60 kg —> 40 mg po bid; < 60 kg —> 30 mg po bid. Dose adjustment for peripheral neuropathy: 20 mg po bid.

Toxicity: Peripheral neuropathy, acute pancreatitis, abnormal liver function tests.

O HN O N HO O

Stent A stent is an object – usually a tiny tube made of a metallic mesh – put inside a blood vessel to keep it open and unblocked.

Stereoisomers (R or S) When a drug substance contains a chiral center (or plane or axis), the center will have two different configurations. If the two configurations are mirror images of each other, the two configurations are enantiomeric. If the two configurations are not mirror image, the two configurations are diastereomeric. Unlike enantiomers, diastereomers can differ in physicochemical properties.

Sterile engineering design (Fermentation) The application of techniques to prevent contamination of a fermentation process by undesirable organisms. It includes three basic phases relating to the operation of the plant. First, the fermenter with the ancillary equipment, pipework, and valves must be brought to a sterile state. Secondly, the fermenter feed must be sterilized, and finally, sterile barriers at the interface between the fermenter and the outside environment must be maintained.

Sterile water For Injection, U.S.P. A form in which water is distributed in sterile packages. Sterile Water for Injection is intended mainly for use as a solvent for parenteral products such as sterile solids that must be distributed dry because of limited stability of their solutions. It must be packaged only in single-dose containers of not larger than 1-liter size.

Sterile water for irrigation, U.S.P. This form of water meets most, but not all, of the requirements for Sterile Water for Injection. The exceptions are with respect of container size (i.e., the container may contain a volume of more than 1 liter), container design (i.e., the container may be designed so as to empty rapidly the contents as a single dose), particulate matter requirements (i.e., need not meet the requirement for Large Volume Injections for single-dose infusions), and labeling requirements (e.g., the designation "For Irrigation Only" and "Not For Injection" appear prominently on the label).

Sterility test A test generally done on finished products which are to be injected. Direct transfer: 40 samples of the product are placed in separate containers of an aerobic growth medium (20 samples) and an anaerobic growth medium (20 samples) and incubated for at least 7 days.Membrane filtration: liquids (typically, the contents of 20containers) are forced, in a closed system, through two separate membrane filters (typically 0.45 μm pore size). Then aerobic and anaerobic growth media are placed on the separate filters and cultured for at least 7 days. No growth is allowed in any of the media.

Sterilization The act or process, physical or chemical, that destroys or eliminates all viable microbes including resistant bacterial spores from a fluid or a solid. Despite being stated as an absolute, the action of sterilization is usually stated in terms of probability. Examples of sterilization methods are: steam treatment at 121°C, dry heat at 450°F, flushing with a sterilizing solution such as Hydrogen Peroxide (H2O2) or ozone (O3), irradiation, and filtration.

Sterilizing filter A filter that, when challenged with the microorganisms Brevundimonas diminuta, at a minimum concentration of 107 organisms per square centimeter of filter surface, produces a sterile effluent.

Steroids Chemical substances that are related in structure and contain the same chemical skeleton. Steroids closely resemble a hormone called cortisol that is produced by your adrenal glands. Used to treat inflammatory diseases and conditions, steroids reduce the immune system's activity and decrease inflammation.

STI-571 (Glivec) Oral tyrosine kinase inhibitor - may well transform treatment of chronic myeloid leukaemia.

Stimulatory neurotransmitter A neurotransmitter that increases electro-chemical activity in the nerve cells. Norepinephrine is a stimulatory neurotransmitter.

Stochastic Involving a random variable; involving chance or probability.

Strain A population of cells all descended from a single cell.

Stratification clinical trials The department of health has been cautious in forwarding any policy on genotyping and clinical trial stratification, while at the same time trying to engage the industry in discussions on the subject.

Strength The concentration of the drug substance (for example, weight/weight, weight/volume, or unit dose/volume basis), and/or the potency, that is, the therapeutic activity of the drug product as indicated by appropriate laboratory tests or by adequately developed and controlled clinical data (expressed, for example, in terms of units by reference to a standard).

Streptomycin

Indications: Treatment of TB in combination with other agents.

Contraindications: Hypersensitivity to aminoglycoside antibiotics.

Dosage: 15 mg/kg IM qd.

Toxicity: Ototoxicity, vestibular toxicity.

Stroke A cerebrovascular event that affects the blood vessels that supply blood to the brain. A stroke occurs when a blood vessel that brings oxygen and nutrients to the brain bursts or is clogged by a blood clot. As a result, part of the brain doesn't get the blood and oxygen it needs, and nerve cells in the affected area of the brain die within minutes, thereby affecting whatever part of the body they control.

Structural testing (Bluhm, Meyers, Hetzel) Examining theinternal structure of the source code. Includes low-level andhigh-level code review, path analysis, auditing of programmingprocedures, and standards actually used, inspection for extraneous"dead code", boundary analysis and other techniques. Requires specific computer science and programming expertise.

Study arm Patients in clinical trials are assigned to one part or segment of a study 'arm'. Each arm receives a different treatment or dose.

Sub contractor Any organisation or individual used by a supplier toprovide material or services which are embodied in the product to be supplied.

Sub program A self contained program unit which forms part of aprogram. Sub-programs are sometimes referred to as procedures,subroutines or functions.

Subinvestigator Any individual member of the clinical trial team designated and supervised by the investigator at a trial site to perform critical trial-related procedures and/or to make important trial-related decisions (e.g., associates, residents, research fellows). (ICH)

Subject identification code A unique identifier assigned by the investigator to each trial subject to protect the subject's identity and used in lieu of the subject's name when the investigator reports adverse events and/or other trial-related data.

Subject People being studied as part of clinical trials or other investigation, including those serving as controls.

Subject/trial subject An individual who participates in a clinical trial, either as a recipient of the investigational product(s) or as a control.

Sublimation The process of vaporizing a solid substance by heat and then condensing it (without its having passed through a liquid state in either direction), a process of purification by separating the nonvaporizable impurities, a process analogous to the distillation of liquids.

Submerged arc welding (SAW) An arc welding process that produces coalescence of metals by heating them with an arc or arcs between a bare metal electrode or electrodes and the work. A blanket of granular, fusible material on the work shields the arc. Pressure is not used and filler metal is obtained from the electrode and sometimes from a supplemental source (welding rod, flux, or metal granules).

Substitutive or replacement therapy Treatment directed toward supplying a material normally present in the body, but absent in a specific patient because of disease, injury, congenital deficiencies, etc. Adrenocortical hormones used in the treatment of a patient with Addison's Disease are used as substitutive therapy.

Substrate A chemical species, the reaction of which with some other chemical reagent is under observation (e. g. a compound that is transformed under the influence of a catalyst). The term should be used with care.

mhment In metals, a rise in the carbon signal at depths from 15 to 20 angstroms (⊕). This indicates that organic material is buried in cracks, crevices, pits, or smeared material. Subsurface carbon is most commonly found in materials having rough morphology generally associated with machining processes.

Sulfadiazine Indications: Treatment of toxoplasmic encephalitis in combination with pyrimethamine.

Contraindications: Known hypersensitivity to sulfonamides.

Dosage: Initial therapy: 1-2 grams po qid x 6 weeks.

Maintenance therapy (secondary prophylaxis): 0.5-1 grams po qid.

Toxicity: Fever, rash, pruritus, bone marrow suppression.

Avoid use at term because of risk of kernicterus in newborn.

Sulfonamides The sulfa-related group of antibiotics, which are used to treat bacterial infection and some fungal infections.

Supernatant The material floating on the surface of a liquid mixture (often the liquid component that has the lowest density).

Superoxide dismutase (SOD) A zinc and copper or manganese containing enzyme which reacts with superoxide radicals to convert them to less dangerous chemical entities.

Superoxide radical A free radical thought to play a central role in arthritis and cataract formation.

Supersensitivity An extreme and high degree of sensitivity to a drug or chemical. Usually a high degree of sensitivity induced by some specific procedure such as denervation, administration of another drug, etc. Sensitivity to a drug, of some degree, is inherent in every organism; supersensitivity is a state that has had to be produced in the organism. In the supersensitive subject, the actions of the drug are qualitatively like those observed in a subject of normal sensitivity, and unlike those produced in a subject who is hypersensitive to the drug.

Supplier Any organisation or individual contracted directly by thecustomer to supply a product.

Supportive therapy Treatment directed toward maintaining the patient's physiological or functional integrity until more definitive treatment can be carried out, or until the patient's recuperative powers function to obviate the need for further treatment. Many drugs can provide supportive therapy; even in a single patient supportive therapy can be provided from agents of such different classes as sedatives, diuretics, anti-hypertensives, etc.

Surface finishes This term shall apply to all interior surface finishes accessible and inaccessible, that directly or indirectly come in contact with the designated product in bioprocessing equipment and distribution system components (ASME BPEa-2000). Final criteria shall be determined by Ra values rather than polishing methods.

Surface iron oxide layer Surface iron oxide layer present when the 316L stainless steel's iron composition signal is higher than its chromium signal at the surface.

Surface residual A foreign substance that adheres to a surface by chemical reaction, adhesion, adsorption, or ionic bonding (for example, corrosion, rouging, and staining).

Surface texture The repetitive or random deviations of the nominal metal surface from the three-dimensional topography of the surface. Surface texture includes roughness, waviness, lay, and flaws.

Surface water Any water where the source is above ground such as rivers, lakes, and reservoirs. Surface waters are usually higher in suspended matter and organic material and lower in dissolved minerals than well water.

Surfactant Any substance that changes the nature of a surface, such as lowering the surface tension of water.

Surgery Treating diseases or other medical conditions by operating on a patient to remove or repair parts of the body.

Surgical Oncology Treating cancers by surgically removing tumors.

Surrogate marker A measurement of a drug's biological activity that substitutes for a clinical endpoint such as death or pain relief.

Survival The proportion of patients who survive for a given period of time.

Suspended solids Undissolved solids that can be removed by filtration. Determined by a filter paper before and after filtration of a water sample.

Suspension A specific category of pharmaceutical product that must be in a colloidal dispersion (suspension) for proper action. For example, Kaolin/Pectin works as an adsorbant because its high surface area in suspension.

Symbiosis The phenomenon of two entities performing a joint function that neither entity can perform alone.

Synapse The gap between nerve cells.

Synergies When compounds are combined and their effects are more than the sum of their individual effects; the compounds are said to have positive synergy. Many of the nootropic compounds have positive synergy effects with each other, they become synergistic.

Synergy A mutually reinforcing drug interaction such that the joint effect of two drugs administered simultaneously is greater than the sum of their individual effects. Synergism is distinguished from additivity, in which the joint effect of two drugs is equal to the sum of their individual effects. If the joint effect is less than the sum of the two drugs' independent effects, the interaction is said to be antagonistic.

Synthesis The production of a substance by the union of chemical elements, groups, or simpler compounds or by the degradation of a complex compound.

Synthetic drugs Are artificially produced substances for the illicit market which are almost wholly manufactured from chemical compounds in illicit laboratories (amphetamine, benzodiazepines).

System An assembly of units consisting of one or more microprocessors, associated hardware and all layers of system andapplication system.

System acceptance test specification Documented verification that theautomated system or subsystemperforms as defined in the Functional Specification throug houtrepresentative or anticipated operating ranges.

System software (ANSI/IEEE) Software designed for a specific computersystem or family of computer systems to facilitate the operation andmaintenance of the computer system and associated programs, forexample, operating systems, compilers, utilities.

System specifications (PMA CSVC proposed) Describes how the systemwill meet the functional requirements.Tester: A person performing the test.

System suitability tests Tests intended to determine whether a 'system' including instruments, analysts, etc., is capable of performing a particular process, test or assay.

Systemic Throughout the entire body.

Systems pharmacology Bioinformatics and genomic approaches are suggesting new targets for study. Hypotheses generated by in vitro studies or by computational biology and systems approaches to the integrative behavior of living systems need to be tested in the actual living organism. The ability to develop genetically modified organisms has outstripped the ability to characterize the phenotypic changes in these organisms. Interest is growing in behavioral and neurobiological phenomena that can only be studied in relatively intact systems and living organisms. Discoveries in the areas of chemistry, genomics, and pharmacogenetics have accelerated the rate of research and have increased the demand for integrative and organ systems pharmacologists in the pharmaceutical industry. Pharmacologists, experienced with in vivo models, form an integral part of every drug discovery and development project and are essential to assuring that only safe and efficacious lead compounds go forward to clinical trials.

Systems toxicology Environmental toxicants can be mutagenic, teratogenic, recombinogenic, clastogenic and carcinogenic, and such toxicants are present in both our endogenous and exogenous environments. The research groups affiliated with this broad based project, entitled Systems Toxicology, are exploring mechanisms by which toxicants disrupt biological systems and, perhaps more importantly, exploring how various cells, tissues and animals ameliorate the potentially devastating consequences of toxicant exposure. The response of a wide variety of model organisms to a limited number of model toxicants is under study, and systematic experiments are carried out at the molecular, cellular, tissue and whole animal (mouse) level.

T

T or τ A point in time or a time interval; frequently a time interval following administration of a drug or the time interval between doses of a drug. The definition of a specific T or τ may be explicit or may be inferred from the context in which it is found. Specific times of interest may be indicated by subscripts, e.g., T0 is the time of drug administration; Tn is the time of administration of the nth dose in a series.

T test A statistical test used to compare the means of two groups of test data.

T½ The "half-life" of a drug; the amount of time required for the concentration of a drug in, e.g., a body fluid such as plasma, serum, or blood, to be halved. The idea of half-life is legitimately applied only to the case of a drug eliminated from body fluid according to the laws of first-order reaction kinetics. t½ = 0.301/b = 0.693/kel, where 0.301 and 0.693 are the logarithms of 2 to the bases 10 and e, respectively.

Tachyphylaxis A decline in the response to repeated applications of agonist, typically occurring over a relatively short time scale (seconds to hours).

Tamoxifen Highly active anti-oestrogen drug effective for breast cancer.

Tangential flow filtration A separation method that transfers components of one system (stream) into another. The stream the product is being extracted from crosses the stream that the product is being transferred to, multiple times.

Target haplotype Pharmacogenomics can reduce risk when used toward identifying the haplotypes of a target gene. For example. there are some beta agonists that have differential effects on haplotypes of the beta-1 receptor. In fact, some have absolutely no effect on at least one haplotype of the receptor. Uncovering such differences can reveal the degree to which a candidate compound will vary in its efficacy, and will help identify sub- populations that may benefit from the drug and others which may not benefit... In the few cases where a haplotype effect has been demonstrated, the discovery was accidental, occurring after the development of the drug.

Target The molecule that a substance or a drug binds to (often targets are proteins).

Target validation Evaluation of a gene's specific function in the disease process.

Taxol Semi-natural chemotherapy drug, initially synthesised from the yew tree. One of the taxane group.

Taxonomy The development of approaches to organize and summarize our knowledge about the variety or organisms that exist.

Taxotere Important taxane agent used to treat several types of cancer.

Tay sachs disease An inherited disease of infancy characterized by profound mental retardation and early death; it is caused by a recessive gene mutation.

T cell (T-lymphocyte) A blood cell, probably originating from bone marrow, but which matures in the thymus. Some T-cells are responsible for cell-mediated immunity and in the production of antibodies.

Telomere The end of a chromosome. This specialized structure is involved in the replication and stability of linear DNA molecules.

Team biologics A partnership between department of health's Office of Regulatory Affairs (ORA) and CBER to focus on inspectional and compliance issues in biologics. Its goal is to ensure the quality and safety of biologic products and resolve inconsistencies.

Temperature A specific degree of heat intensity. There are three temperature designations associated with psychrometrics: 1. Dry Bulb (DB) - The air temperature as measured by a standard thermometer.

2. Wet Bulb (WB) - The air temperature measured by a thermometer with its reservoir bulb wrapped in a moistened cloth wick and exposed to an air stream moving at a velocity of 1,000 feet per minute.

3. Dewpoint temperature (DP) - Also called Saturation Temperature is the temperature at which condensation of moisture begins (air is holding 100% of the moisture it can) when the air is cooled, measured in °F.

Tenofovir Indications: Treatment of HIV infection in combination with other agents. Tenofovir is a nucleotide agent.

Contraindications: Known hypersensitivity.

Dosage: 300 mg po qd.

Toxicity: Gastrointestinal intolerance.

Terminal sterilization The process applied to product sealed in its final container that transforms a non-sterile product into a sterile one.

Terminally Ill For an individual, it means that the subject has a life expectancy of six months or less as stated in writing by his or her attending physician and surgeon.

Test procedure A sequence of activities which when executed successfully provides documentary evidence that part of the system works as specified.

Testing Structural & Functional: Both forms of testing areessential. Neither form of testing can be exhaustive. Structuraltesting should occur chiefly during software development.Test procedure: A procedure which when executed successfully providesdocumentary evidence that part of the automated system works asspecified.

Testing (IEEE) The process of exercising or evaluating a system orsystem component by manual or automated means to verify that itsatisfies specified requirements or to identify differences betweenexpected and actual results. .

Testosterone A "male hormone" — a sex hormone produced by the testes that encourages the development of male sexual characteristics, stimulates the activity of the male secondary sex characteristics, and prevents changes in them following castration. Chemically, testosterone is 17-beta-hydroxy-4-androstene-3-one.

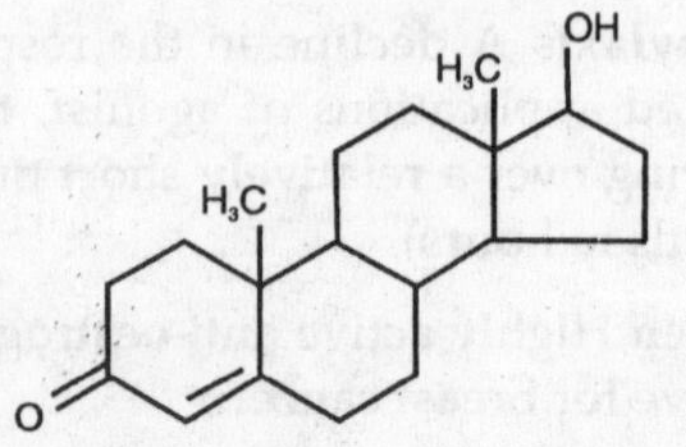

OH
H_3C
H_3C
O

Tetrodotoxin (TTX) A potent neurotoxin from the Japanese puffer fish. It binds to the sodium channel, blocking the passage of action potentials.

TG Trigeminal Ganglion.

Thalidomide (Thalomid) Indications: Treatment of refractory aphthous ulcers; treatment of refractory AIDS wasting syndrome.

Contraindications: Known hypersensitivity, pregnancy.

Dosage: 50-200 mg po qd. Physicians and pharmacists must be registered in the STEPS program (System for Thalidomide Education and Prescribing Safety at 1-888-4-Celgene) to prescribe thalidomide. Female patients must have a negative pregnancy test within 24 hours of starting therapy, weekly pregnancy tests in the first month of therapy, monthly pregnancy tests thereafter, and agree to use two forms of contraception. Male patients must use a condom for contraception.

Toxicity: Peripheral neuropathy, drowsiness, orthostatic hypotension, fever, rash, neutropenia.

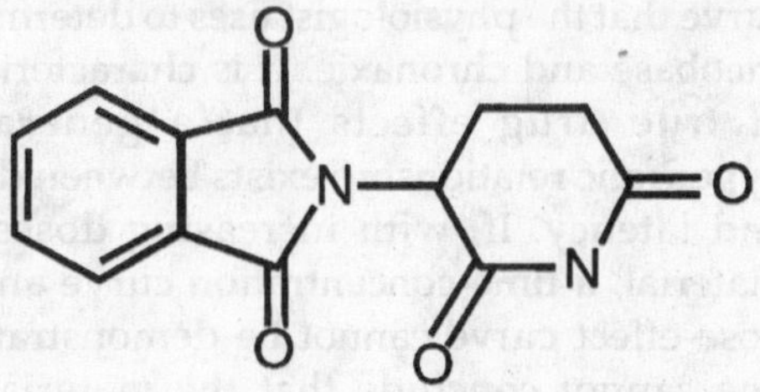

Thalidomide After a disastrous start, this drug is now finding a useful role, e.g. for drug-resistant myeloma.

Theophylline Theophylline is a bronchodilator drug, given by mouth, that widens the airways to the lung. It also is used to prevent attacks of apnea (cessation of breathing) in premature infants and to treat heart failure because it stimulates heart rate and increases urine excretion.

Theoretical yield The quantity that would be produced at any appropriate phase of manufacture, processing, or packing of a particular drug product, based upon the quantity of components to be used, in the absence of any loss or error in actual production.

Therapeutic A pharmaceutical product targeted to treat a specific disease.

Therapeutic equivalency The relative equivalency in the efficacy of different modes of treatment of a disease, most often used to compare the efficacy of different pharmaceuticals to treat a given disease.

Therapeutic index A number, LD50/ED50, which is a measure of the approximate "safety factor" for a drug; a drug with a high index can presumably be administered with greater safety than one with a low index. The therapeutic index is ordinarily calculated from data obtained from experiments with animals. As in comparing ED50s from two different drugs, the comparison of the LD50 and ED50 (therapeutic index) is most meaningful when the dose-effect curves from which the ED50 and LD50 are inferred are parallel.

The therapeutic index is a measure of drug selectivity, and analogous index numbers are frequently computed to measure selectivity that does not involve lethal effects. For example, to measure the selectivity of a drug potentially useful in the treatment of epilepsy, the ED50 for producing ataxia in mice might be compared to the ED50 for abolishing electrically-induced convulsions in mice.

Therapeutic protein A complex organic compound, composed of one or more chains of amino acids, that has been found to have a curative effect.

Therapeutics The science and techniques of restoring patients to health. Properly, therapeutics has many branches, any or all of which may be needed in the treatment of a specific patient. In addition to pharmacotherapeutics or drug therapy, there exist coordinate fields of therapeutics such as surgical therapy, psychotherapy, physical therapy, occupational therapy, dietotherapy, etc. Drugs are commonly considered capable of participating in one or more of the following general kinds of therapy.

Thermophile An organism that grows best at greater than 50ºC (122ºF).

Thermophilic (of a microorganism) With optimum temperature for growth above 45ºC, many thermophilic bacteria exist at high temperatures (greater than 80ºC) and many of their enzymes which posses high thermal stability, are of great commercial interest.

Threshold dose A dose of drug just sufficient to produce a pre-selected effect. Frequently, and improperly, restricted to the dose just sufficient to produce a minimal detectable effect. In fact, an LD50 is a threshold dose if the pre-selected effect is "death in 50% of a population".

Thrombin (blood coagulation factor II) An enzyme (the activated thrombogen) formed in the blood, after this is shed, that converts fibrinogen into fibrin for clot formation. It is formed from conjunction of prothrombin and calcium salts. It is also a sterile protein substance prepared from prothrombin of bovine origin through interaction with thromboplastin in the presence of calcium. Bovine thrombin is often used to aid production of serum from "salvage" plasma.

Thrombolytics Thrombolytics are drugs that dissolve blood clots, such as TPA (tissue plasminogen activator.

Thrombosis Clotting within a blood vessel that may cause infarction of tissues supplied by the vessel.

Throughput volume The amount of solution passed through an exchange bed before the resin is exhausted.

A pyrimidine component of nucleic acid first isolated from the thymus.

Thymus The master gland of the immune system located behind the breastbone.

Thyroid The gland located in the center of the brain responsible (amongst other things) for temperature regulation.

Time concentration curve The graphical representation of the relationship - for a given drug and a given biological system - between concentration (or dose) and latency or latent period: the period of time elapsing between the time the dose is administered and the time a given effect is produced. Time-concentration curves tend to be hyperbolic in form: as dose increases latency decreases and vice versa. Latency is an inverse function of concentration. But the hyperbolic relationship never approaches the axes as asymptotes; there is always a concentration below which the drug is ineffective, regardless of the duration of exposure of the tissue to the drug, and there is always a finite interval between the time of exposure to the drug and the time the response occurs. The time-concentration curve is analogous to the strength-duration curve that the physiologist uses to determine rheobase and chronaxie. It is characteristic of true drug effects that a generally hyperbolic relationship exists between dose and latency. If, with increasing doses of material, a time-concentration curve and a dose-effect curve cannot be demonstrated, one cannot conclude that the material is responsible for the effects observed.

Time stamp A part of the audit trail that clearly documents the sequence of events in human terms, helping to authenticate an electronic signature and minimizing the chances of signer repudiation. A local time stamp correlates with the whereabouts of the signer. With client-server data systems used by international companies and records accessed from remote sites (such as on business trips), time stamps that reflect the local time of only the user might make the sequence of actions for an individual record appear inconsistent. For example, the approval by a peer reviewer could be signed at 9:00 a.m. on a chromatographic analysis that was performed at 11:00 a.m. in a different time zone. Local time stamps should probably be supplemented consistently with the time stamp of a remote server, with one stamp clearly labeled as local.

Time to progression The length of time from the first day of randomization into a clinical trial, until the date progression of the disease is first noted.

Time concentration curve The graphical representation of the relationship - for a given drug and a given biological system - between concentration (or dose) and latency or latent period: the period of time elapsing between the time the dose is administered and the time a given effect is produced. Time-concentration curves tend to be hyperbolic in form: as dose increases latency decreases and vice versa. Latency is an inverse function of concentration. But the hyperbolic relationship never approaches the axes as asymptotes; there is always a concentration below which the drug is ineffective, regardless of the duration of exposure of the tissue to the drug, and there is always a finite interval between the time of exposure to the drug and the time the response occurs. The time-concentration curve is analogous to the strength-duration curve that the physiologist uses to determine rheobase and chronaxie. It is characteristic of true drug effects that a generally hyperbolic relationship exists between dose and latency. If, with increasing doses of material, a time-concentration curve and a dose-effect curve cannot be demonstrated, one cannot conclude that the material is responsible for the effects observed.

Tincture of Iodine A germicidal solution of iodine in aqueous alcohol used primarily as antiseptic on skin and tissue.

Tissue culture Growing mammalian cells in the laboratory in a tissue culture medium (in vitro). For example, this allows researchers to determine the effects of various chemicals on mammalian cells without experimenting directly on live animals or man. Since a molecule of some toxic substances can harm a single mammalian cell, even one part-per-billion of some impurities can affect a tissue culture. Therefore, water used to make up tissue culture media should be extremely pure.

Tissue specific A gene is expressed only in specific tissues of the human body.

Titer A measured sample - the strength of a solution or the concentration of a substance (as an antibody) in solution as determined by titration.

Titration Volumetric analysis by means of the addition of definite amounts of a test solution to a solution of a known amount of the substance analyzed.

TNT (Tumor necrosis therapy) Therapeutic agents that target dead and dying cells found primarily at the core of the tumor.

Tocolytic therapy This therapy works to prevent premature labor by halting contractions and slowing down the birth process.

Toe of weld The junction between the face of a weld and the base material.

Tolerability Describes how much drug is required to elicit an unwanted adverse effect. The toxic response can be expressed as the dose of drug that gives 50% of the maximal toxic effect (i.e., TD50).

Tolerance A condition characterized by a reduced effect of a drug upon repeated administration. In some cases, it may be necessary to increase the dose of the drug to attain the same effect, or the original level of effect may be unattainable. Tolerance typically develops over days to weeks, and is distinguished from tachyphylaxis, a more rapid decline in the effect of a drug. Tolerance can result from multiple mechanisms, including changes in drug metabolism and alteration in the number or responsiveness of receptors . "Tolerance" should not be used to mean "lack of sensitivity" manifested toward a single dose of a drug. A non-habitual drinker who is unaffected by several drinks of whisky downed in rapid succession is probably insensitive to alcohol rather than tolerant to its effects.

Tolerance specification for a formulation A formulation vehicle is usually a mixture of various excipients differing in density and viscosity. The total volume of the final formulation can deviate from the sum of the volumes of the individual excipients, in which case the final concentration of each excipient will deviate from its expected concentration to the same degree. Our tolerance specification for formulations is ± 10%.

Tolerance Tachyphylaxis Continual use of an agent can result in diminished response. In some cases this can appear in mins-hrs or dose to dose and is termed tachyphylaxis (ie. amphetamines). In other cases it appears more gradual over days-months and is termed tolerance. (ie. opioids).

Ton of refrigeration A unit used to indicate the size of a refrigeration unit. One ton of refrigeration effect is equivalent to removing 12,000 Btu/hr of heat, or melting one ton of ice in a 24-hour period.

Tone (Autonomic) Under resting conditions most organs of the body receive a low but steady release of NA or Ach (tonic release) to modulate tissue activity. In the heart the basal release of NA contributes about +5 bpm and the release of Ach about -10 bpm to the resting heart rate. This is why beta-blockers such as propranolol can cause a fall in HR as they prevent the action of the tonic release of NA. Likewise the muscarinic antagonists, such as atropine can cause an increase in HR as it prevents the action of Ach. Usually one division of the autonomic NS dominates under resting conditions, GI-tract, eye, heart (parasympathetic) and vasculature (sympathetic).

Topical Pertaining to a particular surface area. A topical agent is applied to a certain area of the skin and is intended to affect only the area to which it is applied. Whether its effects are indeed limited to that area depends upon whether the agent stays where it is put or is absorbed into the blood stream.

Topical drug A drug designed for local surface application to or action on a body part.

Topical product A pharmaceutical product meant to be applied to the skin or soft tissue in the form of liquid, cream, or ointment, and therefore needs not be aseptic. Sterile ophthalmic products throughout are manufactured aseptically.

Total bacteria count An estimation of the total number of bacteria in a sample based usually on Standard Methods procedures for collecting, incubating, and counting colony-forming units (cfu).

Total Dissolved Solids (TDS) The term used to describe inorganic ions in the water. Usually measured by electrical conductance of the water corrected to 25°C, and expressed as ppm (parts per million).

Total bilirubin The level of pigment in the blood. Elevations can be associated with liver disease or breakdown or red blood cells. Slight increases are sometimes seen without significance. Some people normally have isolated elevations of bilirubin called Gilbert's disease.

Total heat (TH) The sum of sensible heat and latent heat.

Total ionized solids Concentration of dissolved ions in solution expressed in concentration units of Sodium Chloride (NaCl). It determines the operating life of ion exchange resins and is calculated from measurements of Specific Resistance.

Total organic carbon (TOC) A measure of the level of organic impurities in water by their carbon content that determines the operating life of activated carbon beds. This is one of the parameters used to determine the purity of Semiconductor Grade water. Feed water will have TOC measured in ppm (parts per million), and ultrapure water (UPW) will have TOC measured in ppb (parts per billion).

Total parenteral nutrition (TPN) Administration of supplemental nutrition intravenously (through the veins) for patients who are unable to digest or absorb food.

Total protein This is a combination of albumin and globulin, which are proteins. Abnormal values occur in liver disease and poor nutrition.

Total solids Total solids in water include both dissolved and suspended solids. Determined by weighing sample before and after evaporation.

Toxic Poisonous, everything, including water and oxygen is toxic in sufficiently high doses.

Tox chips Developed at NIEHS [National Institute for Environmental Health Sciences, US], which contains copies, or clones, of about 2,000 of the 80,000 genes in the human body. Millions of cloned copies of each gene form a nearly invisible dot that is "arrayed" - hence the name - in a grid pattern on the glass slide.

Toxic effects Responses to drug that are harmful to the health or life of the individual. Almost by definition, toxic effects are "side effects" when diagnosis, prevention, or treatment of disease is the goal of drug administration. Toxic effects are not side-effects in the case of pesticides and chemical warfare agents. Toxic effects may be idiosyncratic or allergic in nature, may be pharmacologic side effects, or may be an extension of therapeutic effect produced by overdosage. An example of the last of these is the apnea produced by an anesthetic agent.

Toxicity The degree to which something causes poisonous effects. It refers to the extent to which a drug adversely affects cancer cells as well as healthy tissue. Toxicity is the dose-limiting factor in the administration of most chemotherapeutic agents.

Toxicogenomics An approach to toxicology measuring how people's genomes respond to environmental stressors or toxicants. Combines genome-wide gene expression profiling with protein expression patterns using bioinformatics to understand the role of gene-environment interactions in disease, understand how chemicals affect the expression of genes, characterize normal genetic and metabolic pathways, and learn how disease occurs when these pathways malfunction.

Toxicokinetics Process of the uptake of potentially toxic substances by the body, the biotransformation they undergo, the distribution of the substances and their metabolites in the tissues, and the elimination of the substances and their metabolites from the body. Both the amounts and the concentrations of the substances are studied. The term has essentially the same meaning as pharmacokinetics, but the latter term should be restricted to the study of pharmaceutical substances.

Toxicology Can be described, according to a U.S. National Library of Medicine online tutorial, as "the study of the adverse effects of chemicals or physical agents on living organisms." Such effects run the gamut from immediate death to subtle effects that manifest only months or years after exposure. Toxic substances may affect various levels of the body, such as a particular organ, cell type, or biomolecule.

Toxicoproteomics Toxicoproteomics is the use of global protein expression technologies to better understand environmental and genetic factors, both in episodes of acute exposure to toxicants and in the long-term development of disease. Integrating transcript, protein, and toxicology data is a major objective of the field of toxicogenomics.

Toxigenomics A compendium of gene expression data enhanced by complete proteomic analysis will enable investigators to probe the complexities of the mechanisms of normal genetic and metabolic pathways, and subsequently, to learn how disease occurs when these pathways malfunction. When combined with information on gene/ protein groups, functional pathways and networks, and human genetic polymorphisms, these data will confer new knowledge of gene-environment interactions and human health risks.

Toxin A substance produced by microorganisms that can inhibit cell growth in tissue culture and may cause temperature rise in animals.

Toxoid An antigenic toxin. Example is tetanus toxoid that is a bacterial vaccine.

TPA (Tissue plasminogen activator) A recombinant drug used in the management of heart attacks to prevent clotting. Produced by Genentech and one of the first successful recombinant DNA drugs to be commercialized.

Trace analysis Analyzing constituents present in ppm and ppb concentrations. Trace analysis requires extremely pure reagents, made with ultrapure Type I reagent grade water.

Traceability A prerequisite for trustworthy records, apart from data security. Traceability is the part of the laboratory data system audit trail that holds the evidence of who did what to a record and when.

Tracer A radioactively labeled nucleic acid component included in a reassociation reaction in amounts too small to influence the progress of reaction.

Tranquilizers Drugs used to treat excessive nervousness and restlessness, having a tranquilizing effect.

Transcription The process by which the genetic information encoded in the gene, represented as a linear sequence of deoxyribonucleotides (DNA), is copied into an exactly complementary sequence of ribonucleotides known as mRNA (messenger RNA).

Transcriptomics In the context of toxicology studies, involves assessing changes in transcription initiation, processing, and degradation after chemical exposure using glass and membrane DNA microarrays and low- output tools, such as ribonuclease protection assays and real-time PCR.

Transduction The transfer of genetic material from one cell to another by means of a viral vector (for bacteria, the vector is Bacteriophage).

Transfection The acquisition of new genetic markers by addition of viral DNA to cells.

Transfer panel A panel to which process and utilities are piped, allowing cross connections between different use points. A jumper spool is used to connect the desired process/utility users and mechanically preclude erroneous connections to other lines.

Transfer RNA (tRNA) A class of RNA having structures with triplet nucleotide sequences that are complementary to the triplet nucleotide coding sequences of mRNA. The role of tRNAs in protein synthesis is to bond with amino acids and transfer them to the ribosomes, where proteins are assembled according to the genetic code carried by mRNA.

Transfer systems Equipment allowing the introduction and removal of material, toxic and/or sterile, with continuous protection to both operator and product.

Transformation A process by which the genetic material carried by an individual cell is altered by incorporation of exogenous DNA into its genome.

Transgene DNA integrated into the germ line of transgenic organisms.

Transgenic models Organisms, such as fruit flies or mice, which carry an extra gene - one that has been over-expressed, providing clues as to the gene's relation to organ development, viability and reproduction.

Transgenics The alteration of a plant or animal's DNA such that it contains a gene from another organism. There are two types of cells in animal and plants, germ line cells (the sperm and egg in animals, pollen and ovule in plants) and somatic cells (all other cells). Transgenic animals have alterations in their germ line DNA so the alterations are passed on to the offspring. That is done to produce therapeutics, to study disease, and to improve farm animals. Transgenic plants have been created for increased resistance to disease and insects as well as to make biopharmaceuticals.

Translation The process in which the genetic code carried by mRNA directs the synthesis of proteins from amino acids.

Transparency Being transparent means making policies and practices open and understandable to customers and members, showing clarity around revenue streams and integrity on intended commitments.

Treatment investigational new drug An Investigational New Drug that makes a promising new drug available to desperately ill patients as early in the drug development process as available. department of health permits the drug to be used if there is preliminary evidence of efficacy and it treats a serious or life-threatening disease, or if there is not comparable therapy available.

Trial Site The location(s) where trial-related activities are actually conducted.

Triglycerides A blood fat related to calories and starch (sweets) in the diet. High levels can impair circulation and lead to hardening of the arteries. Alcohol also will increase the value. Fast overnight test for accurate test results.

Trihalomethanes Compounds present in the feed water that are formed by the reaction of Chlorine and the organic material in the water. Activated carbon and degasification can reduce THMs.

Trimethoprim sulfamethoxazole (TMP SMX, bactrim, septra)

Indications: Treatment and prophylaxis of PCP; primary prophylaxis of toxoplasmosis.

Contraindications: Known hypersensitivity to trimethoprim or sulfonamides, megaloblastic anemia.

Dosage: Treatment of PCP: 5 mg/kg po/IV q8h of trimethoprim component (equivalent to 2 tabs po tid of DS for 65 kg patient) x three weeks.

Prophylaxis of PCP: one DS or SS tablet po qd. Prophylaxis of toxoplasmosis: one DS tablet po qd.

Toxicity: Side effects are common in HIV-infected patients and include gastrointestinal intolerance; rash, urticaria, photosensitivity, Stevens-Johnson syndrome; fever; leukopenia, thrombocytopenia, hemolytic anemia; abnormal liver function tests; renal dysfunction, interstitial nephritis; aseptic meningitis.

Patients with history of mild to moderate drug toxicity should be given retrial of TMP-

SMX or desensitized using an established protocol.

avoid use at term because of risk of kernicterus in newborn.

Triple blind study A study in which knowledge of the treatment is concealed from the people who organize and analyze the data of a study as well as from subjects and investigators.

Trombolytics Drugs used to "dissolve" thrombus.

TRPV Transient Receptor Potential ion channels of the Vanilloid type.

Tryptamines Tryptamines are naturally occurring alkaloids found in a variety of plants and life forms around the world. There exist more than 1500 natural varieties. The basic element of tryptamine is the indol-structure. .

Tryptamines can be also produced either completely synthetically or semi-synthetically. A great number of derivatives are possible and a lot of them are already known .

Tryptamine itself is an endogenous amine found in the human brain. .

Serotonin and Melatonin are two other essential tryptamines present in the human body. They both have the same function as neurotransmitters as the dopamine.

TS Test solution (defined in USP/NF for a particular test)

TTX Tetrodotoxin.

Tube size Tube is sized by its nominal outside diameter. For bioprocessing equipment, tube does not include pipe.

Tumor An abnormal growth of cells. Also defined as a circumscribed growth, not inflammatory in character, arising from preexisting tissue, but independent of the normal rate or laws of growth of such tissue, and subserving no physiological function.

Tumor pathogenesis Morphological and physiological changes associated with tumor growth.

Tumor suppressor genes Genes that normally restrain cell growth but, when missing or inactivated by mutation, allow cells to grow uncontrolled.

Turbidity A suspension of fine particles that obscures light rays but requires many days for sedimentation because of small particle size.

Turnover It is a formal transfer of custody for a system or unit to another group, department, or operating company.

Turnover package (TOP) A collection of pertinent design, construction, vendor, and operational documentation. This collection of documentation is used for the qualification and process validation activity, as well as reference and single source information for the life of any particular system, process, or piece of equipment.

Two bed deionizer Separate beds or layers of cation and anion exchange resins. Results in lower purity than mixed-bed deionization, but provides higher capacity in terms of throughput.

Two state model A simplified model of receptor activation by agonists. The receptor is hypothesized to be in conformational equilibrium between an inactive conformation R and an active conformation R*, with the equilibrium in the absence of agonist normally favoring the inactive state. Agonists bind preferentially (i.e. with greater affinity) to the active state, and by mass action shift the conformational equilibrium such that a greater proportion of receptors are in the active R* conformation. Inverse agonists shift the conformational equilibrium such that a greater proportion of receptors are in the inactive R* conformation.

Type 1 (or Type I) error Error made when a null hypothesis is rejected but is actually true. Also called false positive. (statistics)

Type 2 (or Type II) error Error made when an alternative hypothesis is rejected when it is actually true. Also called false negative. (statistics)

Type 3 (or Type III) error Some statisticians use this designation for an error made when calling the less effective treatment the more effective one. (statistics)

Tyramine MAOIs interaction: certain foods (ie. aged cheese, red wine, figs, fermented and otherwise processed meats, fish and soy products) contain large amounts of the amino acid tyramine which can interact with MAOIs to dramatically raise HP and HR. The tyramine induces the release of large amounts of the stored neurotransmitter, NA from the nerve terminals.

The reaction, which often does not appear for several hours after taking the medication, may also include headache, nausea, vomiting, possible confusion, psychotic symptoms, seizures, stroke and coma.

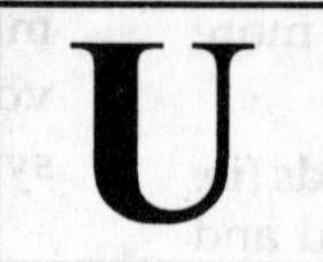

U.S.P. (United states pharmacopeia) A compendium of testing and purity criteria for pharmaceuticals, ancillaries, and raw materials.

Ulcer healing drugs Drugs used mainly in the treatment of gastric and duodenal ulcers.

Ultra low penetration air filters (ULPA) Extended media dry filters in a rigid frame that have a minimum particle-collection efficiency of 99.999% for particles greater than or equal to 0.12μm in size. Most commonly used in microelectronics, few uses in pharmaceuticals.

Ultracentrifugation The separation of macromolecules on the basis of their density and shape using the gravitational field generated in a high-speed centrifuge. It is used in rDNA work for the separation of RNA and DNA, and for purification of plasmids.

Ultrafiltration Molecular sieves; membranes with pores small enough to remove large molecules. Rated in terms of nominal molecular weight cutoff. A 10,000 Dalton (molecular weight) UF membrane, for example, will remove bacterial pyrogens that are typically in the range of 20,000 Daltons.

Ultrafine particle Particle with an equivalent diameter less than 0,1μm. ISO 14644-1.

Ultrapure water Water with a specific resistance higher than 1 megohm-cm. In the laboratory, it usually refers to Type I reagent grade water. Anything in laboratory water that is not H2O is an impurity. Although chemically pure water is not attainable, ultrapure water systems are now capable of reducing impurities down to the limits of detection.

Ultraviolet oxidation Ultraviolet radiation is employed in water purification for the photochemical oxidation of organic impurities resulting in HPLC grade water with organic impurity levels below 0.0005 absorbance units.

Ultraviolet radiation Light in the wavelength region 200-300 nm, used to detect RNA or DNA that has the fluorescent dye, ethidium bromide, bound to it.

Ultraviolet sterilizer Ultraviolet lamps used to kill microorganisms in water.

Ultraviolet TOC reduction An ultraviolet source, which partially oxidizes organic compounds to ionic species that can be removed. It relies on 185 nm (nanometer) radiation from "ozone producing" mercury lamps (along with 254nm germicidal radiation). Generally has a longer contact time than sterilization alone.

Unequal randomization A technique used to allocate subjects into groups at a differential rate; for example, three subjects may be assigned to a treatment group for every one assigned to the control group.

Unexpected Adverse Drug Reaction An adverse reaction, the nature or severity of which is not consistent with the applicable product information (e.g., Investigator's Brochure for an unapproved investigational product or package insert/summary of product characteristics for an approved product) .

Unicellular Composed of only a single cell.

Unidirectional airflow Previously referred as "laminar" airflow, is the "rectified airflow through the entire cross section of a clean zone with a steady velocity and approximately parallel streamlines. This type of airflow results in a directed transport of particles from the clean zone". ISO 14644-4.

Uniform building code (UBC) The most widely adopted model building code in the United States is a performance based document meeting the needs of government units charged with the enforcement of building regulations.

Uniform fire code The premier model fire code in the United States sets forth provisions necessary for fire prevention and fire protection. Published by the International Fire Code Institute (IFCI) and endorsed by the Western Fire Chiefs Association, the International Association of Fire Chiefs, and the International Conference of Building Officials (ICBO), it contains code provisions compatible with the Uniform Building Code, and standards referenced from the code provisions.

Uniform mechanical code A document that provides a complete set of requirements for the design, construction, installation, and maintenance of heating, ventilating, cooling and refrigeration systems; incinerators and other heat-producing appliances.

Uniform resource locator (URL) Address of a Web page—actmagazine.com, for example.

Uniform zoning code A code dedicated to intelligent community development and to the benefit of the public welfare by providing a means of promoting uniformity in zoning laws and enforcement.

Unit Dose Defines an SVP that must be administered in one dose. Unused contents must be discarded.

United states pharmacopoeia (U.S.P.) The United States Pharmacopoeia is a reference volume, published every five years by the U.S. Pharmacopoeial Convention, which describes and defines approved therapeutic agents, as well as sets standards for purity, assay, etc. Agents are included on the basis of their therapeutic value. The U.S.P. is recognized by the F.D.A. as the official standard for the agents described therein.

The purposes of the Pharmacopoeia, as described in the Preface to the first edition in 1820 by Dr. Jacob Bigelow, are to

Select the best, established drugs (those "the utility of which is most fully established and best understood").

Set standards of pharmaceutical quality for them (" form from them preparations and compositions in which their powers may be exerted to the greatest advantage ").

Name them ("distinguish those articles by convenient and definite names, such as may prevent trouble or uncertainty in the intercourse of physicians and apothecaries").

Encourage their use ("the value of a Pharmacopoeia depends upon the fidelity with which it conforms to the best state of medical knowledge of the day. Its usefulness depends upon the sanction it receives from the medical community and the public; and the extent to which it governs the language and practice of those for whose use it is intended:).

Universal precautions Precautions taken when handling, storing, transporting, or shipping items or specimens containing, or contaminated with human blood and body fluids: all such materials are treated as infectious.

Unplanned (Emergency) Change (PMA CSVC) An unanticipated necessarychange to a validated system requiring rapid implementation.

Unsaturated fatty acid A fatty acid containing one or more double bonds.

Unstable (Reactive) material A material other than an explosive, which in the pure state or as commercially produced will vigorously polymerize, decompose, condense or become self-reactive and undergo other violent chemical changes, including explosion, when exposed to heat, friction or shock, or in the absence of an inhibitor or in the presence of contaminants or in contact with noncompatible materials. Unstable, reactive materials are subdivided as follows:

1. Class 4 - Materials that in themselves are readily capable of detonation or of explosive decomposition or explosive reaction at normal temperatures and pressures. This class includes materials that are sensitive to mechanical or localized thermal shock at normal temperatures and pressures.

2. Class 3 - Materials that in themselves, are capable of detonation or of explosive decomposition or explosive reaction but which require a strong initiating source or which must be heated under confinement before initiation. This class includes materials that are sensitive to thermal or mechanical shock at elevated temperatures and pressures.

3. Class 2 - Materials that in themselves are normally unstable and readily undergo violent chemical change but do not detonate. This class includes materials which can undergo chemical change with rapid release of energy at normal temperatures and pressures and which can undergo violent chemical change at elevated temperatures and pressures.

4. Class 1 - Materials that in themselves are normally stable but which can become unstable at elevated temperatures and pressures.

Upward compatibility Refers to software that runs not only on the computer for which it was designed, but also on newer and more powerful models. In the context, compatibility plays an important role in ensuring that legacy data can be moved (copied) accurately and completely to a new system. Without it, legacy systems would have to be maintained as long as the records contained in them are kept.

Uracil A pyrimidine base important as a component of ribonucleic acid (RNA). Uracil is capable of forming a base pair with adenine.

Uric acid A material, which, if in excess, can deposit stones in the kidney or in the joints and cause gout.

Urology Medical specialty dealing with changes and diseases of male and female urinary passages as well as the male sex organs.

Uroselectiv Concerning only the urological organs

URS User Requirements Specification.

Urticaria Urticaria is a skin condition, common known as hives, characterized by the development of itchy, raised white lumps surrounded by an area of red inflammation.

User The pharmaceutical customer or user organisation contracting asupplier to provide a product. In the context of this document it is,therefore, not intended to apply only to individuals who use thesystem, and is synonymous with Customer.

User interface Dials, knobs, operating system commands, graphical display formats, and other devices provided by a computer or a program to allow users to communicate and use the computer or program. A Graphical User Interface (GUI) provides its user with a "picture oriented" way to interact with technology.

Utility software (ANSI/IEEE) Computer programs or routines designed toperform some general support function required by other applicationsoftware, by the operating system, or by system users.

Utility systems Facility wide systems not tailored to a specific process and that do not have contact with the drug substance or potential drug substance.

Utilization review Process in which either an internal or external agency reviews patterns of utilization against norms or policies established by the organization or set by health plans.

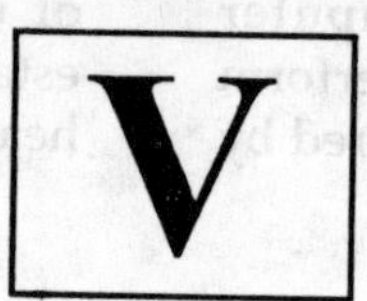

Vaccine A preparation of microbial antigens that provokes an immune response (i.e. the production of antibodies) on injection, thus conferring immunity on the recipient. There are three types of vaccines: 1. Those containing material from a nonvirulent organism that retains its immunogenicity but does not result in infection.

2. Those containing a modified toxin (a toxoid) that has lost its toxic properties but retain its immunogenicity.

3. Those containing live, attenuated organisms (i.e. genetic variants of a virus or bacterium) that are antigenically similar to the original strain but lack virulence.

Recombinant DNA research has allowed the production of new and more specific vaccines. For example, the gene for the B antigen of hepatitis virus has been cloned in E. coli, the protein expressed and a specific anti-B antiserum produced which can be used as a vaccine.

Vacuoles Membrane-bound organelles of low density responsible for food digestion, osmotic regulation, and waste product storage. Vacuoles may occupy a large fraction of cell volume (up to 90% in plant cells).

Vacuum degasification The process of removing dissolved and entrained gases from the Reverse Osmosis (RO) product water by creating a vacuum in a tower through which this water flows. The degasifier may be located before the RO system but the majority of the time will be located after. The most prevalent gas present is Carbon Dioxide (CO_2), which may have been generated during pH adjustment of the RO feed water. The anion exchange resin can remove CO_2 but using the vacuum degasifier can reduce that load. The other gas of concern is Oxygen, which can also be removed by a vacuum degasifier.

Valganciclovir (Valcyte) Indications: Treatment and prophylaxis of CMV infection.

Contraindications: Known hypersensitivity, neutropenia, thrombocytopenia.

Dosage: Initial therapy: 900 mg po bid.

Maintenance therapy (secondary prophylaxis): 900 mg po qd.

Toxicity: Neutropenia, thrombocytopenia, anemia, nausea, abdominal pain, headache, confusion.

Validate, validation Proof of relevance and/or correctness, for example the relevance of a gene for a disease.

Validated cell line In the context of ADME assays, a validated cell line is a cell line that has been demonstrated to produce the proper rank ordering of responses to compounds of known in vivo potency and/or efficacy.

Examples include the proper rank order of permeability compared to human fractional absorption in cultured intestinal epithelial cells and the proper rank order of potency for CYP induction in hepatocytes. The rank order reponses must be reproducible and rugged with respect to typical changes in assay conditions for the cell line to be considered validated.

Validated Means that a method (or instrument, process, etc.) has been tested and shown to do, reliably, what it is supposed to do. For analytical methods, the testing generally covers accuracy, precision, specificity, limit of detection, limit of quantitation, linearity and range, ruggedness, and robustness.

Validation Method validation is the process of establishing the performance characteristics and limitations of a method and the identification of the influences which may change these characteristics and to what extent. It includes accuracy, precision, specificity, sensitivity, reproducibility, stability, predetermined limits for acceptance of data based on QC standards, and extensive documentation. A related process is verification, the confirmation by examination and provision of objective evidence that specified requirements have been fulfilled. Assay parameter optimization is a separate process that precedes assay validation and/or may be iterative with it e.g., assay validation may identify parameters for which the assay should have been optimized; after further optimization, the assay would need to be re-validated.

Validation master plan The documented plan for qualification of a facility or part of a facility that identifies the layout of the operation, the associated utilities and systems, the equipment, and the processes to be validated. The validation master plan also provides preliminary information as to the extent of the qualification and validation (IQ, OQ, PQ), required documentation, SOPs, acceptance criteria and responsibilities. Validation Master Plans should also establish the cross reference of qualification projects by product, system, discipline, etc.

Validation of data Procedure carried out to ensure that the data contained in the final clinical trial report match original observations.

Validation plan A plan created by the customer to define validationactivities, responsibilities and procedures.

Validation protocol (from ICH API) A written plan stating how validation will be conducted and defining acceptance criteria. For example, the protocol for a manufacturing process identifies processing equipment, critical process parameters/operating ranges, product characteristics, sampling, and test data to be collected, number of validation runs, and acceptable test results.

Validation protocol A written plan describing the process to be validated, including production equipment and how validation will be conducted. Such a plan would address objective test parameters, product and process characteristics, predetermined specifications, and factors, which will determine acceptable results.

Validity The degree to which output reflects what it purports to reflect, i.e., input; the degree to which output is a function of known input and it alone. For example, does an essay examination validly measure a student's knowledge of material, or is it invalid, actually measuring his literary skill or the state of the grader's digestion?

Vapor pressure Dalton's Law for a mixture of perfect gases states that the mixture pressure is equal to the sum of the partial pressures of the constituents. The partial pressure of moisture is called vapor pressure, and is expressed as: Total Pressure (Pt) = Partial Pressure of Air (Pa) + Partial Pressure of Moisture (Pv).

Variance A measure of the variability in a sample or population. It is calculated as the mean squared deviation (msd) of the individual values from their common mean. In calculating the msd, the divisor n is commonly used for a population variance and the divisor n-1 for a sample variance.

Vascular targeting agents (VTAs) Multifunctional agents that are home to the capillaries and vessels of solid tumors.

Vasodilator drugs Drugs inducing vasodilation thus enabling greater blood flow; they are used to treat ischemic diseases, hypertension, heart failure, etc.

Vasodilators Vasodilators are drugs that open ("dilate") the arteries, lowering blood pressure; ACE inhibitors are one of the newest class of vasodilators.

Vasopressin Also known as antidiuretic hormone (ADH) or arginine vasopressin (AVP). ADH is secreted by the posterior pituitary and acts on the collecting ducts of the kidneys to cause them to reabsorb water, thereby concentrating the urine. ADH is also a vasoconstrictor. Its overall effect is to increase blood volume and raise blood pressure. Its secretion is stimulated by...

osmoreceptors in the CNS (low osmolarity causes secretion)

low blood pressure as sensed by the baroreceptors.

angiotensin II.

Vd The volume of distribution of a drug; the size of the "compartment" into which a drug apparently has been distributed following absorption. Computed as D/C0 for a one-compartment system, i.e. one yielding a single straight line when log C, or C, is plotted against time after drug administration. Using absolute dose to compute Vd yields Vd in units of volume, i.e. liters. Using relative dose (D/B) to compute Vd yields Vd in relative units, e.g. liters per kilogram, the volume of distribution as a fraction of body weight. When the plot of log C against t yields a biphasic relationship (a two compartment system), Vd is computed by a different method, such as one based on the area under the C vs. t curve.

VEAs (Vasopermeation enhancement agents) A new generation of drugs that increase the uptake of therapeutic agents to solid tumors.

Vegetative Form In bacteria, a stage of active growth, as opposed to a resting state or spore formation.

Vector An agent, such as an insect, that can carry a disease-producing organism from one host to another; the agent used to carry new genes into cells. Plasmids currently are the vectors of choice, though viruses and other bacteria may sometimes be used. These molecules become part of the cell protoplasm.

Vehicle The excipients or matrix, e.g., solvent, in which an active ingredient, e.g., a drug in a pharmaceutical preparation or test compound in research and development is prepared. Ideally, the vehicle should be inert in the context of the particular application, e.g., therapy or research of the active ingredient. In many cases, however, the vehicle in a research experiment may have an effect on the test system. Therefore, a properly controlled experiment includes a vehicle control so that the only difference between the control and test conditions is the absence or presence, respectively, of the test compound.

Venopharmaceuticals Drugs used to treat venous diseases, for example, so-called varices and sometimes also varicophlebitis or haemorrhoids; they are administered generally or locally.

Verification The act of reviewing, inspecting, testing, checking, auditing, or otherwise establishing and documenting whether items, processes, services, or documents conform to specified requirements.

Veterinary Referring to pharmaceuticals or biologicals intended for animal use. Historically veterinary products were made by less than "Good Manufacturing Products". Today, however, the GMP's refer to both human and veterinary products.

VGSC Voltage-gated Sodium Channel.

Viable living Viable Organism Capable of living and reproducing. Thus, nothing is sterile as long as it contains even a single viable organism.

Vial A final container for a parenteral or diagnostic product. Sealed with a rubber closure and over-seal. Generally required to be class I borosilicate glass.

Vincristine Widely used agent, a 'spindle-cell poison' capable of stopping cancer cell division. Other similar agents: vinblastine, vindesine. Originally derived from the common periwinkle Catharantus roseus. Can cause peripheral neuropathy in some patients.

Viral antigens Specific proteins on the capsid of a virus that can act as inducers of antibody formation.

Virion A fully formed, mature virus. Infection is initiated in a cell by a virion.

Virucide An agent that destroys or inactivates viruses.

Virulence The disease-producing power of a microorganism.

Virus A simple, noncellular parasite that can reproduce only inside living cells. The simple structure of viruses is their most important characteristic. Most of them consist only of a genetic material - either DNA or RNA - and a protein coating. Some also have membranous envelopes. Viruses are "alive" in that they can reproduce themselves - although only by taking over a cell's synthetic machinery - but they have none of the other characteristics of living organisms. Viruses cause a large variety of significant diseases in plants and animals, including humans.

Viscosity The tendency of a fluid to resist flowing because of molecular attraction (cohesion).

Vitamin Term coined in 1911 (vita, Latin word for life, and the chemical term amine) by polish biochemist, Casimir Funk, represents one of a group of organic substances, some of which are of unknown composition, present in minute amount in natural foodstuffs which are essential to normal metabolism. A lack of which in the dietary causes deficiency diseases. Vitamins are commonly classified into two groups, the fat-soluble, and the water-soluble. Vitamins A, D, E, and K are fat-soluble. Vitamin C and members of the vitamin B complex group are water-soluble. In general, the vitamins play catalytic and regulatory roles in the body's metabolism. Among the water-soluble vitamins, the B vitamins apparently function as coenzymes. Vitamin's C coenzyme role, if any, has not been established. Part of the importance of vitamin C to the body may result from its strong antioxidant action. The actions of the fat-soluble vitamins are less well understood. Some of them, too, may contribute to enzyme activity, and some of them are essential to the functioning of cellular membranes.

Volume of distribution The volume, in an organism, throughout which a drug appears to have been distributed; the volume into which a drug appears to have been dissolved after administration to an organism. Symbolized by Vd.

Suppose a drug has been completely absorbed from its site of application, has reached an equilibrium in its distribution among the several tissues of the body, and that no biotransformation or excretion of the drug has occurred. If one knew the mass (dose) of drug administered and the average concentration of the drug in the body, the apparent volume into which the drug had been dissolved could be determined from the relationship or definition: concentration = mass/volume. Since these idealized conditions are unobtainable in practice, the volume of distribution of a drug can only be approximated using experimental data.

With the assumption that the concentration of the drug in the plasma (or serum) reflects the average drug concentration in its whole volume of distribution, plasma concentration can be plotted against time after drug administration, and the resulting line can be extrapolated to yield a fictive concentration (C0) "predicted" to have existed at the instant the drug was administered - further assuming instantaneous and complete administration, absorption, and distribution of the drug. Obviously, C0, is the value expected to have occurred at a time when mechanisms of biotransformation and excretion had no significant effect on the amount of drug in the body. Needless to say, it is assumed for proper interpretation of C0, that the drug as measured in the plasma is identical to the agent that was administered, and that the drug underwent no chemical alteration in the course of administration, absorption, or distribution.

When C0 is divided into the mass of the total dose administered, the quotient indicated the volume into which the drug appears to be dissolved. When C0 is divided into dose expressed in terms of body weight (e.g.,mg/kg), the quotient is dimensionless - since kilograms and liters are considered equivalent - and indicates the fraction of body weight into which the drug appears to be dissolved. The volumes, or fractions, can be readily compared with parts of body weight occupied by the various fluid compartments (e.g., intravascular, extracellular, intracellular, etc.), and the approximate locus of drug distribution may be inferable. A volume of distribution corresponding to more than about the volume of total body water is presumptive evidence that the drug is distributed nonuniformly throughout the body, and is concentrated at one or more sites, usually sites of drug storage, biotransformation or elimination, or at a site of drug application when a route of administration other than the intravenous one has been used. Obviously, legitimate and valid interpretation of calculated volume of distribution depends on the degree to which experimental facts are in concordance with the assumption given above. The idealized state is most closely approximated when the drug is given rapidly intravenously, and blood samples for chemical analysis of their drug content are taken at short intervals, beginning very soon after the time of drug administration.

Two more qualifications - first, special account must be taken mathematically, to yield validly interpretable volumes of distribution when binding of drug to plasma protein significantly restricts the mobility of drug molecules. Second, when the plot of plasma concentration against time gives evidence of a system involving two (or more) phases - i.e., two volumes into which drug tends to be distributed to different degrees at different times - special mathematical treatment of the data (more complicated than the treatment described above) is needed to permit calculation of the volumes of the several phases.

VPHP Microbiodecontamination Technology used to decontaminate the exposed, internal surfaces within a sealed isolator and the

exposed, external surfaces of materials and components placed within the sealed isolator. It consists of four distinctive phases:
1. Dehumidification - Lowers humidity and increases temperature

2. Conditioning - "Ramp-up" (VPHP) at or below saturation conditions

3. Sterilization - Steady-State (VPHP) at or below saturation conditions

4. Aeration - Reduces the VPHP to Safe Levels.

VR (VR1) Vanilloid Receptor (Vanilloid Receptor type 1).

VS Volumetric solution (defined in USP/NF for a particular analysis).

Vulnerable subjects Individuals whose willingness to volunteer in a clinical trial may be unduly influenced by the expectation, whether justified or not, of benefits associated with participation, or of a retaliatory response from senior members of a hierarchy in case of refusal to participate. Examples are members of a group with a hierarchical structure, such as medical, pharmacy, dental and nursing students, subordinate hospital and laboratory personnel, employees of the pharmaceutical industry, members of the armed forces, and persons kept in detention. Other vulnerable subjects include patients with incurable diseases, persons in nursing homes, unemployed or impoverished persons, patients in emergency situations, ethnic minority groups, homeless persons, nomads, refugees, minors, and those incapable of giving consent. (ICH)

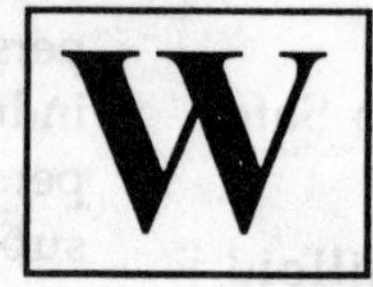

WAN(Wide Area Network) Network with computers far apart, connected by telephone lines or radio waves.LAN (Local Area Network))

Washout period A period in a clinical study during which subjects receive no treatment for the indication under study and the effects of a previous treatment are eliminated (or assumed to be eliminated).

Water hammer A tremendous force produced by rapid interruption of linear flow of a non-compressible fluid. Most commonly occurs when fast acting valves are closed in a high flow liquid system.

Water soluble Able to dissolve in water.

Water treatment Water treatment, also referred to as water conditioning, can consist of adding or removing chemicals to change the properties of water. In water softening, for example, sodium ions are substituted for metallic ions that cause "hardness" thus reducing the scale-forming tendencies of water. Water purification on the other hand, always consists of removing undesirable impurities.

Waviness The more widely spaced component of surface texture. Unless otherwise noted, waviness includes all irregularities whose spacing is greater than the roughness sampling length. Waviness may result from such factors as machine or work deflection, vibration, chatter, heat treatment or warping strains. Roughness may be considered as superimposed on a "wavy" surface.

Web browser A computer program that interprets HTML and other Internet languages and protocols and displays Web pages on your computer monitor.

Web page A single page on a Web site, such as a home page.

Web server A computer program that delivers HTML pages or files. Sometimes the computer on which a server program runs is also referred to as a server.

Web site A collection of Web pages and other files. A site can consist of a single Web page, thousands of pages, or custom-created pages that draw on a database associated with the site.

Weighting An adjustment in a value on the basis of a judgment by the investigator. (statistics)

Well being (of the trial subjects) The physical and mental integrity of the subjects participating in a clinical trial.

Western blot A procedure in which a mixture of proteins is separated on a polyacrylamide gel and then transferred to a nylon membrane. The membrane may then be treated with reagents such as specific antibodies to locate a protein of interest.

Wetted surface The surface(s) of any valve or component that will be exposed to a fluid (liquid or gas) when in service.

WFI (Water for injection), U.S.P. WFI is water purified by distillation or by reverse osmosis, it contains no added substance. WFI meets the purity requirements under Purified Water. Although not intended to be sterile, it meets a test for a limit of bacterial endotoxin. It must be produced, stored, and distributed under Sterile Water for Injection.

White blood cell A blood cell containing no respiratory pigment. In vertebrates it may be a polymorphonuclear leukocyte, a lymphocyte or a monocyte.

Within subject differences In a crossover trial, variability in each patient is used to assess treatment differences. (statistics)

Witness A person observing the test and results.

Working seed lot A culture of microorganism derived from the master seed lot and intended for use in production. Working seed lots are distributed into containers and stored as described above for master seed lots.

Workstation An open or enclosed work surface, usually with direct air supply.

Worst case The highest or lowest value of a given control parameter actually evaluated in a validation exercise.

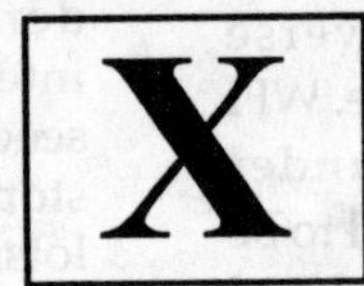

X chromosome A sex chromosome that usually occurs paired in each female cell and single in each male cell in species in which the male typically has two unlike cell chromosomes.

Xenobiotic A key term in toxicology (means foreign substance) is used to identify clearly toxic substances, such as lead, or beneficial therapeutic agents, many of which become toxic at elevated dosage levels.

A compound foreign to an organism. From the Greek xenox = foreign, bios = life. Principal xenobiotics include drugs, carcinogens and various compounds that have been introduced into the environment by artificial means.

XPS(X-Ray photoelectron spectroscopy) or ESCA (Electron spectroscopy for chemical analysis) A surface-sensitive technique capable of detecting all elements with an atomic number greater than that of helium. ESCA provides data on the outermost several atomic layers of a material, and has a sensitivity in the order of 0.5 atomic percent. A primary advantage of ESCA is that it can both determine and quantify the chemical state of the elements detected (i.e. metallic state or oxide state).

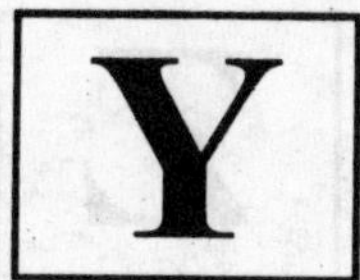

Yeast artificial chromosome A vector used to clone DNA fragments (up to 400 kb); it is constructed from the telomeric, centromeric, and replication origin sequences needed for replication in yeast cells.

Yeasts Unicellular fungi belonging mainly to the Ascomycetes that usually multiply by budding. Their commercial significance lies in their ability to secrete enzymes. For example, in the brewing and baking industries, it is a source of vitamins and proteins. They can also be used as excipients in rDNA technology.

Yield, expected The quantity of material or the percentage of theoretical yield anticipated at any appropriate phase of production based on previous laboratory, pilot scale, or manufacturing data.

Yield, theoretical The quantity that would be produced at any appropriate phase of manufacture, processing, or packing of a particular API (Active Pharmaceutical Ingredient) or intermediate, based upon the quantity of components to be used, in the absence of any loss or error in actual production.

Z

Zalcitabine (ddC, HIVID) Treatment of HIV infection in combination with other agents.

Contraindications: Known hypersensitivity, significant peripheral neuropathy.

Dosage: 0.75 mg po tid.

Toxicity: Peripheral neuropathy, aphthous ulcers of mouth and esophagus, acute pancreatitis, abnormal liver function tests.

Zeolite Naturally occurring or synthetic permutite, a hydrated alkali-aluminum silicate that exhibits limited base exchange. Used as an ion exchange medium for the softening of hard water.

Zero order kinetics Mechanisms of chemical reaction in which the reaction velocity is apparently independent of the concentration of all the reactants. Typically, in biological systems, one reactant (X) is present in a concentration greatly exceeding that of the other (Y), but is capable of undergoing change, while the concentration of Y, in contrast, does not undergo substantial change during the course of the reaction.

For example, consider the inactivation of a drug (X), present in the body in an overwhelming quantity, by an enzyme (Y) present in a limited concentration in cells and having a specific maximum capacity to inactivate X. A sufficiently high concentration of X would "saturate " Y and make the system operate at, effectively, its maximum velocity; the amount of X inactivated per unit time would be constant and would depend on the maximum velocity per mass of Y and the total amount of Y present in the body; modest changes in concentration of X would not detectably change the velocity of the system operating at virtually its maximum rate. (Recollect the shape of the velocity - substrate concentration curve.) The reaction velocity would be independent of the concentrations of both X and Y. Eventually, the concentration of X would decrease to the point that it did not saturate Y, and the inactivation would proceed according to first-order kinetics.

For a zero-order reaction, the plot of C (not ln or log C) against t yields a straight line: $C = C0 - b0\,t$, in which the slope (b0) is in units of concentration per unit time. The amount of change in concentration per unit time is constant; in the case of first-order kinetics, the fractional change in concentration per unit time is constant.

Following administration of a drug eliminated by zero-order kinetics, the linear plot of C against t can be used to infer C0 and C and (if the dose is known) Vd, but no half-life (t1/2) can be determined. The elegant properties of multiple dose regimens (q.v.) for drugs eliminated according to first-order kinetics do not obtain for drugs eliminated by zero-order kinetics: Cmax for "zero-order drugs" does not approach Css,max as an asymptote; for zero-order drugs, Cmax increases progressively without limit with each dose, when equal doses are administered at equal intervals. Drugs that obey first-order kinetics with low doses may obey zero-order kinetics with large doses.

Zeta potential The charge or potential existing at the surface of a particle. It is the positive charge measured at the surface of the membrane across the pH range.

Zidovudine (ZDV, AZT, Retrovir) **Indications**: Treatment of HIV infection in combination with other agents. In addition, ZDV may have specific benefits for patients who have HIV-related thrombocytopenia or encephalopathy.

Prevention of perinatal transmission when given prenatally and during delivery to HIV-infected mother and to infant postpartum.

Contraindications: Known hypersensitivity.

Dosage: Treatment of HIV infection in adults: 300 mg po bid. Also available as Combivir, a fixed dose combination of ZDV 300 mg with 3TC 150 mg; and Trizivir, a fixed dose combination of ZDV 300 mg, 3TC 150 mg, and abacavir 300 mg.

Prevention of perinatal transmission: Pregnancy weeks 14-34 –> 100 mg po 5 times a day; during labor –> 2 mg/kg IV loading dose over 30 minutes to 1 hour, then 1 mg/kg/hr IV through delivery; and infant –> 2 mg/kg syrup q6h for 6 weeks.

Toxicity: Gastrointestinal intolerance, headache, anemia, leukopenia, myopathy, abnormal liver function tests, macrocytosis, fingernail discoloration.

Recommended for pregnant women after the first trimester to prevent vertical transmission.

Zoonosis Any disease in humans acquired from one of the lower animals, rabies is an example.

Zwitterion An ion carrying both a positive and a negative charge in different parts of the molecule, e.g., proteins and some buffers and amino acids near neutral pH.

Zygote Single cell formed from the conjugation of gametes (egg and sperm cells). The zygote has twice as many chromosomes as do gametes.